di Fiore's Atlas of
HISTOLOGY

WITH FUNCTIONAL CORRELATIONS

VICTOR P. EROSCHENKO, Ph.D.

Professor of Anatomy
Department of Biological Sciences
and
WAMI Medical Program,
University of Idaho,
Moscow, Idaho

di Fiore's Atlas of HISTOLOGY

WITH FUNCTIONAL CORRELATIONS

SEVENTH EDITION

1993
LEA & FEBIGER
PHILADELPHIA, LONDON

Lea & Febiger   Executive Editor—George H. Mundorff
Box 3024   Manuscript Editor—Jessica Howie Martin
200 Chester Field Parkway   Production Manager—Thomas J. Colaiezzi
Malvern, Pennsylvania 19355-9725
U.S.A.
(215) 251-2230

     FIRST EDITION, 1957   Reprinted 1958, 1959, 1960, 1961, 1962
   SECOND EDITION, 1963   Reprinted 1964, 1965
    THIRD EDITION, 1967   Reprinted 1968, 1969, 1970, 1971, 1972, 1973
  FOURTH EDITION, 1974   Reprinted 1975, 1976, 1977, 1978, 1979, 1980, 1981
      FIFTH EDITION, 1981 Reprinted 1981, 1982, 1983, 1985, 1987
      SIXTH EDITION, 1989 Reprinted 1989, 1992
SEVENTH EDITION, 1993

Library of Congress Cataloging-in-Publication Data

Eroschenko, Victor P.
      di Fiore's atlas of histology with functional correlations /
   Victor P. Eroschenko. — 7th ed.
         p.   cm.
      Rev. and significantly altered ed. of Atlas de histologia normal.
      Includes index.
      1. Histology—Atlases.   I. Fiore, Mariano S. H. di. Atlas de
   histologia normal.   II. Title.   III. Title: Atlas of normal
   histology with functional correlations.
   QM557.F75513   1993
   611'.018—dc20   92-27341
                                                          CIP

Reprints of Chapters may be purchased from Lea & Febiger in quantities of
100 or more. Contact Sally Grande in the Sales Department.

PRINTED IN THE UNITED STATES OF AMERICA

Print number: 5 4 3 2 1

In Memory of
Dr. Mariano S. H. di Fiore
1900–1991

PREFACE

The publication of the seventh edition of this Atlas, following the death of Dr. di Fiore, marks a change in the authorship, title, and format of the text. This edition represents the first major alteration of the Atlas since it was first published over 35 years ago. Although the format, style, and content of the text have been significantly changed, the original emphasis on presenting composite, precise, and beautiful color drawings of basic histologic structures remains the same. In recognition of the efforts of the late author, the title of this Atlas now bears his name.

One of the most striking and obvious changes in the Atlas is the new format of the print and binding. The text and labels are larger, bolder, and easier to read. In the descriptions of histologic sections, each structure labelled in the illustration is clearly numbered and printed in boldface. This new feature allows the student to see at a glance which structure or part is identified. Also, in designing the new edition, convenience in the histology laboratory was an important consideration; as a result, the spiral binding allows better utilization of the limited laboratory space around the microscope.

Histology is closely correlated with other scientific disciplines, such as cell biology, physiology, pathology, and biochemistry. New information gained from research in these disciplines applies directly to the functions of cells, tissues, and organs that are studied in histology. Because it is imperative in histology to consider both structure and function, a new feature of this Atlas is text on functional correlations. Each new section is preceded by one or more pages of text describing specific and important functions for cells, tissues, or organs that are illustrated. In contrast to previous editions, the current Atlas is dynamic in scope because both structures and the latest information on their functions are closely correlated and considered together. Thus, while examining histology slides in the laboratory, the student has quick access to specific functions of these structures.

Although the functional correlations in this atlas have been designed to reinforce lecture material and make examination of histologic slides more meaningful, their inclusion was not intended to replace textbooks of histology. Thus, functional correlations are presented in brief, summarized formats. Other details not related specifically to histologic structures in the illustrations have been left to textbooks of histology and/or other disciplines.

In previous editions, the most appealing aspect of this Atlas was its correct and precise representation of composite illustrations of different histologic structures. To maintain this feature, the seventh edition has been enriched by the replacement of old figures and text with 17 new, beautiful color illustrations and corresponding text. Thus, with such improvements, the Atlas should continue to appeal to undergraduate students, graduate students, and students in professional schools (medical and veterinary) who are studying histology. All major organs of the body are illustrated, making it a complete treatise on basic histology. As in the sixth edition, new illustrations have been prepared by Amy Werner Carter of Seattle, Washington.

I acknowledge and extend my appreciation to the management of Lea & Febiger Publishers for offering me the authorship of this fine Atlas. In preparing the revision, I sincerely appreciate the efforts of Mr. George H. Mundorff, Mr. Thomas J. Colaiezzi, Mrs. Jessica Howie Martin, and Mr. John F. Spahr, Jr.

Victor P. Eroschenko, Ph.D.

Moscow, Idaho

CONTENTS

T I S S U E S

O R G A N S

THE DIGESTIVE SYSTEM: THE ACCESSORY DIGESTIVE ORGANS 135

THE DIGESTIVE SYSTEM: THE STOMACH 155

THE DIGESTIVE SYSTEM: THE SMALL AND LARGE INTESTINES 175

ABBREVIATIONS ON PLATES

h.s.—horizontal section
l.s.—longitudinal section
o.s.—oblique section
tg. s.—tangential section
t.s—transverse section
v.s.—vertical section

TISSUES

THE EPITHELIAL TISSUE

There are four basic tissue types: epithelial, connective, muscular, and nervous. These tissues exist and function in close association with one another in all organs of the body.

The epithelial tissue or epithelium, consists of sheets of cells. It forms glands and lines all body surfaces, cavities, and ducts. The classification of the epithelium is based on the number of cell layers and the morphology of the surface cells. Based on these criteria, the simple epithelium consists of a single layer of cells; pseudostratified epithelium consists of a single layer of cells in which all cells attach to the basement membrane but not all cells reach the surface; and stratified epithelium consists of two or more cell layers. The epithelium is separated from the connective tissue by a basement membrane.

Some epithelium exhibits cilia, stereocilia, or microvilli on its free surface. The cilia are motile and function by transporting material across the cell surfaces. Ciliated epithelium is found in the uterine tubes and most of the respiratory passages. The stereocilia, on the other hand, are long, nonmotile, branched microvilli found on the surface of cells in the epididymis. The microvilli are usually visible as striated and brush borders on the epithelium of certain digestive organs and proximal convoluted tubules of the kidney. The main function of microvilli and stereocilia is absorption.

The Simple Epithelia

The simple squamous epithelium is common in the body and consists of a single layer of irregular, flattened or squamous cells. In the cardiovascular and lymphatic systems, this epithelium is called the endothelium. In the lining of the peritoneal, pleural, and pericardial cavities, it is called the mesothelium. The cells of the simple epithelium are extremely thin. As a result, its main function is to allow passive transport of fluids, nutrients, or metabolites across the capillaries or gases across the alveoli.

The simple cuboidal epithelium consists of cells that are as tall as they are wide. Its function is secretory or absorptive (proximal and distal convoluted kidney tubules).

The simple columnar epithelium consists of cells that are taller than they are wide. In the digestive organs, it exhibits a striated border, and its major function is absorption of fluids and nutrients; or it is secretory, as in mucous cells of the intestines, trachea, and bronchi secretory cells of the oviduct and uterus.

The pseudostratified columnar epithelium in the respiratory tubes is ciliated, and its major function is to move mucus and dust particles across cell surfaces. In the epididymis, this epithelium contains stereocilia whose main function is absorption of fluids that were produced in the testes.

The Stratified Epithelia

The stratified squamous epithelium contains numerous cell layers. The basal cells are cuboidal to columnar in shape; these give rise to cells that migrate toward the free surface and become squamous. The main function of stratified epithelium is protection, and its multilayered composition is well adopted to withstand wear and tear or abrasion.

There are two types of stratified squamous epithelia: nonkeratinized and keratinized. The nonkeratinized type exhibits live superficial cells with nuclei. It lines the moist cavities of the mouth, pharynx, esophagus, vagina, and anal canal. The keratinized type contains nonliving, keratinized superficial cells and it lines the skin. The major function of the keratinized epithelium is to protect the body from abrasion, desiccation, bacterial invasion, and other similar functions.

The stratified cuboidal epithelium and stratified columnar epithelium have limited distribution in the body. Both types are found in the ducts of larger glands, the pancreas, and the salivary and sweat glands. They usually consist of two or three layers of cells.

The transitional epithelium is designed to change shape when it is stretched. This epithelium can resemble both the stratified squamous and stratified cuboidal epithelia, depending on the degree of stretch. The surface cells are dome-shaped during contraction and squamous during stretching. Transitional epithelium lines the urinary passages (minor and major calyxes, pelvis, ureter, and bladder). Its major function is to allow stretch during urine accumulation and contraction during emptying of the urinary passages without breaking the cell contacts in the epithelium. In addition, the cells of transitional epithelium form an important osmotic barrier between urine and the underlying tissues.

PLATE 1

■ FIG. 1
SIMPLE SQUAMOUS EPITHELIUM: DISSOCIATED SQUAMOUS EPITHELIAL CELLS

The dissociated **simple squamous cells (1, 6, 7)** were obtained by scraping the superficial layers of the oral cavity, which is lined by nonkeratinized stratified epithelium. The collected cells are seen either individually (1, 6), or in sheets (2) in which the cells are firmly attached to each other.

In the surface view, the squamous cells exhibit irregular polygonal shape (1, 6) and distinct **cell membranes (3).** The cell **cytoplasm (4)** is finely granular, and the round or oval **nucleus (5)** assumes either a central or an eccentric position (8) in the cytoplasm. In a lateral view (7), the squamous cells are thin and spindle-shaped and have thin, rod-like nuclei.

■ FIG. 2
SIMPLE SQUAMOUS EPITHELIUM: SURFACE VIEW OF PERITONEAL MESOTHELIUM

To visualize the surface of the simple squamous epithelium, a small piece of mesentery was fixed and treated with silver nitrate and counterstained with hematoxylin. The cells of the simple squamous epithelium (mesothelium) appear flat, adhere tightly to each other, and form a sheet with the thickness of a single cell layer. The irregular **cell boundaries (1)** are highly visible because of silver deposition and form a characteristic mosaic pattern. The blue-gray **cell nuclei (2)** exhibit a central location in the yellow- to brown-stained **cytoplasm (3).**

The simple squamous epithelium is common in the body. It is found lining the surfaces that allow passive transport of gases or fluids and lining the pleural, pericardial, and peritoneal cavities.

■ FIG. 3
SIMPLE SQUAMOUS EPITHELIUM: PERITONEAL MESOTHELIUM (TRANSVERSE SECTION)

Examination of the simple squamous epithelium, the **mesothelium (1)** of jejunum, in transverse section, illustrates that the cells are spindle-shaped with prominent, oval nuclei. Cell boundaries are not seen distinctly but are indicated at **cell junctions (2).** A thin **basement membrane (3)** is observed under the mesothelium (1). In surface view, these cells appear similar to those illustrated in Figure 2.

Mesothelium and the underlying **connective tissue (4)** form the serosa of the peritoneal cavity, which is the outermost layer of the jejunal wall. Serosa is attached to the muscularis externa, which consists of **smooth muscle fibers (6).** In the connective tissue are small blood vessels, lined by a simple squamous epithelium called the **endothelium (5).**

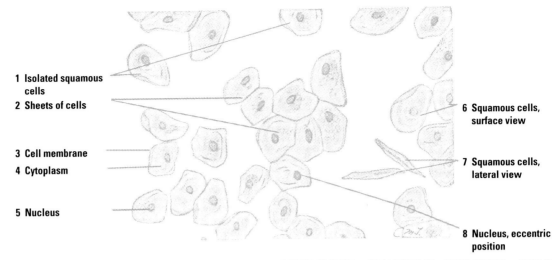

1 Isolated squamous cells
2 Sheets of cells
3 Cell membrane
4 Cytoplasm
5 Nucleus
6 Squamous cells, surface view
7 Squamous cells, lateral view
8 Nucleus, eccentric position

FIG. 1. SIMPLE SQUAMOUS EPITHELIUM. DISSOCIATED SQUAMOUS EPITHELIAL CELLS. Observed in the fresh state. 110×.

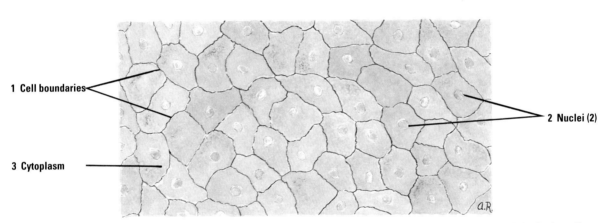

1 Cell boundaries
2 Nuclei (2)
3 Cytoplasm

FIG. 2. SIMPLE SQUAMOUS EPITHELIUM: SURFACE VIEW OF PERITONEAL MESOTHELIUM. Stain: silver nitrate with hematoxylin.

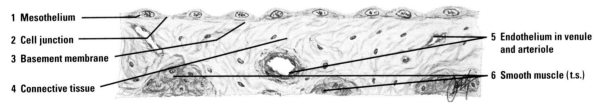

1 Mesothelium
2 Cell junction
3 Basement membrane
4 Connective tissue
5 Endothelium in venule and arteriole
6 Smooth muscle (t.s.)

FIG. 3. SIMPLE SQUAMOUS EPITHELIUM: TRANSVERSE SECTION OF PERITONEAL MESOTHELIUM. Stain: hematoxylin-eosin: 500×.

5

PLATE 2

■ FIG. 1
SIMPLE COLUMNAR EPITHELIUM

In a **simple columnar epithelium (2)**, as seen on the surface of the stomach, the cells are arranged in a single row. Their ovoid nuclei **(7)** are located in the basal region and exhibit a perpendicular orientation. A thin **basement membrane (3)** separates the epithelium from the underlying **connective tissue (4, 10)**, the lamina propria of the gastric mucosa. **Capillaries (5)**, lined with endothelium, are seen in the connective tissue.

In some areas, the epithelium has been sectioned transversely or obliquely. When a plane of section passes close to the free surface of the epithelium, the sectioned apical regions (1) of these cells resemble a mosaic of enucleated polygonal cells. When a plane of section passes through basal regions (6) of the epithelial cells, the nuclei are cut transversely and resemble a stratified epithelium.

The surface cells of the stomach secrete mucus, which protects the stomach lining from its acidic contents. The light appearance of the cell cytoplasm in these cells is caused by the routine preparation of the tissues. The mucigen droplets that filled these cell apices (9) were lost during section preparation. The more granular cytoplasm exhibits a basal location (8) and stains more acidophilically.

Examples of other columnar epithelia may be seen in the lining of the gallbladder (Plate 79:14); the salivary gland ducts (Plate 56:6, 14, IV; Plate 57: 1, 7, III); the bile ducts of the liver (Plate 77, Fig. 1:7, 14); and the interlobular ducts of the pancreas (Plate 80, Fig. 1:19, III).

A simple cuboidal epithelium is illustrated in the smallest ducts of the pancreas (Plate 80, Fig. 1:1, 5, 20, II) and in the follicles of the thyroid gland (Plate 94, Fig. 1:5 and Fig. 2:2).

■ FIG. 2
SIMPLE COLUMNAR EPITHELIUM: CELLS WITH STRIATED BORDERS AND GOBLET CELLS

The intestinal **villi (1)** are lined by simple columnar epithelium, which consists of two types of cells: columnar cells with **striated borders (2, 13, 14)** and **goblet cells (8, 12)**. The striated border (13) is seen as a reddish outer membrane with faint vertical striations; these are the microvilli on the apices of the columnar cells. In an area of contiguous cells, the striated border appears continuous. The cytoplasm of these cells is finely granular and the oval nuclei are in the basal portions of the cells.

The goblet cells (8, 12) are interspersed among the columnar cells. During routine histologic preparation, the mucus was lost and the goblet cell cytoplasm appears clear or only lightly stained (12). Normally, the mucigen droplets occupy the cell apices and the nucleus remains in the basal region of the **cytoplasm (8)**.

The epithelium at the tip of the villus in the lower center of the figure has been sectioned in an oblique plane. As a result, the apices of the columnar cells appear as a mosaic (7) of enucleated cells and the basal regions, where the plane of section passed through the nuclei, appear stratified (7).

The **basement membrane (5)** is more visible than in Fig. 1. In the connective tissue, the **lamina propria (10)**, are seen a lymphatic vessel, the **central lacteal (3)**, a **capillary (9)** lined with endothelium, and **smooth muscle fibers (4, 11)**, seen as either single fibers or small groups of fibers.

Other examples of cells with striated borders and goblet cells may be seen in a section of jejunum-ileum (Plate 69, Fig. 2:1, 2 and unlabeled in Fig. 3).

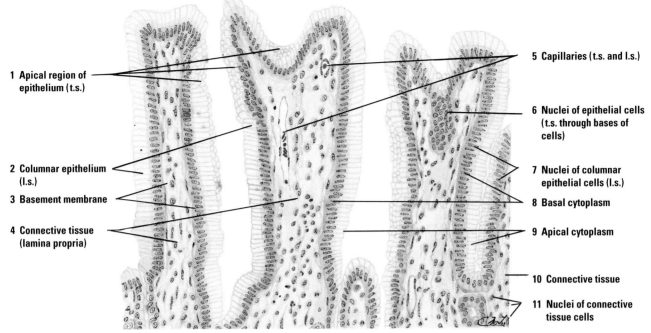

1 Apical region of
  epithelium (t.s.)

2 Columnar epithelium
  (l.s.)

3 Basement membrane

4 Connective tissue
  (lamina propria)

5 Capillaries (t.s. and l.s.)

6 Nuclei of epithelial cells
  (t.s. through bases of
  cells)

7 Nuclei of columnar
  epithelial cells (l.s.)

8 Basal cytoplasm

9 Apical cytoplasm

10 Connective tissue

11 Nuclei of connective
   tissue cells

FIG. 1. SIMPLE COLUMNAR EPITHELIUM. Stain: hematoxylin-eosin. 250×.

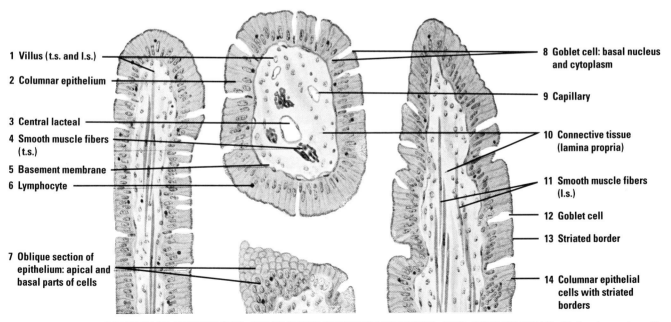

1 Villus (t.s. and l.s.)

2 Columnar epithelium

3 Central lacteal

4 Smooth muscle fibers
  (t.s.)

5 Basement membrane

6 Lymphocyte

7 Oblique section of
  epithelium: apical and
  basal parts of cells

8 Goblet cell: basal nucleus
  and cytoplasm

9 Capillary

10 Connective tissue
   (lamina propria)

11 Smooth muscle fibers
   (l.s.)

12 Goblet cell

13 Striated border

14 Columnar epithelial
   cells with striated
   borders

FIG. 2. SIMPLE COLUMNAR EPITHELIUM: CELLS WITH STRIATED BORDERS AND GOBLET CELLS. Stain: hematoxylin-eosin. 250×.

7

PLATE 3

■ FIG. 1
STRATIFIED SQUAMOUS EPITHELIUM (TRANSVERSE SECTION)

The stratified squamous epithelium is composed of numerous cell layers. Its thickness varies in different regions of the body and, as a result, the cell arrangement is altered.

Illustrated in this figure is an example of a moist, nonkeratinized **epithelium (1)**, which lines the oral cavity, esophagus, vagina, and anal canal. The **basal cells (5)** are cuboidal or low columnar. The cytoplasm is finely granular and the oval, chromatin-rich nucleus occupies most of the cell. Cells in the intermediate layers are **polyhedral (4)** with round or oval nuclei and more visible cell membranes. **Mitoses (7)** are frequently observed in the cells of the deeper layers and the basal cells. Above the polyhedral cells are several rows of **squamous cells (3).** Cells and nuclei become progressively flatter as the cells migrate toward the free surface.

A fine **basement membrane (8)** separates the epithelium (1) from the underlying **connective tissue, the lamina propria (2). Papillae (12)** of connective tissue indent the lower surface of the epithelium (1), giving it a characteristic wavy appearance. The connective tissue contains **collagen fibers (11), fibroblasts (10), capillaries (6, 9, 14)** and **arterioles (13).** Other examples of moist stratified squamous epithelium may be seen on Plates 52, 59, 60, 113, and 114.

When stratified squamous epithelium is exposed to increased wear and tear, the outermost layer, the stratum corneum, becomes thick and keratinized, as illustrated in the epidermis of the palm on Plate 46, Fig. 2.

An example of thin, stratified squamous epithelium without connective tissue papillae indentation is illustrated in the cornea of the eye, Plate 119, Fig. 2; the surface underlying the epithelium is smooth. This type of epithelium is only a few cell layers thick but shows the characteristic arrangement of basal columnar, polyhedral, and squamous cells, the most superficial cells on the cornea.

■ FIG. 2
STRATIFIED SQUAMOUS EPITHELIUM (TANGENTIAL SECTION)

A section made parallel to the surface of the epithelium at line a-a in Fig. 1 passes through several epithelial downgrowths and their connective tissue papillae, both of which are seen in transverse section.

In the connective tissue **papillae (1, 5, 8)** are seen collagen fibers, **fibroblasts (3),** and **capillaries (2, 4).** Basal cells of the epithelium surround the papillae and the polyhedral cells (7) of the intermediate layers occupy the remaining area.

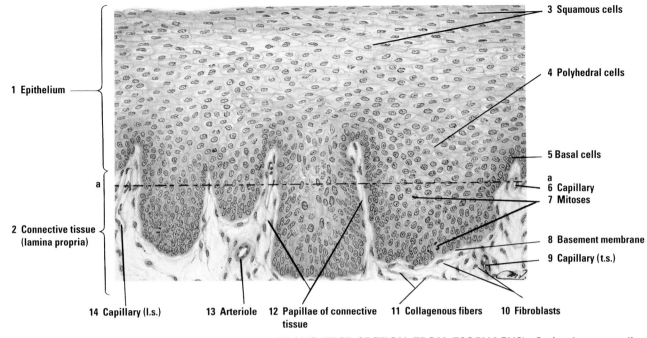

1 Epithelium

3 Squamous cells

4 Polyhedral cells

5 Basal cells

a
6 Capillary
7 Mitoses

2 Connective tissue
(lamina propria)

8 Basement membrane

9 Capillary (t.s.)

14 Capillary (l.s.)   13 Arteriole   12 Papillae of connective   11 Collagenous fibers   10 Fibroblasts
                                         tissue

FIG. 1. STRATIFIED SQUAMOUS EPITHELIUM (TRANSVERSE SECTION FROM ESOPHAGUS). Stain: hematoxylin-eosin. 215×

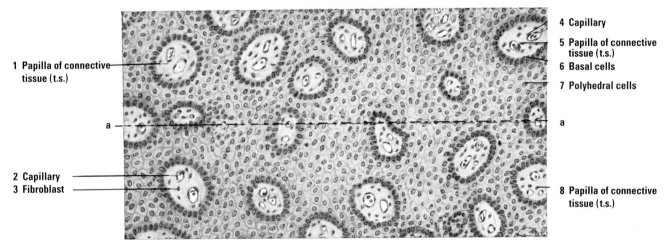

1 Papilla of connective
tissue (t.s.)

4 Capillary

5 Papilla of connective
tissue (t.s.)

6 Basal cells

7 Polyhedral cells

a

a

2 Capillary
3 Fibroblast

8 Papilla of connective
tissue (t.s.)

FIG. 2. STRATIFIED SQUAMOUS EPITHELIUM (TANGENTIAL SECTION FROM ESOPHAGUS). Stain: hematoxylin-eosin. 215×.

9

PLATE 4

■ FIG. 1
PSEUDOSTRATIFIED COLUMNAR CILIATED EPITHELIUM

The **pseudostratified columnar ciliated epithelium (1)** is characteristic of the upper respiratory passages such as the trachea and different-sized bronchi. In this epithelium, the cells appear in several layers because their nuclei are at different levels. Serial sections show that all cells reach the **basement membrane (8)**; however, because the cells are of different shapes and heights, not all reach the surface. For this reason, this type of epithelium is called pseudostratified instead of stratified.

The deeper nuclei belong to the intermediate and short **basal cells (7).** The more superficial, oval nuclei belong to the **columnar ciliated cells (5).** Interspersed among these cells are **goblet cells (6).** The small, round, heavily stained nuclei, without any visible surrounding cytoplasm, are those of **lymphocytes (9),** which migrate from the connective tissue through the epithelium.

The short, motile **cilia (3)** are numerous and closely spaced on the cell apices. Each cilium arises from a **basal body (4),** which is identical to the centriole. The basal bodies are located beneath the cell membrane and adjacent to each other; they often give the appearance of a continuous membrane (4).

The clearly visible **basement membrane (8)** separates the surface epithelium (1) from the underlying connective tissue of the **lamina propria (2, 11).**

In the **connective tissue (11)** are seen collagen fibers, cells (fibroblasts), scattered lymphocytes, and small **blood vessels (10).** Deeper in the connective tissue are found glands with **serous (12)** and **mucous acini (13).**

Other examples of pseudostratified columnar ciliated epithelium are seen on Plate 83:14, and Plate 84, Fig. 1:13, and Fig. 2:5, 6.

■ FIG. 2
TRANSITIONAL EPITHELIUM

The **transitional epithelium (1)** is found exclusively in the excretory passages of the urinary system. This epithelium is stratified and composed of several layers of similar cells (4, 5, 6), which are usually cuboidal with round nuclei. This similarity in cell morphology differentiates this epithelium from the stratified squamous epithelium (which it may resemble during different functional states), in which the cells of various layers have different shapes.

The transitional epithelium (1) has the ability to rearrange the number of cell layers, depending on whether it is in a distended or contracted state. When the epithelium is in a contracted state, the cells may be **cuboidal** or **columnar (4, 5, 6)** and the epithelium exhibits numerous layers. When the epithelium is distended, the number of cell layers is reduced. The cells

in the outer layers are then more elongated or flattened but not to the degree seen in squamous epithelium. (Compare the transitional epithelium with stratified squamous epithelium of the cornea, Plate 119, Fig. 2).

Transitional epithelium (1) rests on a **connective tissue (2, 8)** base, between them is seen a thin **basement membrane (7).** The base of the epithelium is not indented by connective tissue papillae, and it exhibits an even contour. Small **blood vessels (capillaries, venule, arteriole) (9, 10, 11)** are present in the connective tissue. Deeper in the connective tissue are seen **smooth muscle fibers (12),** which indicate a layer of smooth muscle.

Other examples of transitional epithelium are seen in both figures on Plates 90 and 91.

EPITHELIAL TISSUE

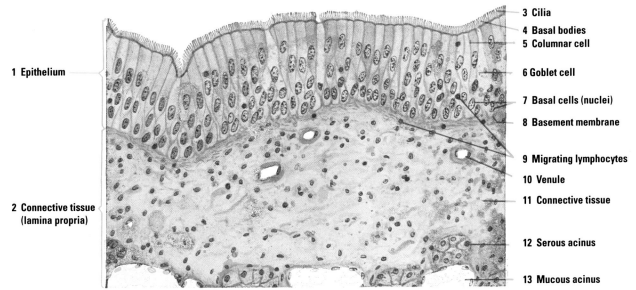

1 Epithelium

2 Connective tissue
(lamina propria)

3 Cilia
4 Basal bodies
5 Columnar cell

6 Goblet cell

7 Basal cells (nuclei)

8 Basement membrane

9 Migrating lymphocytes

10 Venule

11 Connective tissue

12 Serous acinus

13 Mucous acinus

FIG. 1. PSEUDOSTRATIFIED COLUMNAR CILIATED EPITHELIUM. Stain: hematoxylin-eosin. 330×.

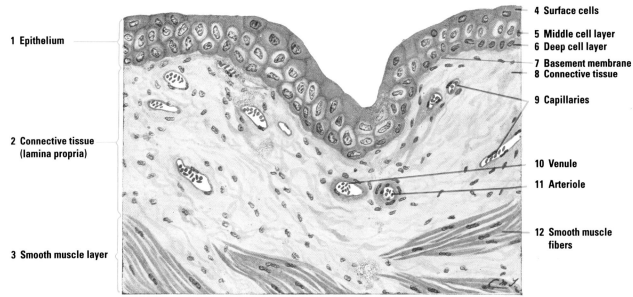

1 Epithelium

2 Connective tissue
(lamina propria)

3 Smooth muscle layer

4 Surface cells

5 Middle cell layer
6 Deep cell layer
7 Basement membrane
8 Connective tissue

9 Capillaries

10 Venule

11 Arteriole

12 Smooth muscle
fibers

FIG. 2. TRANSITIONAL EPITHELIUM. Stain: hematoxylin-eosin. 300×.

11

PLATE 5

SIMPLE BRANCHED TUBULAR GLAND (DIAGRAM)

The diagram illustrates the general structure of a simple branched tubular gland consisting of a long **duct (2)** and a branched terminal portion of four secretory **tubules (3)**, which arise from the basal portion of the duct. There are also variations in structure in different glands.

The **duct (2)** is lined with simple low columnar epithelium with oval basal nuclei; the duct opens onto **surface epithelium (1)** of similar cells. The low columnar epithelium in the duct decreases in height toward the secretory portion of the gland. The **glandular epithelium (3)** is low columnar to cuboidal with flattened basal nuclei, indicating that the cells are filled with secretion.

The diagram in the center illustrates the appearance of sections resulting from cuts that pass at different angles through various parts of the gland.

At **A**, the section was taken at the level of blue line a-a', which passes through the nuclear region of the surface epithelial cells in a plane parallel to the surface. In the center of the section is the orifice or opening of the gland with its wall of **low columnar cells (A-1)**. Surrounding this area are transverse sections of the **surface epithelial cell (A-2)**.

B represents a sagittal section of the same gland along the vertical red line b-b', which extends through the entire length of the gland. At **B-1**, the plane of section passes through the surface epithelium and tangentially through the wall of the duct. As a result, the lumen is not seen and the duct wall appears as a solid column of stratified epithelium. The next plane of section passes through the **lumen of the duct (B-2)** and the lumen of one of the **secretory tubules (B-3)**. At the bottom of the gland, the plane of section passes transversely through the curved basal portion of the adjacent **secretory tubule (B-4)**, which is seen as a circular structure with central lumen surrounded by pyramid-shaped cells.

C represents an oblique section though the duct along the blue line c-c'; the lumen has an elliptical shape **(C-1)**. At both ends of the section, the epithelium has a mosaic appearance **(C-2)** because the oblique plane of section passed through both nucleated and non-nucleated regions of the duct cells.

D represents a sagittal section through the wall of one of the secretory tubules along the blue line d-d'. As a result, the section appears as a solid mass of cells.

E represents an oblique **(E-1)** and a transverse **(E-2)** plane of section through the lumen and wall of a secretory tubule along blue line e-e'.

F illustrates transverse planes of sections through three tubules along the red line f-f'. Each tubule shows a central lumen surrounded by cuboidal or pyramidal cells.

G represents a portion of a secretory tubule sectioned longitudinally along the blue line g-g'. The plane passes through the lumen of the tubule except in the upper region, where the wall was sectioned at an oblique angle.

EXAMPLES

There are probably no tubular glands in the body that have the exact structure represented in the general diagram; however, tubular glands with similar variations occur in several locations of the body.

Unbranched simple tubular glands without ducts are represented by the intestinal glands (crypts of Lieberkühn) of the large intestine (Plate 72:20) and rectum (Plate 75:7). These glands are lined with goblet cells and columnar cells with striated borders.

Similar shorter intestinal glands are found in the small intestine (Plate 69, Fig. 1:3). These glands also contain goblet cells and columnar cells with striated borders. In addition, cells in the bottom of the glands (Paneth cells) are specialized for secretion (Plate 69, Fig. 2).

The simple or slightly branched tubular gastric glands, without ducts, are lined with different, modified columnar cells that are highly specialized for secreting hydrochloric acid and the precursor for the proteolytic enzyme pepsin (Plate 64:5, 14-16). The pyloric glands, in contrast, are coiled tubular glands; their columnar cells secrete mucus and are, therefore, lightly stained (Plate 66:5, 14).

A coiled tubular gland with a long, unbranched duct is a sweat gland, illustrated on Plate 47.

The highly branched tubular glands, lined with mucus-secreting columnar cells, are found in the cervix (Plate 113:2); a narrow constricted portion of the gland serves as a duct.

SIMPLE BRANCHED TUBULAR GLAND (DIAGRAM)

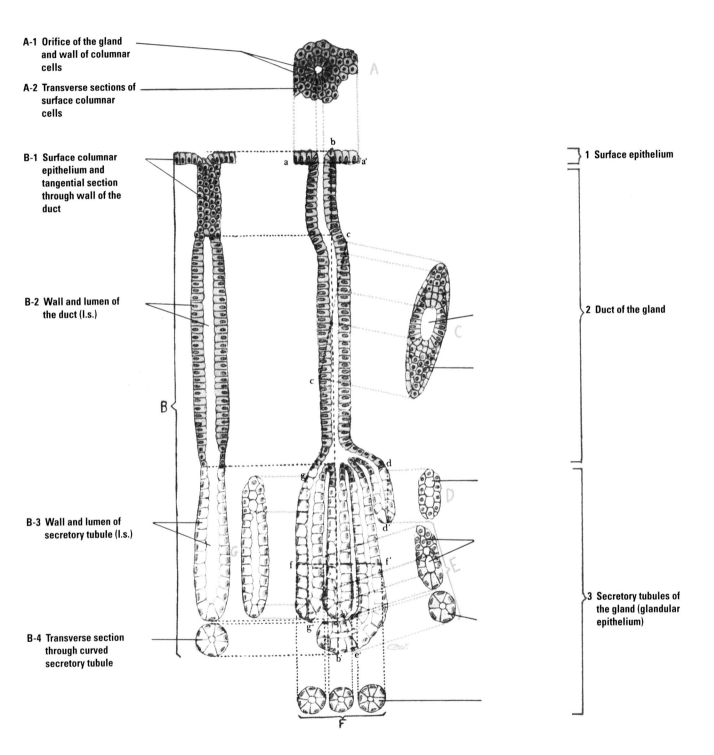

A-1 Orifice of the gland and wall of columnar cells

A-2 Transverse sections of surface columnar cells

B-1 Surface columnar epithelium and tangential section through wall of the duct

B-2 Wall and lumen of the duct (l.s.)

B-3 Wall and lumen of secretory tubule (l.s.)

B-4 Transverse section through curved secretory tubule

1 Surface epithelium

2 Duct of the gland

3 Secretory tubules of the gland (glandular epithelium)

PLATE 6

COMPOUND TUBULOACINAR GLAND (DIAGRAM)

This diagram illustrates a general type of gland that is found in the oral cavity, the digestive system, and the respiratory system. A large **excretory duct (A-1)** opens onto an epithelial surface (not indicated in the diagram). The duct divides or gives off successively **smaller ducts (A-5, A-6)** as it descends toward the secretory portion of the gland. At the terminal portion of the gland are round or elongated secretory units or **acini (C-1, C-2)** with small lumina surrounded by pyramidal or columnar cells. This figure illustrates the general structure of the ducts, their secretory units, and their appearance when the gland is sectioned in various planes.

Area **A** illustrates the appearance of a section when the red dotted line a-a' passes in an oblique plane **(A-2)** through a **large duct (A-1)** and transversely through two **small ducts (A-3)** and two **acini (A-4)**.

In area **B** are illustrated sections of small ducts **(B-1, B-3)** and acini **(B-2, B-4)** when the red dotted line b-b' passes in transverse or oblique planes.

In area **C, C-1** represents the appearance of sections when the blue dotted line c-c' passes through different parts of two acini. Because these acini are round, both sections appear similar. At **C-2**, the same blue line passed longitudinally through two small ducts and the lumen of an acinus which opens into the smallest duct.

EXAMPLES

The histology of the major salivary glands is of this type (Plates 56, 57, 58), composed of masses of acini and ducts of various sizes. The salivary glands contain two major types of secretory acini: serous and mucous acini. Serous acini are described in detail on page 148 and are present in glands illustrated on Plates 56, 57, and 58. Mucous acini are described and compared with serous acini on page 150; they are illustrated on Plates

57 and 58. Ducts are distinct structures; they are lined with cuboidal, columnar, or stratified epithelium, and are named according to their location in the gland.

A less complex tubuloacinar gland, consisting of mucous acini and ducts, is illustrated on Plate 59:11, 12 (esophageal glands). Similar glands consisting of ducts, mucous acini, and serous acini are found in the connective tissue of the trachea (Plate 84).

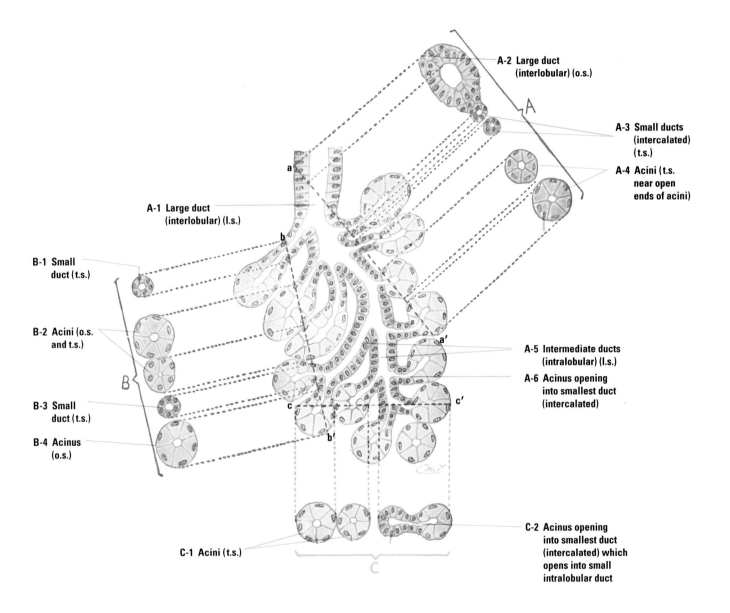

A-2 Large duct (interlobular) (o.s.)

A-3 Small ducts (intercalated) (t.s.)

A-4 Acini (t.s. near open ends of acini)

A-1 Large duct (interlobular) (l.s.)

B-1 Small duct (t.s.)

B-2 Acini (o.s. and t.s.)

B-3 Small duct (t.s.)

B-4 Acinus (o.s.)

A-5 Intermediate ducts (intralobular) (l.s.)

A-6 Acinus opening into smallest duct (intercalated)

C-2 Acinus opening into smallest duct (intercalated) which opens into small intralobular duct

C-1 Acini (t.s.)

PLATE 7

COMPOUND ACINAR GLAND (DIAGRAM)

This is a representative illustration of a gland similar to the mammary gland. The terminal secretory units are the acini. In an active gland, the secretory acini are round sacs with large central lumina surrounded by cuboidal or low columnar cells (**4,6,7**); the **acini** may branch (**6**).

As described previously, the acini open into **small ducts (2, 3)**, which are lined with low columnar cells.

The small ducts then open into successively **larger ducts (1, 5)**. The final excretory duct, which is even larger, is not illustrated.

The blue dotted line a-a' and the red dotted line b-b' pass through the acini and ducts at different planes of section. The resulting appearance of such sections are shown at **A** and **B**.

EXAMPLES

The mammary gland is a good example of this type of gland. It is illustrated in Plates 116 and 117. The lactating mammary gland contains enlarged secretory acini with large lumina that are filled with milk products (Plate 117, Fig. 2).

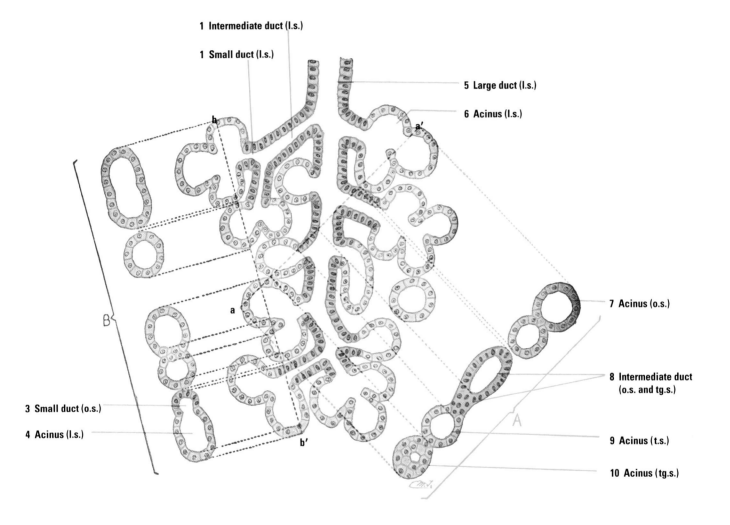

1 Intermediate duct (l.s.)

1 Small duct (l.s.)

5 Large duct (l.s.)

6 Acinus (l.s.)

7 Acinus (o.s.)

8 Intermediate duct
   (o.s. and tg.s.)

3 Small duct (o.s.)

4 Acinus (l.s.)

9 Acinus (t.s.)

10 Acinus (tg.s.)

With the exceptions of blood and lymph, the connective tissue consists of cells and of extracellular material, the matrix. The matrix, in turn, consists of fibers, ground substance, and tissue fluid. The main function of the connective tissue is to bind, anchor, and support various body parts.

Cells of the Connective Tissue

The fusiform-shaped fibroblasts are the most common connective tissue cells; these cells are young and exhibit synthetic activity. The fibrocytes, on the other hand, are the mature cells and are smaller than the fibroblasts. The main function of the fibroblasts is the synthesis of collagen, reticular, and elastic fibers, and of the extracellular matrix.

The macrophages or histiocytes are numerous in the connective tissue regions and may resemble the fibroblasts. The macrophages are phagocytic; their main function is to ingest bacteria, cell debris, and/or other foreign matter in the connective tissue.

The round to oval mast cells contain a cytoplasm filled with small, dark-staining granules. These cells have a wide distribution in the connective tissue of the skin and the digestive and respiratory organs, and are usually associated with blood vessels. The main function of the mast cells is the synthesis and release of heparin and histamine. Heparin is a strong anticoagulant of the blood. Histamine dilates blood vessels, increases their permeability to fluid, and produces edema.

The plasma cells are numerous in the connective tissue regions in the respiratory and digestive tracts. Their main function is the synthesis and secretion of antibodies, which aid the body in defense against bacterial infections.

The white blood cells, or leukocytes, migrate into the connective tissue from the blood vessels. Their main function is the defense of the organism against bacterial invasion or foreign material. The neutrophils are active phagocytes, found in great numbers at the sites of bacterial invasion and infection. The eosinophils increase in number following parasitic infections or allergic reactions. Their main function is the phagocytosis of antigen-antibody complexes formed during allergic reactions. The basophils are filled with basophilic granules, which contain heparin and histamine. Their function is similar to that of the mast cells. The lymphocytes are most numerous in the respiratory and gastrointestinal tracts. Their main function is immunologic in response to invasion by pathogens and/or foreign material.

The adipose (fat) cells store fat and may occur singly or in groups. When adipose cells predominate, the tissue is called adipose tissue. In addition to storing fat, the adipose cells provide packing material in and around numerous organs.

The fibroblasts and the adipose cells are permanent connective tissue cells. On the other hand, leukocytes, plasma cells, mast cells, and macrophages are cells that migrate into the connective tissue regions.

Fibers of the Connective Tissue

There are three types of connective tissue fibers: collagen, elastic, and reticular. The amount, arrangement, and concentration of these fibers depends on the function of the tissues or organs.

The collagen fibers are most abundant and found in almost all types of connective tissue. They exhibit great tensile strength and are found in areas where strong support is needed.

The elastic fibers are thin and small, exhibit branching, and have less tensile strength than the collagen fibers. They exhibit elasticity and, when stretched, return to their original size without deformation. They are found in the lung, bladder, and skin, including large blood vessels and elastic cartilages, where stretching without breaking or distortion is essential for proper function of the organs.

The reticular fibers are thin and form a delicate net-like framework in the liver, lymph nodes, spleen, hemopoietic organs, and other organs. These fibers are normally not visible in organs unless they are stained with silver.

Classification of Connective Tissue

The connective tissue is normally divided into loose connective tissue and dense connective tissue, depending on the amount, type, arrangement, and abundance of cells, fibers, and ground substance.

The loose connective tissue is more abundant in the body. It is characterized by a loose, irregular arrangement of different fibers, and contains all connective tissue cells in its matrix. Although reticular and elastic fibers may be present, collagenous fibers, fibroblasts, and macrophages predominate.

In contrast, the dense connective tissue contains thicker and denser packed collagenous fibers. In addition, there are also fewer types of cells and less ground substance. Dense irregular connective tissue resists pulling forces from all directions because the collagenous fibers are oriented in different directions. Dense regular connective tissue exhibits a parallel arrangement of collagen fibers. As a result, the fibers resist pulling forces from a single direction. Dense regular arrangement of fibers is best seen in the tendons and ligaments.

19

The Ground Substance

The ground substance in the connective tissue is an amorphous, transparent, colorless material with the property of a semifluid gel and high water content. It surrounds the cells and fibers of, and provides structural support for, the connective tissue. The ground substance functions by facilitating diffusion of oxygen, electrolytes, nutrients, fluids, metabolites, waste products, and other products between the cells and the blood vessels. The ground substance also serves as a barrier; it prevents the spread of pathogens from the connective tissue into the bloodstream.

The density of ground substance can vary according to the amount of tissue fluid and/or water content. Mineralization of ground substance changes its density, rigidity, and permeability, as seen in the cartilage and bone.

PLATE 8

■ **FIG. 1**
LOOSE IRREGULAR CONNECTIVE TISSUE (SPREAD)
■ **FIG. 2**
CELLS OF LOOSE CONNECTIVE TISSUE IN SECTIONS

PLATE 8

■ FIG. 1
LOOSE IRREGULAR CONNECTIVE TISSUE (SPREAD)

The plate illustrates subcutaneous connective tissue-from a rat, stained by injection of a dilute solution of neutral red in saline. This solution not only permits the tissue elements to remain in their natural state but also separates them farther from each other than would be seen under normal conditions or when prepared in histologic sections. Under this condition, fibers and cells are readily identified.

The unstained **collagenous fibers (2, 9)** are the most numerous, thickest, and largest. These fibers course in all directions, are thick and somewhat wavy, and exhibit faint longitudinal striations (parts of their component fibrils).

The **elastic fibers (1, 10)** are thin, fine, single fibers that are usually straight; however, after the section is cut, the fibers may become wavy because of release of tension. Elastic fibers form branching and anastomosing networks. Although unstained, the fibers are highly refringent, an appearance in contrast to the dull appearance of collagenous fibers. The fine reticular fibers are also present in loose connective tissue but are not seen in this illustration.

The fixed permanent cells of this and other connective tissue proper are the **fibroblasts (8, I)**. In this preparation, the fibroblasts (8) are illustrated as flattened, branching cells with an oval nucleus in which chromatin is sparse but one or two **nucleoli (14, 15)**

may be present. Fixed **macrophages or histiocytes (4, 11, II)** are always present in varying numbers. When inactive, the macrophages have an appearance of fibroblasts although their processes may be more irregular and their nuclei smaller. Phagocytic inclusions, however, give their cytoplasm a varied appearance. In the illustration, the phagocytic vacuoles in the cytoplasm are filled with neutral red (small vacuoles in 4, larger vacuoles in 11 and II:17).

The **mast cells (7, III)** are also the usual component of loose connective tissue; they are seen as either single cells or grouped along small blood vessels (7). The cells are usually ovoid, with a small, pale, centrally placed **nucleus (18)** and cytoplasm filled with fine, closely packed **granules (7, 19, III)** that stain deep-red with neutral red stain.

Present also are groups of **adipose cells (fat) (3)**. Each cell is a spherical, colorless globule; the small, eccentric nucleus is not visible.

Blood and other connective tissue cells may also be seen in small numbers. These cells are not stained with neutral red; however, **eosinophils (5)** may be identified by lobulated nucleus and coarse, cytoplasmic granules. In the small round **lymphocytes (6),** the nucleus occupies most of the cell.

The faint background stain is the ground substance which has been infiltrated with injected fluid.

■ FIG. 2
CELLS OF LOOSE CONNECTIVE TISSUE IN SECTIONS

This figure illustrates some cells of loose connective tissue as they appear in histologic sections after fixation and hematoxylin-eosin staining.

The free **macrophages (1)** usually appear round with slightly irregular cell outlines. The appearance of macrophages is variable; in the illustration, the macrophage exhibits a small nucleus rich in chromatin and slightly acidophilic cytoplasm. The **fibroblast (2)** is elongated with cytoplasmic projections, an ovoid nucleus with sparse chromatin, and one or two nucleoli. The **fibrocyte (3)** is a more mature, smaller cell without cytoplasmic projections; the nucleus is similar but smaller than that in the fibroblast.

The **large (4)** and **small lymphocytes (5)** are round cells that differ principally in the larger amount of cytoplasm in the former. Their dark-staining nuclei have condensed chromatin clumps but no nucleoli.

The **plasma cells (6)** are distinguished from large lymphocytes (4) by a smaller, eccentrically placed nucleus with condensed, coarse chromatin clumps distributed in a characteristic radial pattern and one central mass. A prominent, clear area in the cytoplasm is seen adjacent to the nucleus.

Eosinophils (7) of the circulating blood are readily distinguished by their large size, a bilobed nucleus, and large, cytoplasmic granules that stain intensely with eosin.

Occasional **pigment cells (8)** may be seen. The **adipose cells (9)** are large cells with a narrow rim of cytoplasm and eccentric nucleus. In histologic sections, the large fat globule in the living cell has been dissolved by reagents used in section preparation, leaving a large, empty space.

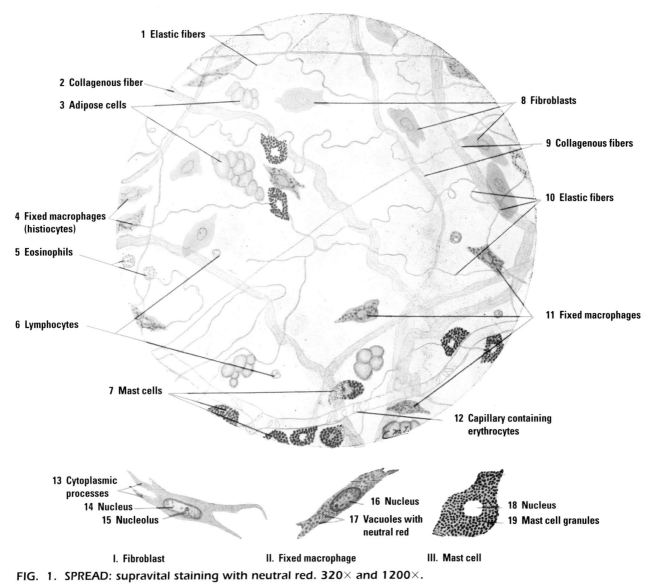

1 Elastic fibers

2 Collagenous fiber

3 Adipose cells

8 Fibroblasts

9 Collagenous fibers

10 Elastic fibers

4 Fixed macrophages (histiocytes)

5 Eosinophils

11 Fixed macrophages

6 Lymphocytes

7 Mast cells

12 Capillary containing erythrocytes

13 Cytoplasmic processes
14 Nucleus
15 Nucleolus

16 Nucleus
17 Vacuoles with neutral red

18 Nucleus
19 Mast cell granules

I. Fibroblast   II. Fixed macrophage   III. Mast cell

FIG. 1. SPREAD: supravital staining with neutral red. 320× and 1200×.

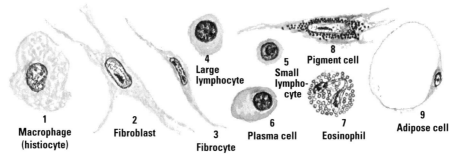

4 Large lymphocyte

5 Small lymphocyte

8 Pigment cell

1 Macrophage (histiocyte)

2 Fibroblast

3 Fibrocyte

6 Plasma cell

7 Eosinophil

9 Adipose cell

FIG. 2. INDIVIDUAL CELLS OF LOOSE CONNECTIVE TISSUE. Stain: hematoxylin-eosin. 1200×.

23

PLATE 9

■ **FIG. 1**
LOOSE IRREGULAR CONNECTIVE TISSUE

Collagen fibers (6) predominate in loose connective tissue, course in different directions, and form a loose meshwork. In the illustration, these fibers are sectioned in various planes, and transverse ends may be seen. Collagen fibers (6) have different diameters and appear longitudinally striated because of their fibrillar structure. The fibers are acidophilic and stain pink with eosin. Thin elastic fibers are also present in loose connective tissue, but are difficult to distinguish with this stain and at this magnification.

The **fibroblasts (1)** are the most numerous cells in the loose connective tissue and may be sectioned in various planes, so that only parts of the cells may be seen. Also, during section preparation, the cytoplasm of these cells may shrink. A typical fibroblast (1) shows an oval nucleus with sparse chromatin and lightly acidophilic cytoplasm with few short processes.

Also present in loose connective tissue are different blood cells such as the **neutrophils (3)** with lobulated nuclei and small **lymphocytes (2)** with dense nuclei and sparse cytoplasm. The **fat or adipose cells (11, 12)** appear characteristically empty with a thin rim of cytoplasm (11) and peripherally displaced flat **nuclei (12)**.

The connective tissue is also highly vascular. **Capillaries (7, 13)** appear cut in different planes and are lined with endothelium. Larger blood vessels, such as the **arterioles (4, 9, 10)** and **venules (5, 8),** sectioned in different planes, are also seen in the loose connective tissue.

Other examples of loose connective tissue in organs are illustrated on Plate 25, Fig. 1:9 and on Plate 90, Fig. 2:6.

■ **FIG. 2**
DENSE IRREGULAR CONNECTIVE TISSUE

This figure illustrates dense irregular connective tissue from the dermis of the skin. The arrangement of fibers and cells is similar to that in loose connective tissue; however, this is modified for areas in the body where more firm support and strength are required.

The **collagen fibers (1, 2)** are large, found typically in thick bundles, and sectioned in different planes because they course in various directions. This type of fiber arrangement is compact. Present here are also thin, wavy **elastic fibers (10),** which form fine networks.

The **fibroblasts (5, 11)** are often found compressed among the collagenous fibers. Also illustrated is an undifferentiated **mesenchymal cell (6)** along a small blood vessel and a few blood cells: **neutrophils (3)** with lobulated nuclei and **lymphocytes (9)** with large round nuclei without visible cytoplasm. **Small blood vessels (4, 8)** are also illustrated.

Additional illustration of dense irregular connective tissue in the dermis of the skin is found on Plate 46, Fig. 1:3.

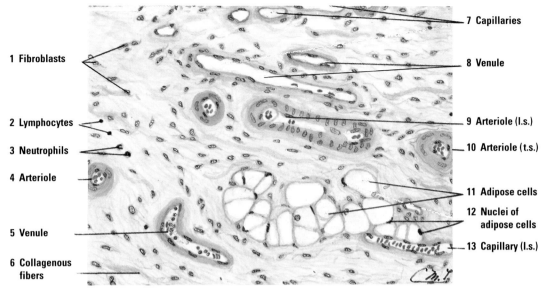

1 Fibroblasts

2 Lymphocytes

3 Neutrophils

4 Arteriole

5 Venule

6 Collagenous fibers

7 Capillaries

8 Venule

9 Arteriole (l.s.)

10 Arteriole (t.s.)

11 Adipose cells

12 Nuclei of adipose cells

13 Capillary (l.s.)

FIG. 1. LOOSE IRREGULAR CONNECTIVE TISSUE. Stain: hematoxylin-eosin. 300×. l.s. = longitudinal section; t.s. = transverse section

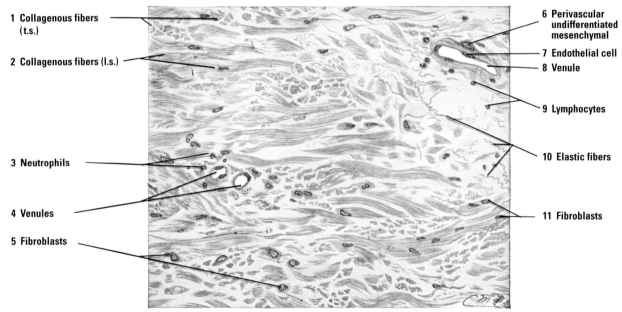

1 Collagenous fibers (t.s.)

2 Collagenous fibers (l.s.)

3 Neutrophils

4 Venules

5 Fibroblasts

6 Perivascular undifferentiated mesenchymal

7 Endothelial cell

8 Venule

9 Lymphocytes

10 Elastic fibers

11 Fibroblasts

FIG. 2. DENSE IRREGULAR CONNECTIVE TISSUE. Stain: hematoxylin-eosin. 300×.

PLATE 10

■ FIG. 1
DENSE REGULAR CONNECTIVE TISSUE: TENDON (LONGITUDINAL SECTION)

Dense regular connective tissue is found where great tensile strength is required, such as in ligaments and tendons. A section of a tendon is illustrated at a higher magnification.

The **collagenous fibers (2, 3)** are arranged in compact, parallel bundles. Between these bundles are thin partitions of looser connective tissue that contain parallel rows of **fibroblasts (1, 4, 5).** These cells have short processes (not visible here) and ovoid nuclei when seen in surface view (4) or rod-like in lateral view (5).

Dense regular connective tissue with less regular fiber arrangement than in the tendon also forms fibrous membranes or capsules around various organs in the body. Examples of such connective tissue are perichondrium around the tracheal cartilage (Plate 84, Fig. 1:2), the dura mater around the spinal cord (Plate 34, Fig. 1:13), and the tunica albuginea surrounding the testis (Plate 97, Fig. 1:1).

■ FIG. 2
DENSE REGULAR CONNECTIVE TISSUE: TENDON (TRANSVERSE SECTION)

A tendon in transverse section is illustrated at a lower magnification than that in Figure 1. Within each large bundle of **collagen fibers (1, 10)** are **fibroblasts (nuclei) (2, 9)** sectioned transversely. The fibroblasts are located between small bundles of collagen fibers. These are better distinguished at the higher magnification in the insert, which shows bundles of collagenous fibers (10) and the branched shape of fibroblasts (9) in transverse section.

Between the large collagenous bundles are thin partitions of **connective tissue (3).** Collagen bundles are grouped into fascicles, between which course larger partitions (septa or trabeculae) of interfascicular **connective tissue (4, 8).** These partitions contain **blood vessels (5),** nerves, and occasionally lamellated **Pacinian corpuscles (6),** which are sensitive pressure receptors. Also illustrated in the figure is a transverse section of **skeletal muscle (7),** which is adjacent to the tendon but separated from it by connective tissue.

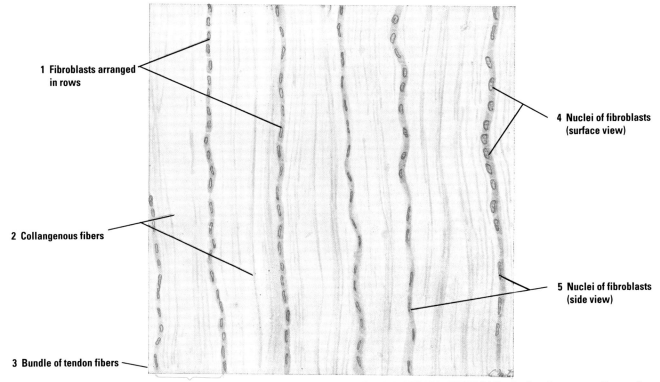

1 Fibroblasts arranged in rows

4 Nuclei of fibroblasts (surface view)

2 Collangenous fibers

5 Nuclei of fibroblasts (side view)

3 Bundle of tendon fibers

FIG. 1. DENSE REGULAR CONNECTIVE TISSUE: TENDON (LONGITUDINAL SECTION). Stain: hematoxylin-eosin. 250×.

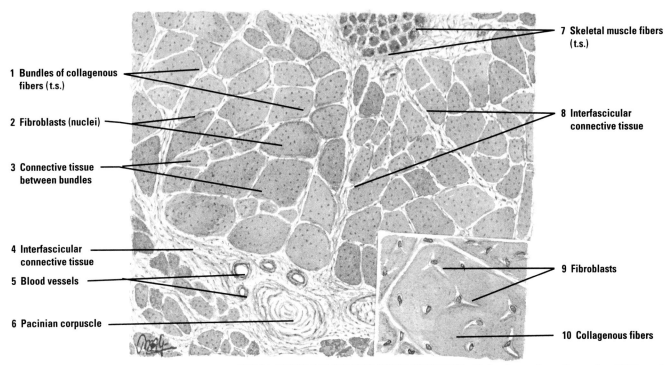

1 Bundles of collagenous fibers (t.s.)

2 Fibroblasts (nuclei)

3 Connective tissue between bundles

4 Interfascicular connective tissue

5 Blood vessels

6 Pacinian corpuscle

7 Skeletal muscle fibers (t.s.)

8 Interfascicular connective tissue

9 Fibroblasts

10 Collagenous fibers

Fig. 2. DENSE REGULAR CONNECTIVE TISSUE: TENDON (TRANSVERSE SECTION). Stain: hematoxylin-eosin. 80× and 300×.

27

PLATE 11

■ **FIG. 1**
DENSE IRREGULAR AND LOOSE CONNECTIVE TISSUE (ELASTIN STAIN)

This figure illustrates an area with dense irregular connective tissue on the left side, a transition zone in the middle, and loose connective tissue on the right.

The **elastic fibers (1, 4)** are selectively stained a deep blue with Verhoeff's method. Using Van Gieson's as a counterstain, acid fuchsin stains **collagenous fibers** red **(2, 5).** Cellular details of fibroblasts are not revealed but the **fibroblast nuclei (3, 6)** stain deep blue.

The characteristic features of dense irregular and loose connective tissues become apparent with this staining technique. In dense irregular connective tissue (2), the collagenous fibers are larger, more numerous, and more concentrated. Elastic fibers are also larger and more numerous (1). In contrast, in the loose connective tissue, both fiber types are smaller (4, 5) and more loosely arranged. Fine elastic networks are seen in both types of connective tissue.

■ **FIG. 2**
ADIPOSE TISSUE

A small section of a mesentery is illustrated in which large accumulations of **adipose (fat) cells (2, 8)** are organized into adipose tissue. The connective tissue of the **peritoneum (6)** serves as a capsule around the adipose tissue.

Adipose cells (2) are closely packed and separated by thin strips of connective tissue, which contains the compressed **fibroblasts (7).** Lobules of adipose tissue are separated by **connective tissue septa (3)** in which are found **blood vessels (1, 4),** nerves, and **capillaries (5).**

Individual adipose cells appear as empty cells (2) because the fat was dissolved by chemicals used during routine histologic preparation of the tissue. Their nuclei (8) are compressed in the peripheral rim of the cytoplasm, and in certain sections, it is difficult to distinguish between fibroblast nuclei (7) and adipose cell nuclei (8).

■ **FIG. 3**
EMBRYONIC CONNECTIVE TISSUE

The embryonic connective tissue resembles the mesenchyme or mucous connective tissue, which is loose and irregular. The difference in ground substance (semifluid versus jelly-like) is not apparent in these sections.

The **fibroblasts (2)** are numerous and fine **collagenous fibers (3)** are found between them, some coming in close contact with fibroblasts. Embryonic connective tissue is also vascular **(1, 4).**

At higher magnification, a primitive **fibroblast (5)** is seen as a large, branching cell with abundant cytoplasm, prominent cytoplasmic processes, an oval nucleus with fine chromatin, and one or more nucleoli. The widely separated **collagenous fibers (6)** are more apparent at this magnification.

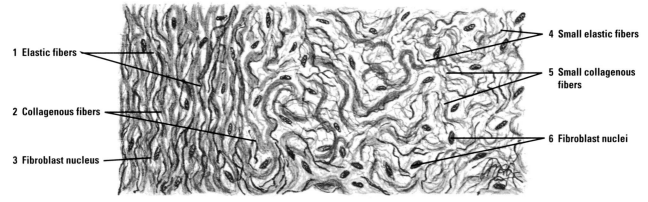

1 Elastic fibers

2 Collagenous fibers

3 Fibroblast nucleus

4 Small elastic fibers

5 Small collagenous fibers

6 Fibroblast nuclei

FIG. 1. DENSE IRREGULAR AND LOOSE CONNECTIVE TISSUE. Stain: Verhoeff's elastin stain and Van Gieson's. 240×.

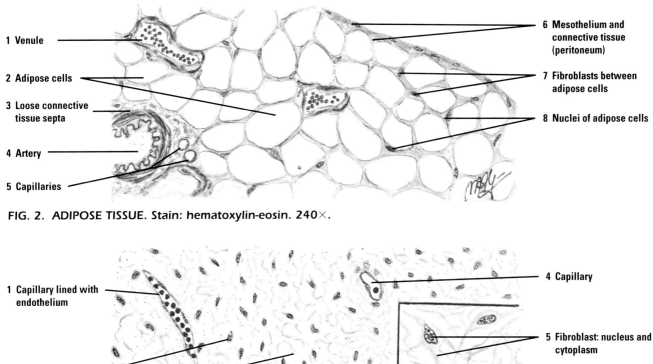

1 Venule

2 Adipose cells

3 Loose connective tissue septa

4 Artery

5 Capillaries

6 Mesothelium and connective tissue (peritoneum)

7 Fibroblasts between adipose cells

8 Nuclei of adipose cells

FIG. 2. ADIPOSE TISSUE. Stain: hematoxylin-eosin. 240×.

1 Capillary lined with endothelium

2 Fibroblast nuclei

3 Collagenous fibers

4 Capillary

5 Fibroblast: nucleus and cytoplasm

6 Collagenous fibers

FIG. 3. EMBRYONIC CONNECTIVE TISSUE. Stain: hematoxylin-eosin. 240× and 900×.

29

THE CARTILAGE

The cartilage is a special form of connective tissue. It consists of cells (chondrocytes and chondroblasts) and matrix (fibers and ground substance). The matrix contains collagen or elastic fibers, which give the cartilage its firmness and resilience. As a result, cartilage exhibits tensile strength, provides structural support, and allows flexibility without distortion.

The cartilage is formed from mesenchymal cells that differentiate into chondroblasts. These cells divide mitotically, grow, and synthesize the cartilage matrix and the extracellular material. Gradually, individual chondroblasts become surrounded by matrix and are trapped in a space called lacuna (lacunae—plural). The trapped cells are the mature cartilage cells and are called chondrocytes. Some lacunae may contain more than one chondrocyte; in that case, these groups of chondrocytes are called isogenous groups. Most cartilage is surrounded by a connective tissue perichondrium. An exception is the cartilage on the articulating surfaces of the bones.

The cartilage is nonvascular but surrounded by vascular connective tissue. As a result, all nutrients enter and metabolites leave the cartilage by diffusion through the matrix. Also, because the matrix is not hard or rigid, cartilage grows by interstitial and appositional means. The interstitial growth involves the mitoses of the chondrocytes within the matrix and the deposition of new matrix between the cells. This process increases the cartilage size from within. The appositional growth occurs peripherally, where the chondroblasts differentiate from the perichondrium and deposit a layer of cartilage that is apposed to the existing cartilage layer.

Types of Cartilage

There are three types of cartilage in the body: hyaline, elastic, and fibrocartilage. This classification is based on the amount and types of fibers present in the matrix.

The hyaline cartilage is the most common type and, in the embryo, it functions as a skeletal model for most bones. In adults, the hyaline cartilage functions as structural and flexible support on the articular bone surfaces, ends of ribs (costal cartilage), nose, larynx, trachea, and bronchi.

The elastic cartilage is similar to the hyaline except for the presence of elastic fibers in its matrix. This type of cartilage allows increased flexibility as well as support. Elastic cartilage is found in the external ear, the walls of the auditory tube, and the larynx. A layer of connective tissue, the perichondrium, surrounds the elastic cartilage.

The fibrocartilage contains irregular, thick bundles of collagen fibers. It is found in the intervertebral disks, symphysis pubis, and certain joints. The fibrocartilage serves an important function in the areas of the body where durability, tensile strength, and resistance to compression is needed.

PLATE 12

■ FIG. 1
FETAL CARTILAGE: DEVELOPING HYALINE CARTILAGE

This figure illustrates a cartilage model of a bone in an early stages of development. Most of the model consists of young **chondroblasts (1)** that still resemble mesenchymal cells, having spherical nuclei and cytoplasmic processes. Lacunae have not developed at this stage. The chondroblasts are numerous, crowded into a specific area, and randomly distributed in the cartilage without forming isogenous groups. At this stage of development, cartilage **matrix (3)** is secreted.

On the periphery of the cartilage model (left side),

mesenchymal cells are concentrated and exhibit a parallel arrangement **(2).** The nuclei of these cells are elongated and flattened, and the cell membranes are not distinct. This peripheral area of the cartilage develops into perichondrium, a sheath of dense connective tissue that surrounds hyaline and elastic cartilage. The inner portion of perichondrium is the chondrogenic layer from which chondroblasts (2) develop; there is some indication of such transition in the illustration.

■ FIG. 1A
FETAL CARTILAGE (SECTIONAL VIEW)

A higher magnification of a region from the middle of Fig. 1 illustrates early **chondroblasts (2)** with round nuclei and cytoplasmic processes. Some of the **chondroblasts (1)** from the superficial portion of the cartilage exhibit more elongated nuclei and indistinct cell outlines.

In a routine histologic preparation, the collagenous fibers in the **matrix (3)** are not visible and the matrix (3) appears homogeneous; however, it is more acidophilic in the superficial zone.

■ FIG. 2
MATURE HYALINE CARTILAGE

This section illustrates an interior or central region of the hyaline cartilage. Distributed throughout the homogeneous ground substance, the **matrix (5, 6)**, are ovoid spaces called **lacunae (2)** with mature cartilage cells, the **chondrocytes (1)**. In the intact cartilage, chondrocytes fill the lacunae. Each cell has a granular cytoplasm and a **nucleus (3)**. During histologic preparations, however, the chondrocytes (1) shrink and the lacunae (2) are seen as clear spaces. Cartilage cells in

the matrix are observed either singly or in isogenous groups.

The **matrix (6)** appears homogeneous and is usually basophilic; however, this condition can vary. The matrix between cells or groups of cells is called **interterritorial matrix (6)**. The more basophilic matrix around the cartilage cells is the **territorial matrix (5)**. Around each of the lacunae, the matrix forms a thin **cartilage capsule (4)**.

■ FIG. 3
NEWLY FORMED HYALINE CARTILAGE OF THE TRACHEA

A plate of hyaline cartilage from the trachea illustrates lacunae with either single **chondrocytes (12)** or **isogenous groups (13)**. Because the chondrocytes fill their lacunae, only margins of lacunae, the **cartilage capsule (16)**, are visible. Lacunae and chondrocytes in the middle of the cartilage are large and spherical (12, 13), but become progressively flatter in the periphery; these flat cells are young chondrocytes **(11)**.

The **interterritorial** (intercellular) **matrix (14)** stains lighter, whereas the **territorial matrix (15)** stains deeper.

A **perichondrium (4, 9, 18)** of dense connective tissue surrounds the entire cartilage plate. Its inner layer is **chondrogenic (10)** where the chondrocytes are formed by proliferation and differentiation of mesenchymal cells **(17)**.

Other examples of hyaline cartilage are illustrated in Plates 83 and 84.

HYALINE CARTILAGE

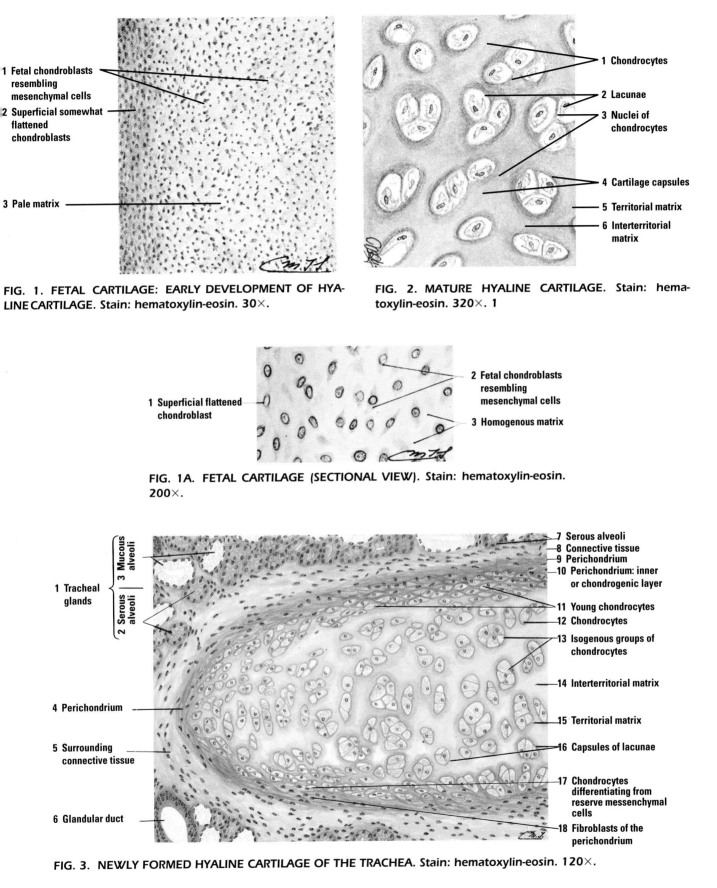

1 Fetal chondroblasts resembling mesenchymal cells

2 Superficial somewhat flattened chondroblasts

3 Pale matrix

FIG. 1. FETAL CARTILAGE: EARLY DEVELOPMENT OF HYALINE CARTILAGE. Stain: hematoxylin-eosin. 30×.

1 Chondrocytes

2 Lacunae

3 Nuclei of chondrocytes

4 Cartilage capsules

5 Territorial matrix

6 Interterritorial matrix

FIG. 2. MATURE HYALINE CARTILAGE. Stain: hematoxylin-eosin. 320×. 1

1 Superficial flattened chondroblast

2 Fetal chondroblasts resembling mesenchymal cells

3 Homogenous matrix

FIG. 1A. FETAL CARTILAGE (SECTIONAL VIEW). Stain: hematoxylin-eosin. 200×.

1 Tracheal glands

3 Mucous alveoli

2 Serous alveoli

4 Perichondrium

5 Surrounding connective tissue

6 Glandular duct

7 Serous alveoli

8 Connective tissue

9 Perichondrium

10 Perichondrium: inner or chondrogenic layer

11 Young chondrocytes

12 Chondrocytes

13 Isogenous groups of chondrocytes

14 Interterritorial matrix

15 Territorial matrix

16 Capsules of lacunae

17 Chondrocytes differentiating from reserve messenchymal cells

18 Fibroblasts of the perichondrium

FIG. 3. NEWLY FORMED HYALINE CARTILAGE OF THE TRACHEA. Stain: hematoxylin-eosin. 120×.

33

PLATE 13

■ FIG. 1
FIBROUS CARTILAGE: INTERVERTEBRAL DISK

In fibrous cartilage, the **matrix (6)** is permeated with **collagenous fibers (5),** which frequently exhibit parallel fiber arrangement as seen in tendons. Small **chondrocytes (2, 4)** in **lacunae (1)** are usually distributed in **rows (3)** within the fibrous matrix and not at random or in isogenous groups as is usually seen in hyaline or elastic cartilage. All chondrocytes and lacunae are of similar size; there is no gradation from larger central chondrocytes to smaller and flatter peripheral cells.

A perichondrium, normally present around hyaline and elastic cartilage, is absent because fibrous cartilage usually forms a transitional area between hyaline cartilage and tendon or ligament.

The proportion of collagenous fibers to matrix, the number of chondrocytes, and their arrangement may vary. The collagenous fibers may be so dense that matrix becomes invisible; in such cases, chondrocytes and lacunae appear flattened. Fibers within a bundle may be parallel, but different fibers may course in different directions.

■ FIG. 2
ELASTIC CARTILAGE: EPIGLOTTIS

Elastic cartilage differs from hyaline cartilage principally by the presence of **elastic fibers (1, 3)** in its matrix. These can be demonstrated, as deep purple fibers, after staining the cartilage with orcein (3). The fibers enter the cartilagenous matrix from the **perichondrium (4),** usually as small fibers, and are distributed in the interior as branching and anastomosing fibers of varying size (3); some of the fibers exhibit considerable thickness (3, middle leader). The density of fibers in the matrix varies in different elastic cartilages as well as in different areas of the same cartilage.

As in hyaline cartilage, larger **chondrocytes (2, 5)** in lacunae are seen in the interior of the plate. The smaller ones are more peripheral; the latter finally become fibroblasts in the perichondrium (4).

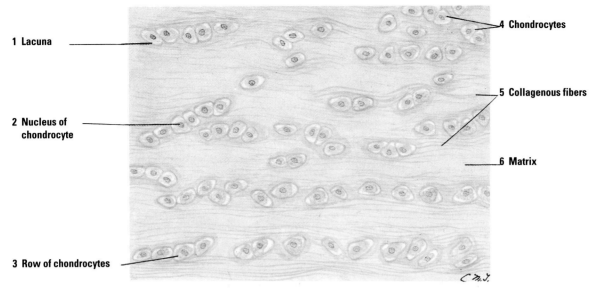

1 Lacuna

2 Nucleus of
   chondrocyte

3 Row of chondrocytes

4 Chondrocytes

5 Collagenous fibers

6 Matrix

FIG. 1. FIBROUS CARTILAGE: INTERVERTEBRAL DISC. Stain: hematoxylin-eosin. 320×.

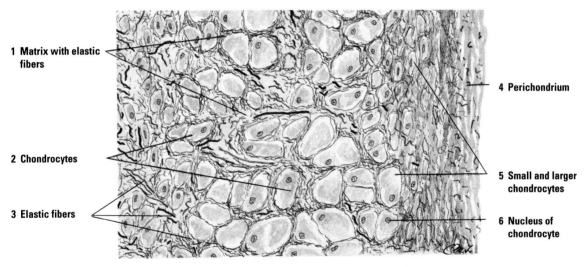

1 Matrix with elastic
   fibers

2 Chondrocytes

3 Elastic fibers

4 Perichondrium

5 Small and larger
   chondrocytes

6 Nucleus of
   chondrocyte

FIG. 2. ELASTIC CARTILAGE: EPIGLOTTIS. Stain: hematoxylin-eosin. 320×.

The bone is also a special form of connective tissue. Like other connective tissues, the bones consist of cells, fibers, and matrix. However, because the bone matrix is mineralized, the bones become hard, dense, and rigid. As a result of their mineral composition, the bones provide a rigid support for the body and form a protective cover for soft organs. In addition, the bones function as reservoirs for calcium, phosphate, and other minerals.

The minerals can be either stored in the bones or released into the body fluids when it becomes necessary to maintain proper mineral homeostasis. The bones are also dynamic structures; they are continually being renewed and/or remodeled in response to mineral needs of the body, mechanical stresses, and bone thinning during aging.

The Bone Cells

The developing and adult bones contain four different types of cells: osteogenic (osteoprogenitor) cells, osteoblasts, osteocytes, and osteoclasts.

The osteogenic cells are the undifferentiated, pleuripotential stem cells that are derived from mesenchyme. During bone development, the osteogenic cells proliferate by mitosis and differentiate into osteoblasts. In mature bones, the osteogenic cells are found in the external periosteum and in the single layer of the internal endosteum. The periosteum and endosteum provide a continuous supply of new osteoblasts for growth, remodeling, and/or repair of the bones.

The osteoblasts are the immature bone cells, present on the surfaces of bone tissue. Their main function is to synthesize, secrete, and deposit the organic compo-nents of the new bone matrix called osteoid. Osteoid is uncalcified, newly formed bone matrix that does not contain any minerals; however, after its deposition, it undergoes rapid mineralization and becomes bone.

The osteocytes are the main cells of the bone. Like the chondrocytes in the cartilage, they are trapped in their surrounding bone matrix and lie within lacunae; however, only one osteocyte is found in each lacuna. The osteocytes are responsible for the maintenance of the bone matrix.

Osteoclasts are large, multinucleated cells. Their main function is to resorb and remodel bone. Osteoclasts are often located in shallow depressions on the resorbed bone surface called Howship's lacunae. It is currently believed that osteoclasts originate from the circulating blood monocytes.

The Bone Matrix

Because the mineralized bone matrix is much harder than cartilage, the nutrients and metabolites cannot freely diffuse through it to the bone cells. Consequently, the bones become highly vascular and exhibit a unique system of canals called canaliculi. Cytoplasmic processes from the osteocytes extend into the canaliculi, which radiate in all directions from the lacunae. The canaliculi contain extracellular fluid and the extensions allow the osteocytes to communicate with adjacent osteocytes and with materials in the blood vessels of the bone matrix. In this manner, gaseous exchange takes place, nutrients are supplied to the osteocytes, and the metabolic wastes of osteocytes are eliminated.

PLATE 14

■ **FIG. 1**
COMPACT BONE, DRIED: DIAPHYSIS OF THE TIBIA (TRANSVERSE SECTION)

The characteristic feature of a compact bone is the arrangement of mineralized bone matrix into layers called lamellae, which exhibit various shapes. These are thin plates of bony tissue containing osteocytes or bone cells in almond-shaped **lacunae (11, 15)** from which radiate in all directions small canals, the **canaliculi (12).** These penetrate the lamellae and anastomose with canaliculi from other lacunae. Some of the canaliculi open into **Haversian canals (2)** and marrow cavities of the bone.

The outer wall of the compact bone (beneath the periosteum) is formed of **external circumferential lamellae (10),** which run parallel to each other and to the long axis of the bone. The inner wall (along the marrow cavity) is composed of **internal circumferential lamellae (6).** Between the internal and external cir-

cumferential lamellae are the **osteons (Haversian systems) (4, 8),** which are illustrated in transverse or oblique sections. The small irregular areas of bone between osteons are **interstitial lamellae (7, 9).**

The osteons or Haversian systems are the structural units of bone. Each osteon (4, 8) consists of a number of **concentric lamellae (3)** that surround a central **Haversian canal (2, 14).** In the living bone, the Haversian canal contains reticular connective tissue, blood vessels, and nerves (a miniature marrow cavity). The boundary between each osteon is sharply outlined by a refractile line called the **cement line (5),** which consists of modified matrix. Connections or anastomosis between central canals in the bone are frequently visible **(13).**

■ **FIG. 2**
COMPACT BONE, DRIED: DIAPHYSIS OF THE TIBIA (LONGITUDINAL SECTION)

The figure represents a small area of a longitudinal section from the diaphysis of a compact bone. Because the **Haversian canals (3)** course longitudinally in the bone, each canal (3) is seen as a tube, often branched, sectioned parallel to the long axis of the bone. It is surrounded by numerous **lamellae**

(1), within or between which are the **lacunae (4)** from which radiate the **canaliculi (6).** Lamellae, lacunae, and the osteon boundaries [the **cement lines (2)**] are generally parallel to the corresponding Haversian canals (3). The cement lines (2) indicate the extent of an osteon, as seen in longitudinal section.

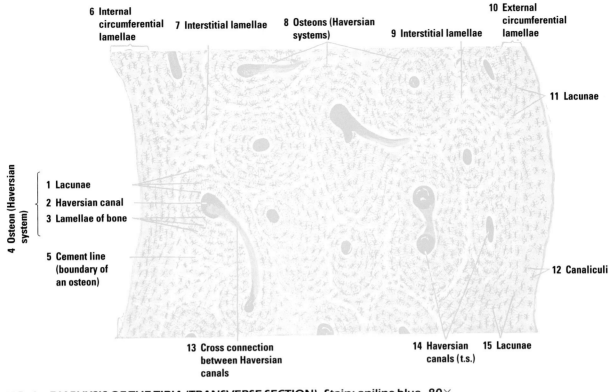

6 Internal circumferential lamellae

7 Interstitial lamellae

8 Osteons (Haversian systems)

9 Interstitial lamellae

10 External circumferential lamellae

11 Lacunae

4 Osteon (Haversian system)

1 Lacunae

2 Haversian canal

3 Lamellae of bone

5 Cement line (boundary of an osteon)

12 Canaliculi

13 Cross connection between Haversian canals

14 Haversian canals (t.s.)

15 Lacunae

FIG. 1. DIAPHYSIS OF THE TIBIA (TRANSVERSE SECTION). Stain: aniline blue. 80×.

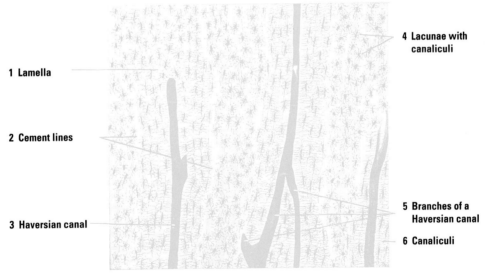

4 Lacunae with canaliculi

1 Lamella

2 Cement lines

3 Haversian canal

5 Branches of a Haversian canal

6 Canaliculi

FIG. 2. DIAPHYSIS OF THE TIBIA (LONGITUDINAL SECTION). Stain: aniline blue. 80×.

PLATE 15

■ **FIG. 1**
CANCELLOUS BONE: ADULT STERNUM (TRANSVERSE SECTION, DECALCIFIED)

Cancellous bone consists primarily of slender, bony **trabeculae (6),** which ramify, anastomose, and enclose irregular **marrow cavities (5)** of various sizes. Peripherally, these trabeculae merge with a thin shell of **compact bone (3)** which contains scattered **osteons (Haversian systems) (4, 7).** The surrounding **periosteum (2)** may descend into the bone at intervals and merge with adjacent loose **connective tissue (1),** which is rich in blood vessels.

Except for concentric lamellae in the osteons (4, 7), the **peripheral bone (3)** and the trabeculae exhibit **par-** **allel lamellae (8),** which (in this figure) are more apparent on the margins of bony areas. Lacunae with **osteocytes (9)** are visible in all regions of the bone.

The reticular connective tissue in the marrow cavities is obscured by **adipose cells (10)** and **hemopoietic (blood-forming) tissue (11).** Arteries are clearly visible in this illustration but sinusoids are too small to distinguish. The marrow fills the cavities; however, a thin, inner layer of cells, the **endosteum (12),** becomes visible when marrow separates from the bone.

■ **FIG. 2**
INTRAMEMBRANOUS OSSIFICATION: MANDIBLE OF FIVE-MONTH FETUS (TRANSVERSE SECTION, DECALCIFIED)

In the upper part of the illustration is the gum that covers the developing mandible. The mucosa of the gum consists of **stratified squamous epithelium (1)** and a wide **lamina propria (2)** containing blood vessels and nerves.

Below the lamina propria (2) is seen the developing bone. The **periosteum (3)** is differentiated, and numerous anastomosing trabeculae constitute the bone. These trabeculae surround the primitive **marrow cavities (14)** of various sizes, which consists of embryonic connective tissue, blood vessels, and nerves **(16).** Peripherally, collagenous fibers of the inner periosteum are in continuity with the fibers of the embryonic connective tissue of adjacent **marrow cavities (6)** and with collagenous fibers within the **bony trabeculae (10).**

Osteoblasts (7, 15) are associated with bone deposition and are seen in linear arrangement along the developing trabeculae. **Osteoclasts (5, 8)** are multinucleated giant cells and are associated with bone resorption and remodeling. The bony **osteocytes (4, 9)** are located in lacunae of the trabeculae.

Although collagenous fibers embedded in the bony matrix are obscured, the continuity with fibers of embryonic connective tissue in the marrow cavities may be seen at the margins of numerous trabeculae **(13).**

Formation of new bone is not a continuous process. Inactive areas appear where ossification has temporarily ceased: osteoid (newly synthesized bony matrix) and osteoblasts are not present. In some of the primitive marrow cavities, fibroblasts enlarge and differentiate into **osteoblasts (12).** In other areas, **osteoid (11, 17)** is seen on the margins of bony trabeculae; osteoblasts may (11) or may not be present (17).

CANCELLOUS BONE AND INTRAMEMBRANOUS OSSIFICATION

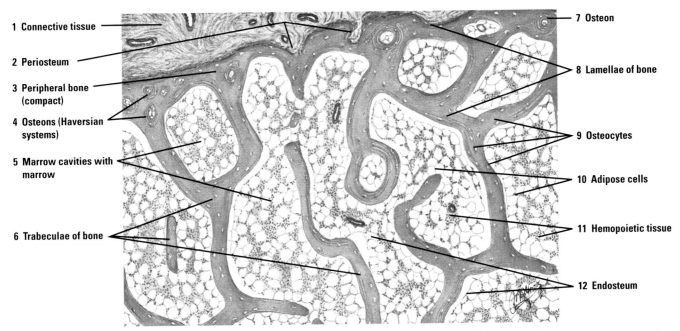

1 Connective tissue

2 Periosteum

3 Peripheral bone (compact)

4 Osteons (Haversian systems)

5 Marrow cavities with marrow

6 Trabeculae of bone

7 Osteon

8 Lamellae of bone

9 Osteocytes

10 Adipose cells

11 Hemopoietic tissue

12 Endosteum

FIG. 1. CANCELLOUS BONE: ADULT STERNUM (TRANSVERSE SECTION, DECALCIFIED). Stain: hematoxylin-eosin. 35×.

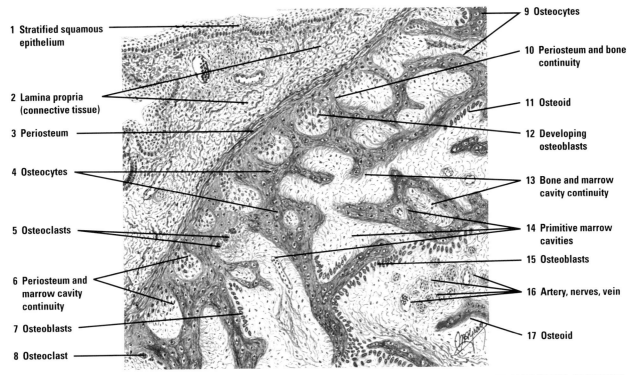

1 Stratified squamous epithelium

2 Lamina propria (connective tissue)

3 Periosteum

4 Osteocytes

5 Osteoclasts

6 Periosteum and marrow cavity continuity

7 Osteoblasts

8 Osteoclast

9 Osteocytes

10 Periosteum and bone continuity

11 Osteoid

12 Developing osteoblasts

13 Bone and marrow cavity continuity

14 Primitive marrow cavities

15 Osteoblasts

16 Artery, nerves, vein

17 Osteoid

FIG. 2. INTRAMEMBRANOUS OSSIFICATION: MANDIBLE OF FIVE-MONTH FETUS (TRANSVERSE SECTION, DECALCIFIED) Stain: Mallory-azan. 50×.

PLATE 16

ENDOCHONDRAL OSSIFICATION: DEVELOPING METACARPAL BONE (PANORAMIC VIEW, LONGITUDINAL SECTION)

This illustration depicts endochondral ossification, in which the future bone is first formed as model of embryonic hyaline cartilage. The cartilage model is then gradually replaced by a deposition of bone. In the center of the illustrated model, this process has already occurred. In addition, most of the original spongy bone so formed has been replaced and resorbed to form the central marrow cavity, leaving only scattered, thin spicules of bone of **endochondral origin (11, 30)**. **Red marrow (13)** fills the cavity of newly formed bone. The reticular connective tissue is obscured by masses of developing erythrocytes, granulocytes, **megakaryocytes (14)**, numerous **sinusoids (12)**, capillaries, and other blood vessels.

The process of endochondral ossification can be followed from the upper part of the illustration downward to the central marrow cavity. In the uppermost region is seen the zone of **reserve hyaline cartilage (17)**, in which the **chondrocytes in lacunae (2)** are distributed singly or in small groups. Chondrocytes then proliferate rapidly and become arranged in **columns (3, 18)**; cells and lacunae increase in size toward the lower area of this **zone of proliferating cartilage (18)**. The chondrocytes then **hypertrophy (19)** because of the swelling of nucleus and cytoplasm. The lacunae enlarge **(4)**, the cells then degenerate and the thin parti-

tions of intervening matrix calcify **(20)**. The calcified cartilage stains a deep purple.

Tufts of **vascular marrow (5)** invade the area of **calcifying cartilage (20)**, erode the lacunar walls and the calcified cartilage (20), and form new, small marrow cavities. Osteoprogenitor cells differentiate into osteoblasts and deposit osteoid and bone around the remaining **spicules (6)** of calcified cartilage. This region is the **zone of ossification (21)**.

The lower, lateral two thirds of the illustration shows the development of periosteal bone. Osteoblasts differentiate from osteoprogenitor cells in the inner layer of the **periosteum (9)** and form a **bone collar (10)** by the intramembranous method. Formation of new **periosteal bone (22)** keeps pace with formation of new endochondral bone. The bone collar increases in thickness and compactness as development of bone proceeds. The thickest portion of the collar is seen in the central part of the diaphysis at the initial site of **periosteal bone (29)** formation around the primary ossification center.

Surrounding the shaft of the developing bone are soft tissues: **muscle (7)**, **subcutaneous connective tissue** and **dermis of skin (15, 25)** with **hair follicles (26)**, **sebaceous glands (28)**, **sweat glands (16)**, and the **epidermis (24)**.

ENDOCHONDRAL OSSIFICATION: DEVELOPING METACARPAL BONE
(PANORAMIC VIEW, LONGITUDINAL SECTION)

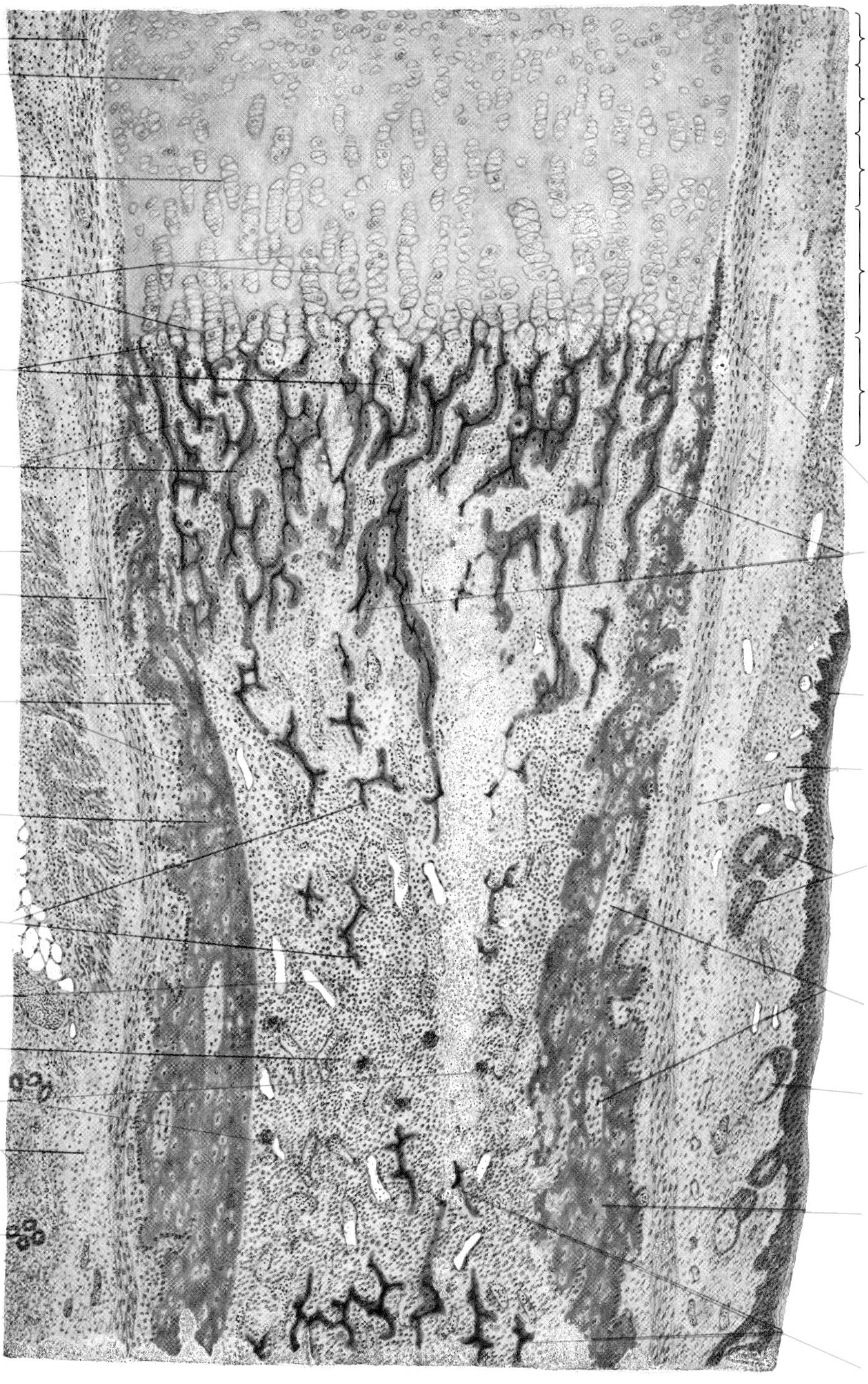

1 Perichondrium

2 Chondrocytes in lacunae

3 Column of chondrocytes

4 Hypertrophied chondrocytes and calcified matrix

5 Vascular tufts of osteogenic marrow

6 Osteoid and bone tissue around a spicule of calcified cartilage

7 Muscle

8 Periosteum (outer layer)

9 Periosteum (inner layer with osteoblasts)

10 Periosteal bone (bone collar)

11 Spicules of bone of endochondral origin

12 Sinusoid

13 Red bone marrow with myeloid elements

14 Megakaryocytes

15 Subcutaneous connective tissue and dermis

16 Sweat gland

17 Zone of reserve cartilage

18 Zone of proliferating cartilage

19 Zone of hypertrophying cells and lacunae

20 Zone of calcifying cartilage

21 Zone of erosion and ossification

22 Newly formed periosteal bone

23 Younger and older bony spicules

24 Epidermis

25 Dermis and subcutaneous layer

26 Hair follicles

27 Primitive marrow cavities in periosteal bone

28 Sebaceous gland

29 Periosteal bone

30 Spicules of bone of endochondral origin

Stain: hematoxylin-eosin. 60×.

43

PLATE 17

ENDOCHONDRAL OSSIFICATION (SECTIONAL VIEW)

This preparation shows in greater detail the processes of endochondral ossification at the zone of ossification and adjacent areas which correspond approximately to labels 3 through 6 in Plate 16.

Proliferating **chondrocytes (2, 10)** are arranged in columns. The cells in the lower part of this zone hypertrophy because of increased glycogen accumulation in the cytoplasm and nuclear swelling; lacunae also hypertrophy simultaneously. The cytoplasm of **hypertrophied chondrocytes (3)** then exhibits vacuolations, the nuclei become pyknotic, and the thin partitions of cartilagenous matrix become **calcified (4, 11).**

Tufts of **vascular marrow (5)** invade this area and form the zone of erosion. **Osteoblasts (14)** are formed and line up along remaining spicules of calcified carti-

lage, and lay down **osteoid (15)** and bone. Osteoblasts trapped in the osteoid or bone become **osteocytes (7).**

The **bone marrow (17)** contains cells belonging to the **erythrocytic (18)** and **granulocytic (19)** series as well as **megakaryocytes (8).** Multinucleated **osteoclasts (16),** which lie in shallow depressions called the **Howship's lacunae (16),** are situated adjacent to bone which is being resorbed.

On the right side of the illustration is an area of **periosteal cancellous bone (13)** with osteocytes and bone marrow cavities. The new bone is added peripherally by osteoblasts which develop from osteoprogenitor cells of the inner **periosteum (12).** The outer layer of periosteum continues superiorly over the cartilage as the **perichondrium (9).**

ENDOCHONDRAL OSSIFICATION (SECTIONAL VIEW)

1 Basophilic matrix

2 Columns of chondrocytes

3 Hypertrophied
chondrocytes
(vacuolized cytoplasm,
pyknotic nuclei)

4 Degenerating chondrocytes
surrounded by calcified
matrix

5 Invading capillaries
and embryonic bone
marrow in zone of
erosion

6 Spicules of calcified
cartilage surrounded
by osteoid

7 Newly formed
osteocytes

8 Megakaryocytes

9 Perichondrium

10 Columns of
chondrocytes

11 Calcified cartilage

12 Periosteum, outer
layer, and inner layer
with osteoblasts

13 Periosteal bone with
osteocytes

14 Osteoblasts

15 Osteoid

16 Osteoclasts in
Howship's lacunae

17 Hematogenous bone
marrow (red marrow)

18 Nests of erythroblasts

19 Group of myelocytes

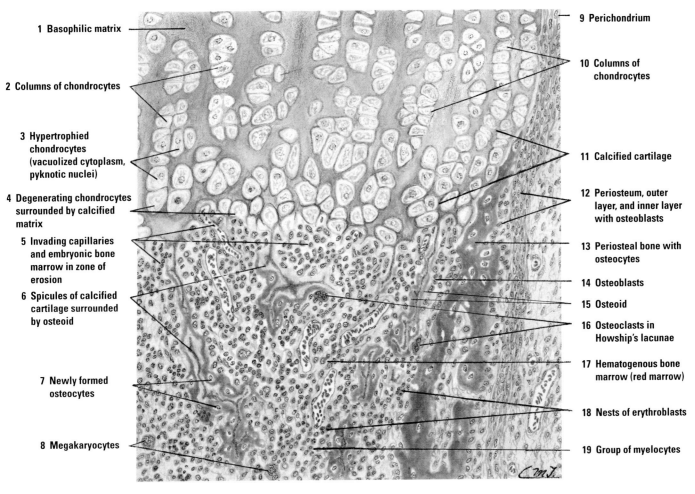

Stain: hematoxylin-eosin. 200×.

PLATE 18

FORMATION OF BONE: DEVELOPMENT OF OSTEONS (HAVERSIAN SYSTEMS) (TRANSVERSE SECTION, DECALCIFIED)

This illustration represents a late stage in the development of compact bone. Primitive osteons (Haversian systems) have already formed and others are in the process of development. In a metacarpal bone, such as seen in Plate 16, or in a long bone, the first compact bone is formed by deposition in the subperiosteal region (Plate 16:29). Vascular tufts of connective tissue from periosteum or endosteum erode this bone and form primitive osteons, as seen in this illustration. Bone reconstruction continues by breakdown of these first and later osteons and formation of new ones.

This plate illustrates a section of immature compact bone whose **matrix (11)** is stained deep with eosin. Primitive osteons are seen in transverse sections, with large **Haversian canals (8)** surrounded by a few **concentric lamellae (3)** of bone and **osteocytes (1)**. The Haversian canals (8) contain primitive connective tissue and **blood vessels (6, 8).** Bone deposition is contin-

uing in some of these osteons, as indicated by the presence of **osteoblasts (9)** along the Haversian canal (8) periphery and the margin of the innermost bone lamella. In some of the primitive osteons, the **osteoclasts (2)** are resorbing and remodeling the bone.

A longitudinal channel of **osteogenic connective tissue (10)** passes through the bone. From it arise tufts of vascular connective tissue which give rise to **Haversian canals (4).** Osteoblasts already line the periphery of the canal.

In the lower part of the figure is a large **bone marrow cavity (14)** in which hemopoiesis is in progress; this is the red marrow. Also present in the red marrow are developing erythrocytes and granulocytes, **megakaryocytes (16), blood vessels (6), bone spicule (15),** and **osteoclasts (13)** in **Howship's lacunae (12)** along the wall of the bone.

FORMATION OF BONE: DEVELOPMENT OF OSTEONS (HAVERSIAN SYSTEMS) (DECALCIFIED, TRANSVERSE SECTION)

1 Osteocytes

2 Osteoclast

3 Concentric lamellae

4 Haversian canals in process of formation from tufts of vascular connective tissue

5 Inactive area

6 Blood vessel in a Haversian canal

7 Sinusoids in the bone marrow

8 Haversian canals with primitive connective tissue and blood vessels

9 Osteoblasts

10 Osteogenic connective tissue

11 Bone matrix

12 Howship's lacunae

13 Osteoclasts

14 Bone marrow with myeloid elements

15 Spicule of bone

16 Megakaryocytes

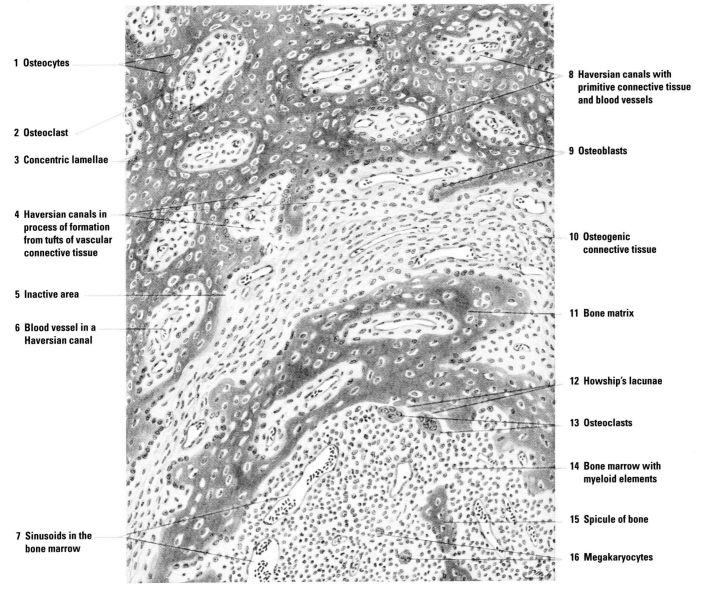

Stain: hematoxylin-eosin. 140×.

PLATE 19

FORMATION OF BONE: SECONDARY (EPIPHYSEAL) OSSIFICATION CENTERS (LONGITUDINAL SECTION, DECALCIFIED)

The cartilaginous epiphyseal ends (articular cartilages) of two fetal bones are illustrated. Both bones contain a secondary center of ossification (2, 6). The **ossification center (2)** in the upper bone exhibits an earlier stage of development than that in the lower bone **(6).** Located between the two developing cartilage models is the **synovial** or **joint cavity (5, 11).**

In the upper epiphysis is seen the peripheral or superficial zone of cartilage with flattened **chondrocytes** and **lacunae (3).** Toward the center of the cartilage, the chondrocytes and lacunae are rounder **(1).** Deeper and at the margin of the established center of calcification, the chondrocytes show **hypertrophy (10)** in preparation for ossification. Small spicules of red-stained **bone (2)** and primitive marrow cavities are seen in the center.

Similar structural components are also seen in the secondary center of ossification **(6, 13-15)** in the lower bone. **Bony spicules (13)** are larger and more numerous than above. A small area of **metaphysis (9),** a transitional zone where cartilage is being replaced by bone, illustrates typical features of the **zone of ossification (8, 9, 16, 17). Periosteum (18)** is seen on the right side and on the left side (unlabeled) **(8, 9).**

The synovial or joint cavity (5, 11) is covered by a joint capsule (a diarthritic joint). A portion of the outer fibrous layer of the **articular capsule (7)** is illustrated. The inner synovial membrane of flattened cells lines the cavity except over the articulating cartilages. The synovial membrane, together with the connective tissue of the capsule, may extend into the joint cavity as simple **projections (12)** or more complex **synovial folds (4).**

FORMATION OF BONE: SECONDARY (EPIPHYSEAL) OSSIFICATION CENTERS (DECALCIFIED, LONGITUDINAL SECTION)

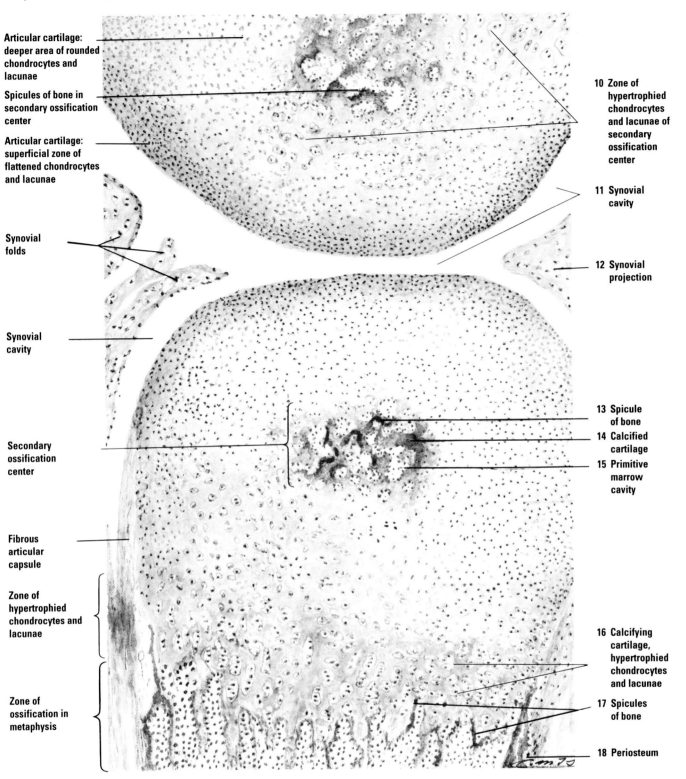

Articular cartilage: deeper area of rounded chondrocytes and lacunae

Spicules of bone in secondary ossification center

Articular cartilage: superficial zone of flattened chondrocytes and lacunae

Synovial folds

Synovial cavity

Secondary ossification center

Fibrous articular capsule

Zone of hypertrophied chondrocytes and lacunae

Zone of ossification in metaphysis

10 Zone of hypertrophied chondrocytes and lacunae of secondary ossification center

11 Synovial cavity

12 Synovial projection

13 Spicule of bone

14 Calcified cartilage

15 Primitive marrow cavity

16 Calcifying cartilage, hypertrophied chondrocytes and lacunae

17 Spicules of bone

18 Periosteum

FETAL FINGERTIP: EPIPHYSES OF TWO ADJACENT BONES IN EARLY STAGES OF OSSIFICATION. Stain: hematoxylin-eosin. 20×.

The blood is a specialized form of connective tissue. It consists of various cell types or formed elements suspended in a liquid medium called plasma. The blood performs numerous important functions. It transports gases, nutrients, waste products, hormones, antibodies, cells, various chemicals, and other substances in the liquid medium to different parts of the body.

Blood Cells

The blood cells are formed by a process called hemopoiesis. In this process, pluripotential stem cells multiply, differentiate, and develop into various types of mature blood cells. In a developing and maturing organism, hemopoiesis occurs in different sites of the body, depending on the stage of development. In the embryo, hemopoiesis occurs in the yolk sac. Later in the development, hemopoiesis takes place in the liver, spleen, and lymph nodes. After birth, hemopoiesis continues almost exclusively in the red marrow of different bones. In adults, the red marrow is found in the flat bones of the skull, sternum and ribs, vertebrae, and pelvic bones.

Microscopic examination of a blood smear reveals the formed elements. These are the erythrocytes or red blood cells, leukocytes or white blood cells, and platelets. The erythrocytes and platelets perform their major functions in the blood vessels. The leukocytes, on the other hand, perform their major functions outside the blood vessels. These cells leave the blood vessels through the capillary walls and enter the connective tissue, lymphatic tissue, and bone marrow.

The mature erythrocytes are highly specialized to transport oxygen and carbon dioxide. The ability to transport these respiratory gases depends on the presence of the protein hemoglobin in the erythrocytes. The hemoglobin binds with oxygen and most of the oxygen in the blood is carried to the tissues in the form of oxyhemoglobin. The carbon dioxide from the cells and tissues is carried to the lungs partly dissolved in the blood and partly in combination with hemoglobin, as carbaminohemoglobin. During the maturation process, the erythrocytes synthesize large amounts of hemoglobin. Also, before the erythrocytes are released into the systemic circulation, the nucleus is extruded from the cytoplasm and the mature erythrocytes assume a biconcave shape. This shape provides more surface area for carrying respiratory gases. Thus, the mature mammalian erythrocytes in the circulation are non-nucleated biconcave disks surrounded by a membrane and containing hemoglobin and some enzymes.

The leukocytes function primarily as a defense system of the organism against foreign material. Because most of the leukocytes are concentrated in the connective tissue, the specific functions of different leukocytes were described in detail in the connective tissue section.

Platelets

The platelets or thrombocytes are the smallest formed elements in the blood. They are non-nucleated cytoplasmic fragments of megakaryocytes, which are the large, multilobed cells found in the bone marrow. The platelets are produced when small portions of the cytoplasm separate or fragment from the peripheries of the megakaryocytes. The main function of platelets is to promote blood clotting. When the wall of the blood vessel is broken or damaged, the platelets adhere to the damaged wall and release chemicals that initiate the complex process of blood clotting. After a blood clot is formed and the bleeding ceases, the aggregated platelets contribute to the clot retraction.

PLATE 20

PERIPHERAL BLOOD SMEAR

The circular area in the illustration represents an idealized blood smear, stained with May-Grunwald-Giemsa stain. Erythrocytes, leucocytes, and blood platelets are shown.

The **erythrocytes (6)** are enucleated cells that stain pink with eosin. They are uniform in size, measure about 7.5 μm in diameter, and can be used as a size reference for other cell types.

The **blood platelets (7),** the smallest of the formed elements, are irregular masses of basophilic cytoplasm containing azurophilic granules. Platelets tend to form clumps in blood smears.

The leukocytes are subdivided into different categories according to the shape of their nucleus, the absence or presence of cytoplasmic granules, and the staining affinities of their granules.

Leukocytes with numerous granules and a lobulated nucleus are polymorphonuclear granulocytes, of which the **neutrophils (3)** are most numerous. Their cytoplasm contains fine violet or pink granules. The nucleus consists of several lobes connected by narrow chromatin strands; the presence of fewer lobes indicates less mature cells.

The **eosinophils (1)** have large, bright pink granules that fill the cytoplasm. The nucleus is typically bilobed, but a small, third lobe may be present. The granules in the **basophils (2)** are not as numerous as in the eosinophils; however, they are more variable in size, less densely packed, and stain dark blue or brown. The nucleus is not markedly lobulated and stains pale basophilic.

The agranular leukocytes have few or no cytoplasmic granules and round to horseshoe-shaped nuclei. **Lymphocytes (4)** exhibit more variation in size, ranging from cells smaller than erythrocytes to almost twice as large. The nucleus occupies a large portion of the cytoplasm and stains intensely with the chromatin, which is arranged in dense blocks intermingled with less dense areas. The narrow rim of basophilic cytoplasm is agranular but may contain a few azurophilic granules.

The **monocytes (5)** are the largest leukocytes. The nucleus varies from round or oval to indented or horseshoe-shaped and stains lighter than in lymphocytes. The chromatin is more finely dispersed; the abundant cytoplasm is lightly basophilic and often contains a few fine azurophilic granules.

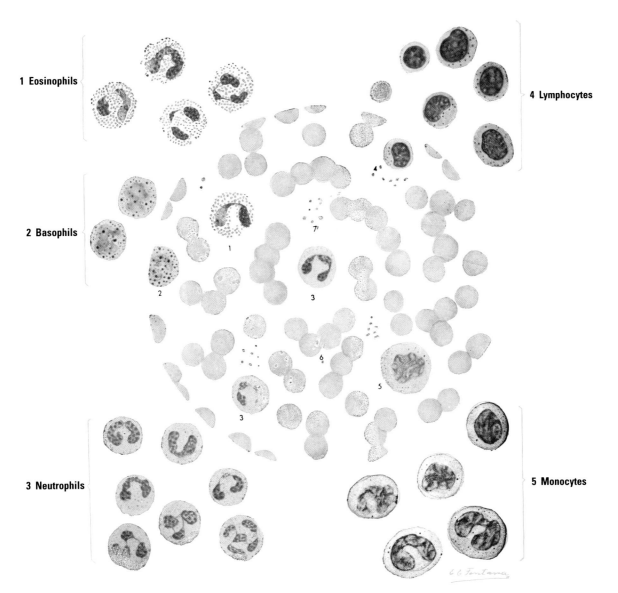

1 Eosinophils

4 Lymphocytes

2 Basophils

3 Neutrophils

5 Monocytes

Stain: May-Grünwald-Giemsa. 1100×.

PLATE 21

■ **FIG. 1**
BLOOD CELLS: SUPRAVITAL STAINS

The phagocytic vacuoles within leukocytes can be easily demonstrated with certain stains. A dilute solution of neutral red stain is placed on a slide, a drop of blood is added, and a cover slip placed over the solution. In 15 to 50 minutes, **phagocytic vacuoles (1, 2, 3:a)** of different sizes appear in the cytoplasm. The smallest and slowest vacuoles to appear are in the cytoplasm of the small lymphocytes (2:a).

The presence of mitochondria in leukocytes are demonstrated by essentially the same technique by applying the Janus green stain. The **mitochondria (1, 2, 3:b)** stain a bluish green in the cell cytoplasm.

In reticulated erythrocytes, which are the youngest erythrocytes after extrusion of the nucleus, the reticulum can be demonstrated by placing a drop of blood on a slide on which a solution of cresyl blue has dried. The **reticulum (4:c)** is then seen as a filamentous network of dark-staining granular material.

■ **FIG. 2**
BLOOD SMEARS: PAPPENHEIM'S AND CELANI'S STAINS

The various types of blood cells can be clearly differentiated by staining a blood film with Pappenheim's stain (May-Grunwald's stain followed by Giemsa's stain). Nuclear structures, the more or less intense basophilic nature of the cytoplasm, and the various types of **granules (a)** are well demonstrated by this method.

Benzidine is oxidized by hydrogen peroxide activated by the peroxides in the blood cells (Celani's stain). Granules that have oxidases stain blue. Polymorphs and monocytes in circulating blood have **peroxidases (b)** and the lymphocytes do not.

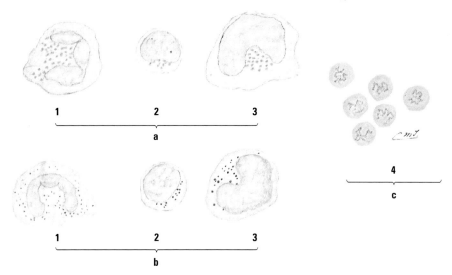

FIG. 1. SUPRAVITAL STAIN: blood cells.
1. Neutrophilic granulocyte; 2. lymphocyte; 3. monocyte; 4. erythrocytes
   a) Vacuoles stained with neutral red.
   b) Mitochondria stained with Janus green.
   c) Reticulum stained with cresyl blue.

BLOOD SMEARS: PAPPENHEIM'S AND CELANI'S STAINS

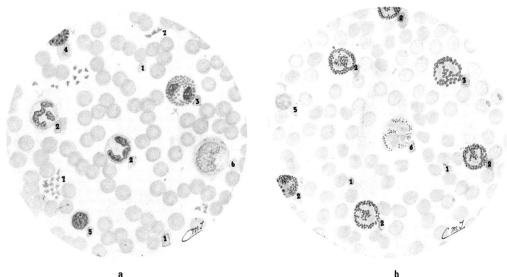

a   b

FIG. 2. PAPPENHEIM'S AND CELANI'S STAINS: blood smears.
a) Pappenheim's method (May-Grünwald and Giemsa stains). Nuclei: reddish violet; basophilic cytoplasm: blue of varying intensity according to degree of basophilia; acidophilic cytoplasm: more or less deep red; neutrophilic granules: violet; eosinophilic granules: orange-red; basophilic granules: dark violet; azurophilic granules: brilliant purple.
b) Peroxidase reaction. Celani's technique. Nuclei: light red; cytoplasm of leukocytes: pale pink; erythrocytes: yellow; granules with peroxidases: blue.
1. erythrocytes; 2. neutrophilic granulocyte; 3. eosinophil granulocyte; 4. basophil granulocyte; 5. lymphocyte; 6. monocyte; 7. platelets.

PLATE 22

■ **FIG. 1**
HEMOPOIETIC BONE MARROW

In a section of red bone marrow, it is difficult to distinguish all types of developing blood cells. The cells are densely packed and different cell types are intermixed, although some of the erythrocytic forms often occur in groups or "nests" **(6, 20)**. Structural details of different cells are not as apparent as in a blood smear because of cell shrinkage during section preparation; only parts of cells, rather than entire cells, may be present.

This section is stained with hematoxylin-eosin. At low magnification, little differentiation of cytoplasm is visible, except for bright staining **eosinophilic granules (4)**. The individual blood cells from a marrow smear are illustrated below the figure at a higher magnification to show more details.

The reticular connective tissue stroma of the marrow is largely obscured by hemopoietic cells. In less dense areas, the reticular **connective tissue (8)** can be seen and the elongated **reticular cells (24)** often recognized. Different types of **blood vessels (9, 10, 19, 25)** are also seen. Also conspicuous in the bone marrow are large **adipose cells (14)**, each containing a large vacuole (because of fat removal during section preparation) and small, peripheral cytoplasm surrounding the **nucleus (2)**. Other cells easily identified in the bone marrow are the large **megakaryocytes (5, 23)** with varied nuclear lobulation.

Erythrocytes (12) are abundant in the marrow. The most easily recognizable of the earlier erythrocytic cells are the **normoblasts (20)**, which are characterized by small, dark-staining nuclei (as in **f**); numerous normoblast cells also exhibit **mitotic activity (18)**. **Polychromatophilic erythroblasts (22)** may also occur in groups or "nests." These cells are larger than normoblasts, with a larger nucleus exhibiting a more evident "checkerboard" distribution of the chromatin (as in **e**). **Basophilic erythroblasts (3)** are still larger cells exhibiting a large, less dense nuclei and basophilic cytoplasm (as in **d**).

In the granulocytic series, the most easily recognizable cells are the **polymorphonuclear heterophils (16)** (corresponding to neutrophils in man) and eosinophils. Their earlier forms, the **metamyelocytes (21)**, have bean or horseshoe-shaped nuclei (as in **c**). **Heterophilic myelocytes (1, 4, b)** have larger, round or ovoid nuclei. Less easily recognizable in a section are the pale-staining primitive **reticular cells (11)** and **hemocytoblasts (13, 17, a)**.

An alternate terminology for the developing erythrocytic forms, in wide use clinically, is as follows:

Proerythroblast = rubriblast
Basophilic erythroblast = prorubricyte
Polychromatophilic erythroblast = rubricyte
Normoblast (orthochromatophilic erythroblast) = metarubricyte

■ **FIG. 2**
BONE MARROW OF A RABBIT, INDIA INK PREPARATION

Illustrated is a section of a hemopoietic bone marrow from a rabbit, injected with India ink.

Carbon particles have been ingested by the **stromal macrophages (1, 8)** and by **fixed macrophages (3)** situated adjacent to the endothelium which lines the sinusoids. Dense carbon inclusions in some phagocytic cells can obscure the nucleus (1).

Reticular cells (12) of the connective tissue may be seen occasionally, but are frequently obscured by developing blood cells. Various cells of the **erythrocytic** and **granulocytic series (4, 6, 7, 11, 13)** as well as **megakaryocytes (10)** can be identified.

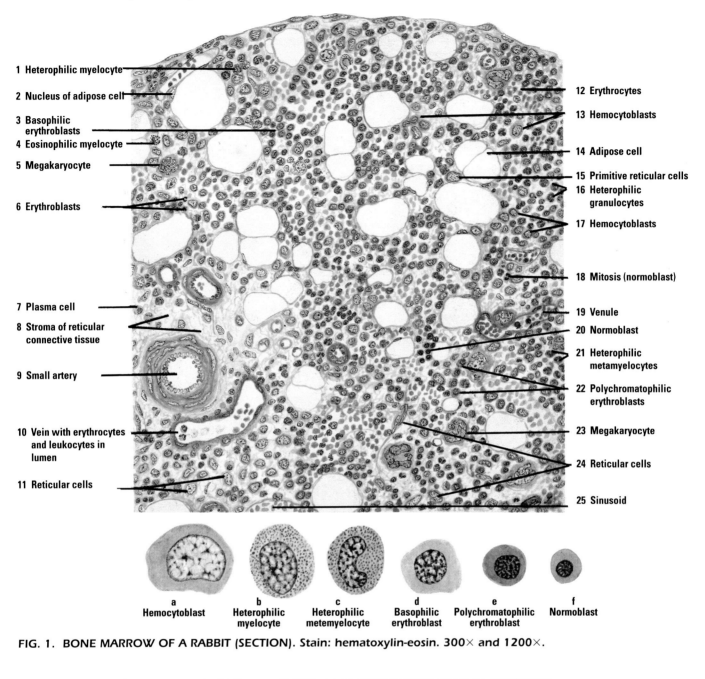

1 Heterophilic myelocyte
2 Nucleus of adipose cell
3 Basophilic erythroblasts
4 Eosinophilic myelocyte
5 Megakaryocyte
6 Erythroblasts
7 Plasma cell
8 Stroma of reticular connective tissue
9 Small artery
10 Vein with erythrocytes and leukocytes in lumen
11 Reticular cells

12 Erythrocytes
13 Hemocytoblasts
14 Adipose cell
15 Primitive reticular cells
16 Heterophilic granulocytes
17 Hemocytoblasts
18 Mitosis (normoblast)
19 Venule
20 Normoblast
21 Heterophilic metamyelocytes
22 Polychromatophilic erythroblasts
23 Megakaryocyte
24 Reticular cells
25 Sinusoid

a	b	c	d	e	f
Hemocytoblast	Heterophilic myelocyte	Heterophilic metemyelocyte	Basophilic erythroblast	Polychromatophilic erythroblast	Normoblast

FIG. 1. BONE MARROW OF A RABBIT (SECTION). Stain: hematoxylin-eosin. 300× and 1200×.

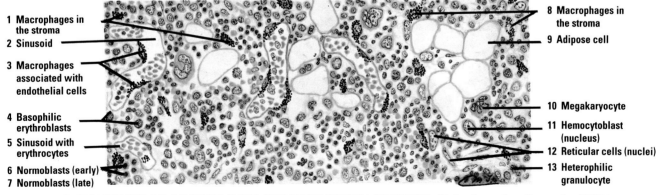

1 Macrophages in the stroma
2 Sinusoid
3 Macrophages associated with endothelial cells
4 Basophilic erythroblasts
5 Sinusoid with erythrocytes
6 Normoblasts (early)
7 Normoblasts (late)

8 Macrophages in the stroma
9 Adipose cell
10 Megakaryocyte
11 Hemocytoblast (nucleus)
12 Reticular cells (nuclei)
13 Heterophilic granulocyte

FIG. 2. BONE MARROW OF A RABBIT, INDIA INK PREPARATION (SECTION). Stain: hematoxylin-eosin. 250×.

PLATE 23

BONE MARROW: SMEAR

In the center of the illustration is a representative microscopic field of human bone marrow smear obtained by sternal puncture. Around the periphery are illustrated in greater detail the typical bone marrow cells. The formed elements that are normally found in the blood are easily recognized: **erythrocytes (18, 31)**, granulocytes **(eosinophil, 32; neutrophil, 33)**, and **platelets (24)**.

Recent evidence indicates that a common, free pluripotential stem cell is capable of differentiating into stem cells that give rise to different hemopoietic cell lines such as the erythrocytes, granulocytes, lymphocytes, and megakaryocytes. Because the existence of this stem cell was first demonstrated on the basis of colonies in the spleen, this cell has been termed colony forming unit (CFU). It is currently believed that these stem cells appear similar to a large lymphocyte. In adults, the greatest concentration of such stem cells is found in the bone marrow.

In the erythrocytic series, the precursor cell is the **proerythroblast**[*] (3, 8), which measures about 20 to 30 μm in diameter and contains a thin rim of basophilic cytoplasm and a large, oval nucleus that occupies most of the cell. Azurophilic granules are absent in all cells of this series. The chromatin is uniformly dispersed, and two or more nuclei may be present. Early proerythroblast undergoes a series of divisions to produce smaller basophilic erythroblasts whose size varies from 15 to 17 μm.

Basophilic erythroblasts (4, 7) exhibit less intensely basophilic cytoplasm; however, sufficient basophilia is present in the cytoplasm to obscure the small amount of hemoglobin that is being synthesized by these cells. The nucleus has decreased in size; the chromatin is coarse and exhibits the characteristic "checkerboard" pattern. Nucleoli are either inconspicuous or absent. The progeny of mitotic divisions of basophilic erythroblasts are the **polychromatophilic erythroblasts (5, 13, 14)**. These cells are recognized by their smaller size (12 to 15 μm in diameter). Their cytoplasm becomes progressively less basophilic and more acidophilic as a result of increased hemoglobin accumulation. The nuclei are smaller and exhibit the coarse "checkerboard" pattern.

When the cells acquire an acidophilic cytoplasm because of an increased amount of hemoglobin, they are called **normoblasts (6, 11)** and their size is about 8 to 10 μm. Initially, the nucleus still exhibits a concentrated "checkerboard" chromatin pattern (6, 11), and the cell division continues. The nucleus then decreases in size, becomes pyknotic, and is extruded from the cytoplasm. The resulting flattened cell is the **reticulocyte (9, 16, 17)** or a young erythrocyte, exhibiting a bluish-pink cytoplasm. With special supravital staining, a delicate reticulum is demonstrated in the cyto-

plasm (see Plate 21, Fig. 1, 4c). Mature **erythrocytes (18, 31)** are smaller and have a homogeneous acidophilic cytoplasm.

The granulocytes also originate from the pluripotential stem cell or the colony-forming unit (CFU), and the **myeloblast (2, 25)** is the first recognizable precursor in the granulocytic series. The myeloblast is a relatively small cell (10 to 13 μm in diameter) with a large nucleus containing two or three nucleoli and a distinctly basophilic cytoplasm that lacks specific granules. In its further development, the cell enlarges, acquires azurophilic granules, and is now called a **promyelocyte (19,** early, **23,** later). The cell measures about 15 to 20 μm in diameter. The chromatin in the oval nucleus exhibits a dispersed pattern, and multiple nucleoli are still evident. In more advanced promyelocytes, the cells are smaller, nucleoli become inconspicuous, azurophilic granules increase, and there is an appearance of specific granules with different staining properties in the perinuclear region **(23, neutrophilic promyelocyte)**.

Myelocytes are smaller than promyelocytes. The nucleus is eccentric and the chromatin more condensed. The cytoplasm is less basophilic, with few azurophilic granules evident, and there is an increase of specific granules **(neutrophilic early myelocyte, 26; basophilic early myelocyte, 20)**. More **mature myelocytes (12, 21, 22, 27, 29, 34, 35)** have an abundance of specific granules, slightly acidophilic cytoplasm, and a smaller nucleus. The myelocyte is the last cell of granulocytic series capable of mitosis; myelocytes then mature into metamyelocytes.

In the **metamyelocytes,** the configuration of the nucleus changes from an oval, eccentric nucleus to that of deep indentation that is seen in mature cells; the greatest change takes place in the **neutrophilic** forms (in succession: **30** and **36, 28, 33)**. Similar structural alterations in **eosinophils** and **basophils** can be also followed in the illustrations: **(27** lower leader, **27** upper leader, **32, 20, 12)**.

Megakaryoblasts (37) are large cells that measure about 40 to 60 μm in diameter. The cytoplasm is basophilic and largely free of specific granules. The voluminous nucleus is ovoid or indented, and exhibits a loose chromatin pattern and poorly defined nucleoli. The mature cells, **megakaryocytes (15, 38),** are giant cells approximately 80 to 100 μm in diameter, and have a larger volume of slightly acidophilic cytoplasm filled with fine azurophilic granules. The nucleus of these cells is large and convoluted, with the multiple, irregular lobes interconnected by constricted regions. The chromatin is condensed and coarse, and there are no visible nucleoli. In mature megakaryocytes (38) plasma membrane invaginates the cytoplasm and forms demarcation membranes. This delimits the areas of the megakaryocyte cytoplasm that is then shed into the bloodstream in the form of **platelets (39)**.

[*]For alternate terminology, see page 56, Fig. 1, paragraph 9.

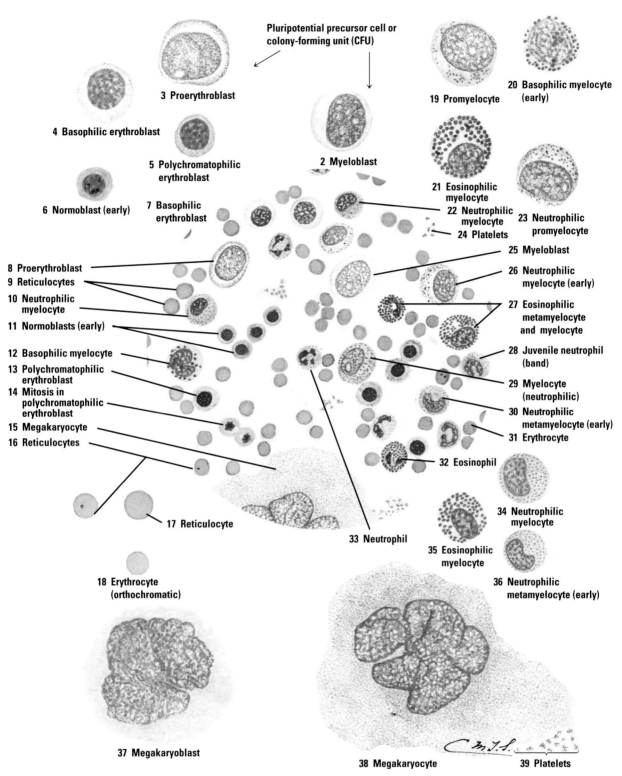

Pluripotential precursor cell or colony-forming unit (CFU)

3 Proerythroblast

4 Basophilic erythroblast

5 Polychromatophilic erythroblast

2 Myeloblast

6 Normoblast (early)

7 Basophilic erythroblast

8 Proerythroblast
9 Reticulocytes
10 Neutrophilic myelocyte
11 Normoblasts (early)
12 Basophilic myelocyte
13 Polychromatophilic erythroblast
14 Mitosis in polychromatophilic erythroblast
15 Megakaryocyte
16 Reticulocytes

17 Reticulocyte

18 Erythrocyte (orthochromatic)

19 Promyelocyte

20 Basophilic myelocyte (early)

21 Eosinophilic myelocyte
22 Neutrophilic myelocyte
23 Neutrophilic promyelocyte
24 Platelets
25 Myeloblast
26 Neutrophilic myelocyte (early)
27 Eosinophilic metamyelocyte and myelocyte
28 Juvenile neutrophil (band)
29 Myelocyte (neutrophilic)
30 Neutrophilic metamyelocyte (early)
31 Erythrocyte
32 Eosinophil

33 Neutrophil

34 Neutrophilic myelocyte

35 Eosinophilic myelocyte

36 Neutrophilic metamyelocyte (early)

37 Megakaryoblast

38 Megakaryocyte

39 Platelets

Stain: May-Grünwald-Giemsa. 800× and 1200×.

The major function of the muscle tissue is to produce motion. Externally, this is seen as movement of limbs; internally, as the beat of the heart, intestinal peristalsis, and other motions. The muscle tissue consists of elongated cells called fibers, and the cytoplasm of these fibers contains different amounts of the contractile protein filaments called actin and myosin.

There are three types of muscle tissue in the body. Based on its location, structure, and function, the muscle tissue is divided into three general categories: skeletal muscle, cardiac muscle, and smooth muscle. Each muscle category has certain structural and functional similarities as well as differences with each other.

A special terminology is used to describe the organelles in the cytoplasm of the muscle fiber. The plasma membrane in the muscle fiber is called the sarcolemma, the cytoplasm is called sarcoplasm, and endoplasmic reticulum is called sarcoplasmic reticulum.

The Skeletal Muscle

The major type of muscle tissue in the body is the skeletal muscle. The skeletal muscles attach to and move different bones of the skeleton. Other skeletal muscles attach to and move the facial skin, tongue, eyeball, or deep fascia. The skeletal muscles are voluntary because they contract and relax as a result of a conscious control. In the skeletal muscle cytoplasm, the arrangement of contractile protein filaments actin and myosin is regular. As a result, the contractile filaments form distinct cross-striations, which are seen with the light microscope as the light I bands and the dark A bands across each muscle fiber. Because of these striations, the skeletal muscles are also called striated muscles.

The skeletal muscle fibers are long and multinucleated. They exhibit longitudinal and parallel arrangements that are held together by connective tissue. The skeletal muscles are also richly innervated by large motor nerves or axons. As a large terminal of the motor nerve nears the skeleton muscle, it branches, and each smaller axon branch then innervates a single muscle fiber. As a result of such innervation, each skeletal muscle fiber contracts only when stimulated by the nerve.

Each skeletal muscle fiber exhibits a specialized site where the nerve branch terminates. This is called the neuromuscular junction or motor end-plate, a site where the impulse from the nerve is transmitted to the skeletal muscle. The terminal end of each axon exhibits numerous vesicles; these vesicles contain the neurotransmitter chemical acetylcholine. Between the nerve terminal and the muscle fiber is a shallow trough that separates the two structures. This trough is called the synaptic cleft.

The arrival of a nerve impulse or the action potential at the axon terminal causes the release of acetylcholine from the vesicles into the synaptic cleft. The released acetylcholine then diffuses across the synaptic cleft, combines with acetylcholine receptors on the muscle fiber membrane, and stimulates the muscle fiber. This produces the skeletal muscle contraction. An enzyme called acetylcholinesterase, located on the membrane of the muscle fiber, inactivates the released acetylcholine. This prevents further muscle stimulation and contraction until the arrival of the next impulse.

Located within all skeletal muscles are the sensitive stretch receptors called neuromuscular spindles. These spindles consist of special muscle fibers called intrafusal fibers and nerve endings, which are surrounded by a connective tissue capsule. The main function of the neuromuscular spindles is to detect changes in length of the muscle fibers. An increase in the length of these muscle fibers stimulates the neuromuscular spindle and causes a conduction of impulses to the spinal cord. This produces a muscle reflex, which causes a contraction and shortening of the stretched muscle. A decrease in muscle length then decreases or ceases the stimulation of the neuromuscular spindle.

The proper function of the skeletal muscles depends on the intact nerve supply. If the nerve to a given muscle is severed or damaged, the muscle can eventually undergo atrophy and degeneration unless proper therapy is initiated.

The Cardiac Muscle

The cardiac muscle is found primarily in the walls and septa of the heart, and in the walls of the large vessels that are attached to the heart. Like the skeletal muscles, the cardiac muscles exhibit distinct cross-striations because the contractile protein filaments actin and myosin have a similar distribution patterns. In contrast to the skeletal muscle, however, the cardiac muscle is involuntary and contracts rhythmically and automatically during the life of the individual. The rate of this rhythm, however, is influenced by the innervation of the nerve fibers from the autonomic nervous system and different hormones.

The cardiac muscles usually have one or two nuclei that are centrally located. The cardiac muscle fibers are also shorter than the skeletal muscle fibers and exhibit branching; this forms a complicated network of muscle fibers. The terminal ends of adjacent cardiac muscle fibers form distinct end-to-end junctions called the intercalated disks. The main function of these disks is to functionally couple all cardiac muscle fibers and allow a rapid spread of stimuli for contraction of the heart. As a result of this coupling, the cardiac muscle fibers act as a functional syncytium.

In contrast to the skeletal muscles, the impulse-generating and impulse-conducting system in the cardiac muscles is located within the heart wall itself. This system consists of specialized cardiac muscle fibers that are found in the sinoatrial (SA) node and atrioventricular (AV) node, bundle of His, and the Purkinje fibers. The cardiac cells in the SA node exhibit the most rapid rhythm of producing stimuli for the heart contraction. As a result, the SA node sets the pace for the heart rate and is, therefore, the pacemaker of the heart.

The Purkinje fibers are thicker and larger than the cardiac muscle fibers and contain increased amount of glycogen. Also, they contain fewer contractile filaments. Purkinje fibers deliver the stimulatory impulses from the nodes to the rest of the heart musculature that produces ventricular contraction and ejection of blood.

Both the parasympathetic and sympathetic division of the autonomic nervous system innervate the heart in the vicinity of the nodes. The nerve fibers of the parasympathetic division, by way of the vagus nerves, slows down the heart and decreases the blood pressure. The nerve fibers of the sympathetic produce the opposite effect; they increase the rhythm of the pacemaker and, consequently, the heart rate and blood pressure.

The Smooth Muscle

The smooth muscle fibers do not contain any visible cross-striations. The contractile protein filaments in the smooth muscle fibers are not arranged in the same pattern as in the skeletal or the cardiac muscles. As a result, the cross-striations are not visible, and the muscles appear smooth or nonstriated. The smooth muscle fibers are small, fusiform in shape, and contain a single nucleus. The smooth muscles are also involuntary and are predominantly found lining the visceral organs and blood vessels. Generally, the smooth muscles occur in large sheets, as in the walls of the hollow viscera such as the digestive tract, uterus, ureters, and others. In the blood vessels, the smooth muscle fibers are arranged in a circular pattern and participate in controlling the blood pressure by altering the size of the lumina.

The smooth muscles usually have spontaneous activity in a wave-like fashion that passes in slow, sustained contraction over the entire muscle. This type of action produces a continuous contraction of low force. The smooth muscles make contact with each other by specialized zones of contact, the gap junctions. These gap junctions provide close contacts between individual cells and allow the passage of stimuli between them. The smooth muscles are also innervated by nerves from the sympathetic and parasympathetic divisions of the autonomic nervous system; these innervations enhance their contractility.

PLATE 24

■ **FIG. 1**
SMOOTH MUSCLE FIBERS

■ **FIG. 2**
SKELETAL (STRIATED) MUSCLE FIBERS (DISSOCIATED)

PLATE 24

■ FIG. 1
SMOOTH MUSCLE FIBERS

This illustration represents the wall of a distended toad bladder, in which the **smooth muscles (2, 5)** are distributed in small bundles of various sizes. Individual muscle fibers can be distinguished in some of the small bundles (2). Each smooth **muscle fiber (3)** is a spindle-shaped cell with deeply stained cytoplasm (sarcoplasm) and an elongated or ovoid nucleus in the center.

In the loose connective tissue around bundles of muscle fibers are **fibroblasts (1, 6)** and a **capillary with erythrocytes (4).** In amphibians, mature erythrocytes remain nucleated.

Single and small groups of smooth muscle fibers are also illustrated on Plate 2, Fig. 2 (4, 11).

■ FIG. 2
SKELETAL (STRIATED) MUSCLE FIBERS (DISSOCIATED)

In this illustration, the muscle fibers have been separated and stained with hematoxylin-eosin. The skeletal **muscle fibers (1)** are much longer and larger in diameter than the smooth muscle fibers. Skeletal muscles are multinucleated, with the **nuclei (6)** situated peripherally and immediately below the sarcolemma. (Sarcolemma is not illustrated in the figure.) Each skeletal muscle fiber shows distinct cross-striations, which are visible as alternating dark or **A bands (4)** and light or **I bands (5).** With higher magnification, additional details of the cross striations are more readily visible in Plate 25, Fig. 4.

A dissociated skeletal muscle fiber exhibits thin bundles of **myofibrils (2).** Each myofibril also exhibits the characteristic cross-striation pattern which are aligned adjacent to each other in the myofibrils. This gives the appearance of continuous cross-striations across the entire muscle fiber.

Numerous **capillaries (3)** are present in the connective tissue (endomysium) that surrounds each muscle fiber.

MUSCLE TISSUE

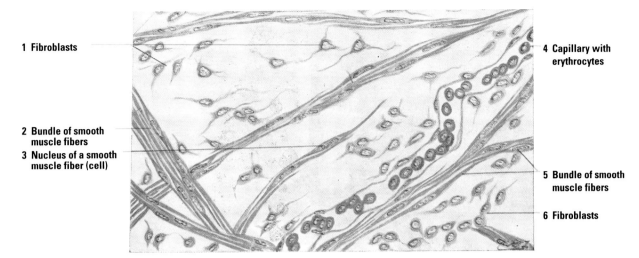

1 Fibroblasts

2 Bundle of smooth muscle fibers

3 Nucleus of a smooth muscle fiber (cell)

4 Capillary with erythrocytes

5 Bundle of smooth muscle fibers

6 Fibroblasts

FIG. 1. SMOOTH MUSCLE FIBERS. Stain: hematoxylin-eosin. 360×.

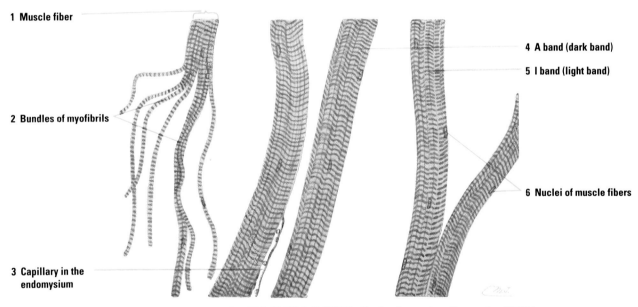

1 Muscle fiber

2 Bundles of myofibrils

3 Capillary in the endomysium

4 A band (dark band)

5 I band (light band)

6 Nuclei of muscle fibers

FIG. 2. SKELETAL (STRIATED) MUSCLE FIBERS (DISSOCIATED). Stain: hematoxylin-eosin. 250×.

PLATE 25

■ FIG. 1
SKELETAL MUSCLES OF THE TONGUE

Skeletal muscles of the tongue course in different directions. A section from the central part of the tongue shows skeletal muscle fibers cut **longitudinally (3, 5)** or **transversely (4, 7)**. The fibers are aggregated into **fascicles (3, 5)** and are bound by **connective tissue (9)**. The connective tissue sheath around each muscle fascicle is the **perimysium (2)**. From the perimysium, thin partitions of connective tissue, called the **endomysium (1,**

11), extend into each fascicle and invest individual muscle fibers. Small **blood vessels (6)** are present throughout the connective tissue sheaths.

The muscle fibers that have been sectioned longitudinally show **cross-striations (5)**; fibers sectioned transversely exhibit cross-sections of **myofibril bundles (4, 7)**. The **nuclei of skeletal muscle fibers (8, 10)** are located peripherally as seen in transverse sections.

■ FIG. 2
SMOOTH MUSCLE LAYERS OF THE INTESTINE

In the upper muscle layer, the **smooth muscle fibers (1)**, were cut longitudinally exhibiting the spindle shape of individual fibers. The **nucleus (2)** is located in the widest part of each smooth muscle fiber. The muscle fibers in this compact layer are arranged in such a manner that the wide portions of some fibers are adjacent to the tapered ends of others.

In the lower muscle layer, the fibers were cut transversely **(5)**. The cross sections of smooth muscles exhib-

it different diameters, depending on whether the plane of section passed through the central or the tapering ends of each fiber. The widest sections of the fiber contain nuclei, as seen in the transverse section (5, upper leader).

Fine reticular and elastic fibers envelop individual muscle fibers, whereas larger amounts of **connective tissue (3)** are seen between the muscle layers and around blood vessels **(4)**.

■ FIG. 3
CARDIAC MUSCLE: MYOCARDIUM

The cross-striations of the cardiac muscles resemble the skeletal muscles; however, the cardiac muscle fibers branch without much change in diameter. **Cross-striations (1)** and **intercalated disks (2)** are visible in fibers sectioned longitudinally. The intercalated disks are irregular and wider than the normal cross-striations, and represent specialized junctions between cardiac muscle fibers. These disks are characteristic features of cardiac muscle.

Nuclei (5, 8) of cardiac muscle fibers are centrally located and are clearly visible in fibers sectioned transversely **(8)**. A clear zone of **perinuclear sarcoplasm (9)**, free of myofibrils, may be seen in some sections.

Numerous **small blood vessels (6, 7)** lie in the interfascicular **connective tissue (4)**, and capillaries are abundant in the endomysium.

■ FIG. 4
SKELETAL MUSCLE (LONGITUDINAL SECTION)

High magnification of muscle fibers clearly demonstrates the cross striations. The anisotropic or **A bands (2)** are the prominent, dark-staining bands; a lighter, middle region, the H band, is not visible. The isotropic or I bands are equally prominent and are lightly stained acidophilic bands. Crossing each central portion of the I bands are distinct, narrow lines, the **Z lines (3)**.

The closely arranged parallel myofibrils give a longitudinally striated appearance to the muscle fibers.

Where the **myofibrils (6)** are separated because of rupture of the sarcolemma, the A, I, and Z lines are visible on the myofibrils, aligned next to each other on adjacent myofibrils.

Slender ovoid or **elongated nuclei (4)** of muscle fibers are seen peripherally. In the **endomysium (1)** between muscle fibers are seen **fibroblasts (5)** and a **capillary (7)**.

■ FIG. 5
CARDIAC MUSCLE (LONGITUDINAL SECTION)

Comparison of cardiac muscle with skeletal muscle at the same magnification and the same stain clearly illustrates the similarities and differences between the two types of muscles.

Branching **cardiac fibers (3)** are in distinct contrast to individual skeletal fibers. **Cross striations (2, 5)** are similar in both but less prominent in cardiac muscle fibers. The prominence of the **intercalated disks (7)** and their irregular structure are better seen at higher

magnification. The area between two intercalated disks represents one cardiac muscle cell.

Large, oval **nuclei (1)**, usually one per cell, occupy the central position and much of the width of the cardiac fibers, in contrast to the many elongated peripheral nuclei of the skeletal fibers. The **perinuclear sarcoplasm (6)** region is distinct. **Endomysium (4)** fills the spaces between fibers.

MUSCLE

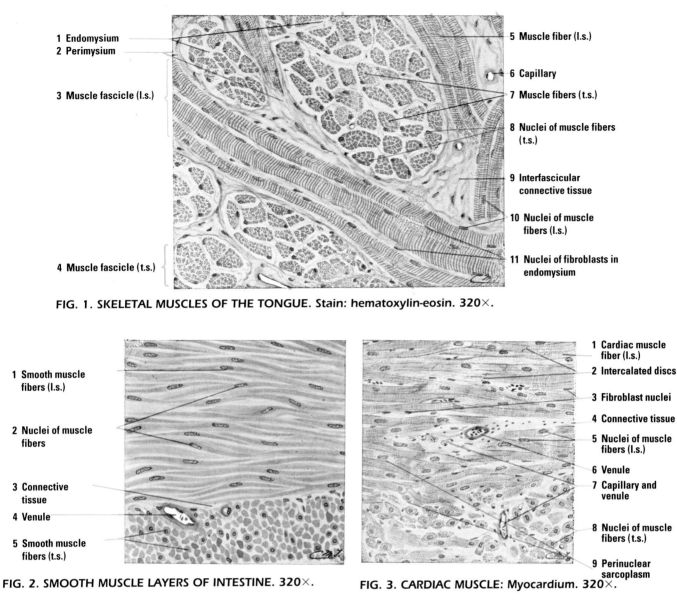

1 Endomysium
2 Perimysium

3 Muscle fascicle (l.s.)

4 Muscle fascicle (t.s.)

5 Muscle fiber (l.s.)

6 Capillary

7 Muscle fibers (t.s.)

8 Nuclei of muscle fibers (t.s.)

9 Interfascicular connective tissue

10 Nuclei of muscle fibers (l.s.)

11 Nuclei of fibroblasts in endomysium

FIG. 1. SKELETAL MUSCLES OF THE TONGUE. Stain: hematoxylin-eosin. 320×.

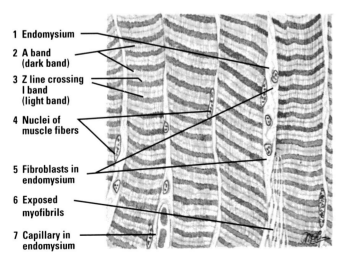

1 Smooth muscle fibers (l.s.)

2 Nuclei of muscle fibers

3 Connective tissue

4 Venule

5 Smooth muscle fibers (t.s.)

FIG. 2. SMOOTH MUSCLE LAYERS OF INTESTINE. 320×.

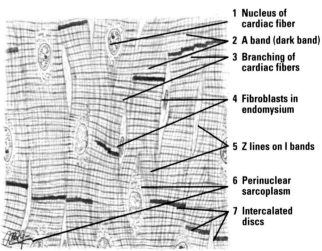

1 Cardiac muscle fiber (l.s.)

2 Intercalated discs

3 Fibroblast nuclei

4 Connective tissue

5 Nuclei of muscle fibers (l.s.)

6 Venule

7 Capillary and venule

8 Nuclei of muscle fibers (t.s.)

9 Perinuclear sarcoplasm

FIG. 3. CARDIAC MUSCLE: Myocardium. 320×.

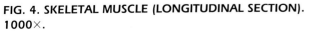

1 Endomysium

2 A band (dark band)

3 Z line crossing I band (light band)

4 Nuclei of muscle fibers

5 Fibroblasts in endomysium

6 Exposed myofibrils

7 Capillary in endomysium

FIG. 4. SKELETAL MUSCLE (LONGITUDINAL SECTION). 1000×.

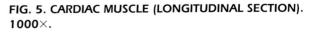

1 Nucleus of cardiac fiber

2 A band (dark band)

3 Branching of cardiac fibers

4 Fibroblasts in endomysium

5 Z lines on I bands

6 Perinuclear sarcoplasm

7 Intercalated discs

FIG. 5. CARDIAC MUSCLE (LONGITUDINAL SECTION). 1000×.

Stain: Iron hematoxylin-eosin.

67

PLATE 26

■ FIG. 1
NERVE TERMINATIONS IN SKELETAL MUSCLE: SKELETAL MUSCLE AND MUSCLE SPINDLE (TRANSVERSE SECTION)

A transverse section of the skeletal muscle shows individual **muscle fibers (1)** grouped into fascicles by interfascicular connective tissue septa, the **perimysium (2).** In one of such septa is seen a **muscle spindle (3)** and a **very small artery (4),** in transverse section. The muscle spindle is an encapsulated sensory end organ.

When viewed at a higher magnification, the muscle spindle is surrounded by an ovoid connective tissue **capsule (5),** which is derived from the **perimysium (9).** The capsule encloses several components of the spindle, all of which are surrounded by loose connective tissue. The specialized muscle fibers called the **intrafusal fibers (7)** are surrounded by the capsule. The intrafusal muscle fibers are smaller in diameter and stain somewhat lighter (more sarcoplasm) than the ordinary muscle fibers, the **extrafusal fibers (10).** Small **nerves (6)** associated with the muscle spindles represent incoming myelinated and terminal unmyelinated fibers (axons). Very small blood vessels are also present in the capsule of the muscle spindle. These come from the nerves and blood vessels that are located in the connective tissue septa of the muscle proper.

■ FIG. 2
NERVE TERMINATIONS IN SKELETAL MUSCLE: MOTOR END PLATES

Illustrated is a portion of a skeletal muscle sectioned **longitudinally (4, 7).** The distal part of the **motor nerve (somatic efferent) (1)** courses over the muscle and distributes its axonal branches. These subdivide and terminate on individual muscle fibers as specialized junctional regions called the **motor end plates (2, 6).** The round structures seen in the motor end plates represent terminal axonal expansions and muscle nuclei which accumulate in this region but remain separated from the axon terminals.

Also seen in this figure are an **end plate (5)** whose terminal fibril is in another plane of section and an **axon terminal (3)** whose end plate is not present in this section.

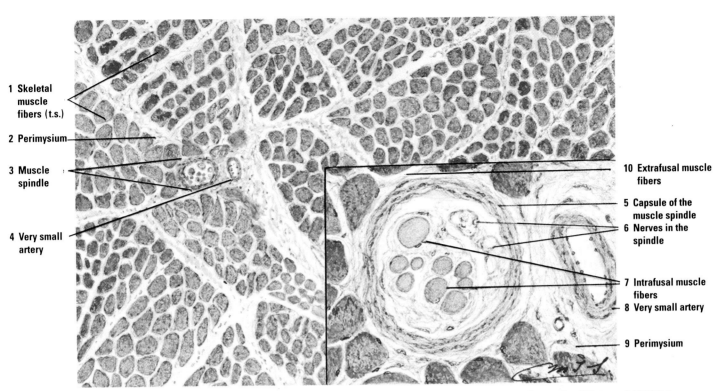

1 Skeletal muscle fibers (t.s.)

2 Perimysium

3 Muscle spindle

4 Very small artery

10 Extrafusal muscle fibers

5 Capsule of the muscle spindle

6 Nerves in the spindle

7 Intrafusal muscle fibers

8 Very small artery

9 Perimysium

FIG. 1. SKELETAL MUSCLE AND MUSCLE SPINDLE (TRANSVERSE SECTION). Stain: hematoxylin-eosin. 90× and 5000×.

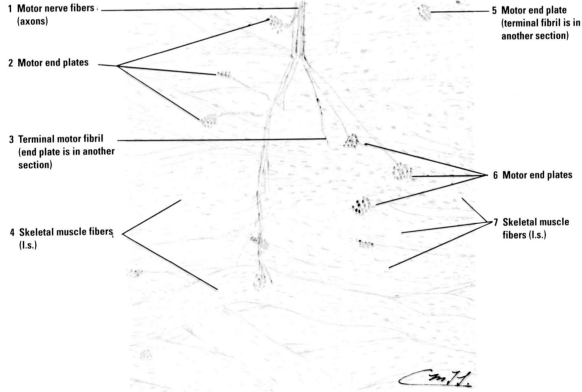

1 Motor nerve fibers (axons)

2 Motor end plates

3 Terminal motor fibril (end plate is in another section)

4 Skeletal muscle fibers (l.s.)

5 Motor end plate (terminal fibril is in another section)

6 Motor end plates

7 Skeletal muscle fibers (l.s.)

FIG. 2. MOTOR END PLATES. Stain: methylene blue. 180×.

69

The perception of internal and external stimuli is the primary function of the cells in the nervous tissue and nervous system. Anatomically, the nervous system is divided into the central nervous system (CNS) and the peripheral nervous system (PNS). The CNS consists of the brain and the spinal cord and is the integrating and communicating center of the body. The PNS consists of the nervous tissue that is located outside of the CNS. Its function is to interconnect all other nervous tissue with the CNS.

The Neuron

The nervous tissue consists of two principal cell types: the nerve cells or neurons and the supporting cells or the neuroglia. The structural and functional cells of the nervous tissue are the neurons. The neurons form the highly complex intercommunicating network of cells that receive and conduct impulses along their neural pathways or axons to the CNS for analysis, integration, and response. The appropriate response to a given stimuli is then provided by the action of the muscles and/or glands of the body.

Functionally, the neurons are classified as sensory (afferent), motor (efferent), or interneurons. The sensory neurons conduct impulses from internal or external receptors to the CNS. The motor neurons convey impulses from the CNS to the effector muscles or glands. The interneurons serve as intermediary cells and are located between sensory and motor neurons in the CNS. Anatomically, there are three major groups of neurons: multipolar, bipolar, and unipolar or pseudounipolar. Their anatomic classification is based on the number of dendrites and axon processes that originate from the cell body.

The multipolar neurons are the most common type in the CNS and include the motor neurons and the interneurons of the brain and spinal cord. The bipolar neurons are not as common and are purely sensory neurons. The bipolar neurons are the receptor cells found in the retina of the eye, the inner ear, and the olfactory epithelium of the nose. Most neurons in adults that exhibit only one process leaving the cell body were originally bipolar. The unipolar or pseudounipolar neurons are also sensory and are found in the numerous craniosacral ganglia of the body.

The neurons are highly specialized cells for irritability and conductivity. During a stimulus, these specializations allow the neurons to react (irritability) and to transmit (conductivity) the information to other neurons in other parts of the nervous system. Strong impulses create a wave of excitation or nervous impulses that are then self-propagated along the entire nerve fiber over a long distance.

The Neuroglia

The neuroglia are the supportive, non-neural cells in the CNS that are located between the neurons. These cells do not conduct impulses and are morphologically and functionally different from the neurons. There are three types of neuroglia cells: astrocytes, oligodendrocytes, and microglia.

Astrocytes are the largest neuroglia cells and are of two types: fibrous astrocytes and protoplasmic astrocytes. In the CNS, both types of astrocytes are attached to the walls of the capillaries. The astrocytes are believed to support the neurons, repair the CNS tissue, and form scar tissue after neural damage. In addition, the astrocytes may be involved in supporting metabolic exchanges between neurons and the capillaries of the CNS.

The oligodendrocytes function by forming myelin sheaths around the axons in the CNS. Because the oligodendrocytes have several processes, a single cell can surround and myelinate numerous axons. This same function of myelination of the axons in the PNS is carried out by a different type of supporting cells called the Schwann cells.

The microglia are considered the macrophages of the CNS and are found throughout the CNS. When the nervous tissue is injured or damaged, microglia proliferate, become phagocytic, and remove the dead tissue.

The Nerve: Myelinated and Unmyelinated Axons

The nerves contain axons of various sizes and their surrounding sheaths. In the PNS, all axons are surrounded by Schwann cells, which extend along the length of the axon, from its origin at the neuron to its termination in the muscle or gland. In the CNS, the cells that surround the axons of different size are the oligodendrocytes.

The smaller axons, such as those of the autonomic nervous system, are surrounded only by the cytoplasm of the Schwann cell. Such axons do not have a myelin sheath around them and are considered unmyelinated. As the axons become progressively larger in diameter, they become surrounded or sheathed by increased number of successive layers of the plasma membrane of the Schwann cell. These membranes then form the myelin sheath that surrounds and insulates the axon. Axons that are surrounded by a myelin sheath are considered myelinated. There are small gaps in the myelin sheath between individual Schwann cells. These gaps are the nodes of Ranvier, and in these regions, the axon is exposed to the extracellular environment.

Myelination of the axons and the nodes of Ranvier performs an important role in the conduction of the nerve impulse along the axon. Small unmyelinated axons conduct nerve impulses at a slower rate than the larger, myelinated axons. In larger, myelinated axons, the nerve impulse jumps from node to node, resulting in a much faster conducting velocity. This type of conduction is called saltatory conduction. In an unmyelinated axon, the impulse travels along the entire length of the axon and, as a result, its velocity of conduction is reduced. Thus, the larger, heavy myelinated axons have the highest velocity of impulse conduction. This rate of conduction depends directly on the axon size and the myelin sheath.

PLATE 27

■ **FIG. 1**
GRAY MATTER: ANTERIOR HORN OF THE SPINAL CORD

■ **FIG. 2**
GRAY MATTER: ANTERIOR HORN OF THE SPINAL CORD (CAJAL'S METHOD)

PLATE 27

■ **FIG. 1**
GRAY MATTER: ANTERIOR HORN OF THE SPINAL CORD

The large, multipolar anterior horn cells or **motor neurons (2)** of the anterior gray matter of the spinal cord have a proportionately large central **nucleus (7, 14)**, a prominent **nucleolus (6, 13)**, and several radiating cell processes, the **dendrites (8, 9)**. A single **axon (1)** arises from a clear area of the cell, the **axon hillock (5)**.

The cytoplasm or perikaryon of the neuron contains numerous clumps of coarse, granular substance (basophilic masses), the **Nissl bodies (12)**, which stain a deep blue with basic aniline of Nissl's method. The Nissl bodies extend into the dendrites (8, 9) but not into

the axon hillock (5) or into the axon (1). The nucleus (7, 14) is distinctly outlined and stains light because of uniform dispersion of the chromatin in fine network often described as "vesicular." The nucleolus (6, 13) is large and dense, and stains deep.

Nuclei of neuroglia cells are stained, whereas the small amount of cytoplasm remains unstained. **Protoplasmic astrocytes (3, 17)** have spherical nuclei with a somewhat loose chromatin network. **Nuclei of oligodendrocytes (16)** are smaller and round, and stain deeper. **Microglia (11)** have elongated dark nuclei.

■ **FIG. 2**
GRAY MATTER: ANTERIOR HORN OF THE SPINAL CORD (CAJAL'S METHOD)

This section was prepared by silver impregnation (Cajal's method) to demonstrate neurofibrils. In the large anterior horn cells or motor neurons, typical neurofibril arrangements are seen in the nerve **cell bodies (2, 3, 6, 11, 13)** and the **dendrites (7, 12)**. Axons are not illustrated, but neurofibrils would be seen in parallel arrangement.

Other details of cell structure are not revealed with

silver impregnation technique. The nucleus of the **neuron (14,** and in neurons 3 and 11) is seen as a lightly stained or almost clear space. The **nucleolus** may stain either slightly (11) or deep **(15)**. In the intercellular areas are seen many fibrillar processes, some of which are anterior horn neurons or associated neuroglia.

Neuroglial **nuclei** are stained **(1, 4, 5, 8, 9, 10)** and show the same characteristics as described in Figure 1.

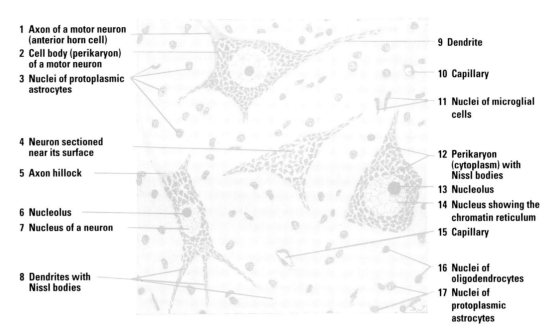

1 Axon of a motor neuron (anterior horn cell)
2 Cell body (perikaryon) of a motor neuron
3 Nuclei of protoplasmic astrocytes
4 Neuron sectioned near its surface
5 Axon hillock
6 Nucleolus
7 Nucleus of a neuron
8 Dendrites with Nissl bodies

9 Dendrite
10 Capillary
11 Nuclei of microglial cells
12 Perikaryon (cytoplasm) with Nissl bodies
13 Nucleolus
14 Nucleus showing the chromatin reticulum
15 Capillary
16 Nuclei of oligodendrocytes
17 Nuclei of protoplasmic astrocytes

FIG. 1. GRAY MATTER: ANTERIOR HORN OF THE SPINAL CORD. Nissl's method for chromophilic substance (Nissl bodies). 350×.

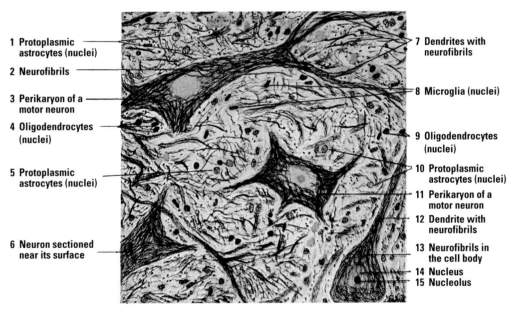

1 Protoplasmic astrocytes (nuclei)
2 Neurofibrils
3 Perikaryon of a motor neuron
4 Oligodendrocytes (nuclei)
5 Protoplasmic astrocytes (nuclei)
6 Neuron sectioned near its surface

7 Dendrites with neurofibrils
8 Microglia (nuclei)
9 Oligodendrocytes (nuclei)
10 Protoplasmic astrocytes (nuclei)
11 Perikaryon of a motor neuron
12 Dendrite with neurofibrils
13 Neurofibrils in the cell body
14 Nucleus
15 Nucleolus

FIG. 2. GRAY MATTER: ANTERIOR HORN OF THE SPINAL CORD. Cajal's method for neurofibrils. 350×.

75

PLATE 28

■ FIG. 1
GRAY MATTER: ANTERIOR HORN OF THE SPINAL CORD (GOLGI'S METHOD)

With Golgi's method of silver impregnation, **neurons (4)**, their **processes (2)**, and their finest branches stain a homogeneous dark color. Structural details of different cells as seen in Plate 27, however, are not well demonstrated with this method.

Protoplasmic astrocytes (1, 3) are also stained. The small cell body and numerous short, thick, branching processes are characteristic features of these cells.

■ FIG. 2
GRAY MATTER: ANTERIOR HORN OF THE SPINAL CORD (MORDANTED SECTIONS AND HEMATOXYLIN STAIN)

This staining method, using mordanted sections and hematoxylin, demonstrates different nerve fibers (axons). In the gray matter, nerve fibers of different sizes course in various directions. The myelin in the **myelinated nerve fibers (2)** stains deep blue or reddish-blue.

The **neurons (1, 4)** are visible in the section but without structural details. They appear shrunken and retracted, and stain only pale yellow or green. The **nucleus (3)** outline is visible but shows shrinkage.

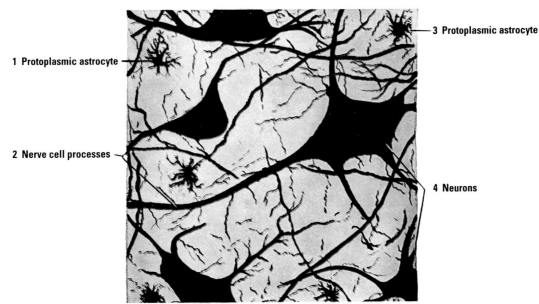

1 Protoplasmic astrocyte

3 Protoplasmic astrocyte

2 Nerve cell processes

4 Neurons

FIG. 1. GRAY MATTER (ANTERIOR HORN OF THE SPINAL CORD). Golgi's method. 350×.

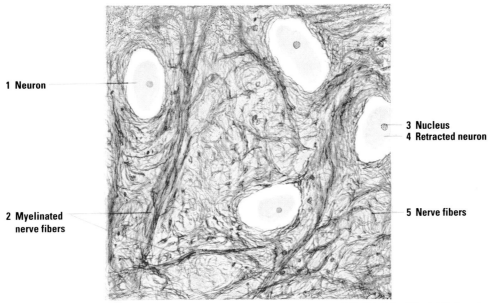

1 Neuron

3 Nucleus
4 Retracted neuron

2 Myelinated
nerve fibers

5 Nerve fibers

FIG. 2. GRAY MATTER (ANTERIOR HORN OF THE SPINAL CORD). Modified Weigert-Pal's method. 350×.

PLATE 29

■ **FIG. 1**
FIBROUS ASTROCYTES OF THE BRAIN

A section of nervous tissue, stained by Del Rio Hortega's method for macroglia (i.e., astrocytes and oligodendrocytes), demonstrates their cell outline, processes, and glial fibers.

In the center of the figure is a **fibrous astrocyte (5).** It exhibits a small cell body, a large nucleus, and numerous long, smooth, slightly branched processes extending in all directions. One of these processes terminates on a blood vessel as a **vascular pedicle (4)** or foot plate.

In the upper left portion of the figure, the **processes (2)** of another **fibrous astrocyte (1)** are seen associated with a blood vessel.

■ **FIG. 2**
OLIGODENDROCYTES OF THE BRAIN

This section has been stained with Del Rio Hortega's modification of Golgi's method.

A **protoplasmic astrocyte (4)** is seen with its small cell body, large nucleus, and numerous, thick branched processes.

The **oligodendrocytes (2, 5)** have smaller oval cell bodies and nuclei than the astrocytes, and exhibit few, thin, short processes without excessive branching. The processes may be either extremely thin (5), or somewhat thicker (2).

The oligodendrocytes are found in both the gray and white matter of the central nervous system. In the white matter, the oligodendrocytes form myelin sheaths around numerous **axons (6),** and are analogous to the Schwann cells on the peripheral nerves.

The **neuron (1)** provides a size contrast with the astrocytes and oligodendrocytes.

■ **FIG. 3**
MICROGLIA OF THE BRAIN

In this section, Del Rio Hortega's method demonstrates the **microglia (1, 4).** Their cell bodies are extremely small, vary in shape, and often exhibit irregular contours. The small, deeply stained nucleus almost fills the entire cell. The cell processes are few, short, slender, tortuous, and covered with small **"spines" (5).** The **neuron (3),** located superiorly in the figure, provides a size contrast with the microglia.

Microglia are normally not numerous, but are found in both the white and gray matter of the central nervous system (CNS). They are the main source of phagocytic cells in the CNS. It is also believed that microglia may represent a variety of oligodendrocyte.

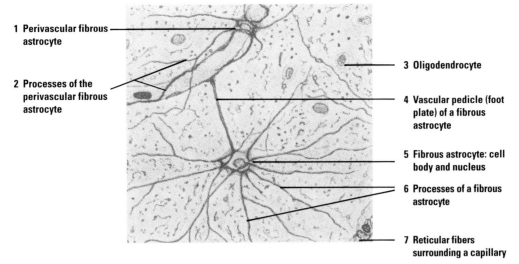

1 Perivascular fibrous astrocyte

2 Processes of the perivascular fibrous astrocyte

3 Oligodendrocyte

4 Vascular pedicle (foot plate) of a fibrous astrocyte

5 Fibrous astrocyte: cell body and nucleus

6 Processes of a fibrous astrocyte

7 Reticular fibers surrounding a capillary

FIG. 1. FIBROUS ASTROCYTES OF THE BRAIN. Del Rio Hortega's method.

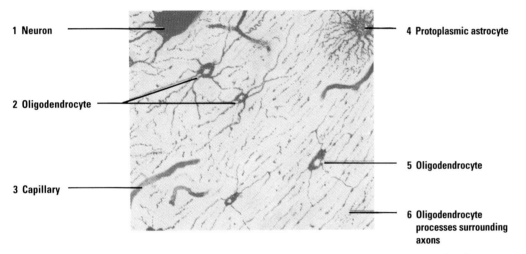

1 Neuron

2 Oligodendrocyte

3 Capillary

4 Protoplasmic astrocyte

5 Oligodendrocyte

6 Oligodendrocyte processes surrounding axons

FIG. 2. OLIGODENDROCYTES OF THE BRAIN. Modified Del Rio Hortega's method.

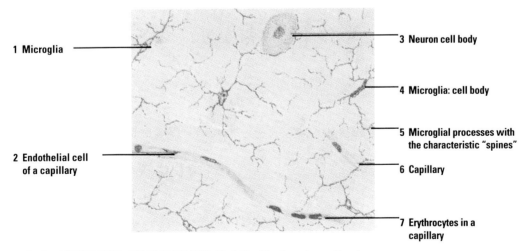

1 Microglia

2 Endothelial cell of a capillary

3 Neuron cell body

4 Microglia: cell body

5 Microglial processes with the characteristic "spines"

6 Capillary

7 Erythrocytes in a capillary

FIG. 3. MICROGLIA OF THE BRAIN. Del Rio Hortega's method.

PLATE 30

■ **FIG. 1**
MYELINATED NERVE FIBERS

The Schwann cells surround the axons of the peripheral nerves and form a myelin sheath. To illustrate the myelin sheath, the nerve fibers are fixed with an osmic acid; this preparation stains the lipid in the myelin sheath black. In this illustration, a portion of the peripheral nerve has been prepared in a longitudinal section (upper figure) and in a cross section (lower figure).

In the longitudinal section, the **myelin sheath (1)** appears as a thick, black band surrounding a lighter, central **axon (2).** At intervals of a few microns, the myelin sheath exhibits discontinuity between adjacent Schwann cells. This region represents the **node of Ranvier (4).**

A group of nerve fibers or fascicle is also illustrated. The fascicle is surrounded by a light-appearing connective tissue layer called the **perineurium (3, 5, 8).** Each individual nerve fiber or axon, in turn, is surrounded by a thin layer of connective tissue called the **endoneurium (7, 11).**

In cross section, different sizes of myelinated axons are seen. The **myelin sheath (9)** appears as a thick, black ring around the light, unstained **axon (13),** which in most fibers is seen in the center.

The connective tissue surrounding individual nerve fibers or the fascicle exhibits a rich supply of **blood vessels (6, 12)** of different sizes.

■ **FIG. 2**
PERIPHERAL NERVE (TRANSVERSE SECTION)

Several **bundles (fascicles) (1)** of nerve fibers have been sectioned in transverse **(1)** or oblique **(8)** planes. Each nerve fascicle is surrounded by a connective tissue sheath, the **perineurium (2),** which merges with surrounding **interfascicular connective tissue (17).** Perineurial septa may separate larger nerve fascicles. From these or directly from the perineurium, delicate connective tissue strands surround individual nerve fibers in a fascicle and form the **endoneurium (5).**

Numerous nuclei are seen between individual nerve fibers. Most of these are **Schwann cell nuclei (3);** others are **fibroblast nuclei of the endoneurium (5).** (See Plate 31, Fig. 2).

Numerous **blood vessels (9–12, 16)** that course in the interfascicular connective tissue send branches into each fascicle that ultimately divide into capillaries in the endoneurium (5).

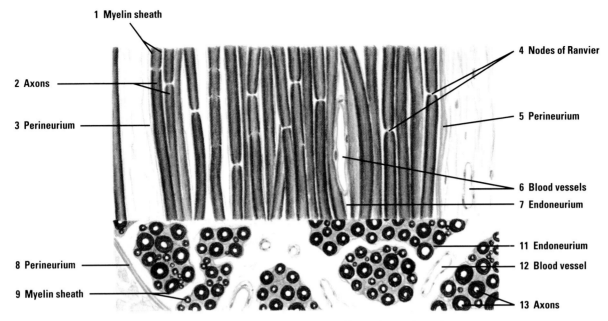

1 Myelin sheath

4 Nodes of Ranvier

2 Axons

5 Perineurium

3 Perineurium

6 Blood vessels

7 Endoneurium

11 Endoneurium

8 Perineurium

12 Blood vessel

9 Myelin sheath

13 Axons

FIG. 1. NERVOUS TISSUE: NERVE FIBERS AND NERVES. Myelinated: osmic stain.

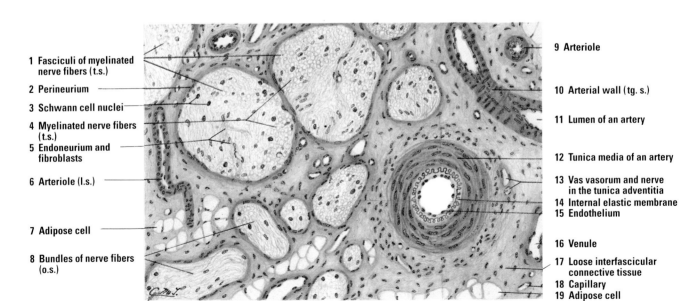

1 Fasciculi of myelinated nerve fibers (t.s.)

2 Perineurium

3 Schwann cell nuclei

4 Myelinated nerve fibers (t.s.)

5 Endoneurium and fibroblasts

6 Arteriole (l.s.)

7 Adipose cell

8 Bundles of nerve fibers (o.s.)

9 Arteriole

10 Arterial wall (tg. s.)

11 Lumen of an artery

12 Tunica media of an artery

13 Vas vasorum and nerve in the tunica adventitia
14 Internal elastic membrane
15 Endothelium

16 Venule

17 Loose interfascicular connective tissue
18 Capillary
19 Adipose cell

FIG. 2. NERVE (TRANSVERSE SECTION). Stain: hematoxylin-eosin. 250×.

PLATE 31

■ **FIG. 1**
NERVE, SCIATIC (PANORAMIC VIEW, LONGITUDINAL SECTION)

A portion of sciatic nerve is illustrated at a low magnification, as it appears in a routine histologic preparation stained with hematoxylin-eosin. The complete outer layer of dense connective tissue, the epineurium, is not shown in the illustration. The deeper part of the epineurium contains **adipose tissue (2)** and **blood vessels (1). Extensions of the epineurium (3)** surround large **nerve fascicles (5). Perineurium (4)** is the connective tissue sheath that surrounds individual nerve fascicles. The numerous nuclei that are arranged along nerve fibers are the Schwann cell nuclei (neurolemma nuclei) or fibroblast nuclei of the endoneurium connective tissue. It is not possible to differentiate between the Schwann cells and fibroblasts at this magnification.

■ **FIG. 2**
NERVE, SCIATIC (LONGITUDINAL SECTION)

A small portion of the nerve illustrated in Figure 1 is shown at a higher magnification. The **axons (1)** appear as slender threads stained lightly with hematoxylin. The surrounding myelin sheath has been dissolved as a result of routine histologic preparation, leaving a distinct **neurokeratin network (3)** of protein. The **sheath (4)** of Schwann cells is not always distinguishable from the surrounding connective tissue; however, in certain areas it is seen as a thin, peripheral boundary and at the **node of Ranvier (2)** as it descends toward the axon. Two **Schwann cell nuclei (5)** and the connective tissue **endoneurium (7)** are seen in the illustration. The **fibroblasts (6)** in the endoneurium are distinguished from the Schwann cell nuclei (5).

■ **FIG. 3**
NERVE, SCIATIC (TRANSVERSE SECTION)

The transverse section of sciatic nerve, as seen in Figure 2, illustrates the central **axons (2)**, the **neurokeratin network (3)** of protein as peripheral radial lines, and the peripheral **Schwann cell sheath (4). Schwann cell nucleus (1)** appears to encircle the axon (2).

Collagenous fibers of the endoneurium are faintly distinguishable; however, the **fibroblasts (5)** are clearly seen. **Perineurium (6)** surrounds a fascicle of nerve fibers and contains a small **venule (7).**

■ **FIG. 4**
NERVE, SCIATIC (LONGITUDINAL SECTION, PROTARGOL AND ANILINE
BLUE STAIN)

This section is stained with Protargol and aniline blue. The **axons (1)**, stained black, are prominent because of silver impregnation of the neurofibrils. The scattered black droplets probably represent remnants of neurofibrils remaining after axon shrinkage. The neurokeratin network is not stained. Other visible structures are the **nodes of Ranvier (4, 8), Schwann cell nuclei (7)**, and **fibroblast nuclei (5)** in the **endoneurium (6).**

■ **FIG. 5**
NERVE, SCIATIC (TRANSVERSE SECTION, PROTARGOL STAIN)

As described in Fig. 4, Protargol stains the **axons (1)** black, as seen in cross section. The surrounding gray area and small, black droplets probably indicate the original axon diameter. The **endoneurium (4, 6)** is well demonstrated by aniline blue staining of the collagenous fibers. Other visible structures are **Schwann cell sheath (3)** and **fibroblasts (5).**

■ **FIG. 6**
NERVE: BRANCH OF THE VAGUS (TRANSVERSE SECTION)

This figure illustrates still another staining method for nerve fibers and shows myelinated axons of varying size in a branch of the vagus nerve. The **fibroblast (1)** and **Schwann cell (6)** nuclei, **axons (3)**, and **neuro**keratin network (4) stain red with azocarmine. The **endoneurium (7)** is clearly demonstrated, especially in areas where axons are close together and within groups of **small nerve fibers (8).**

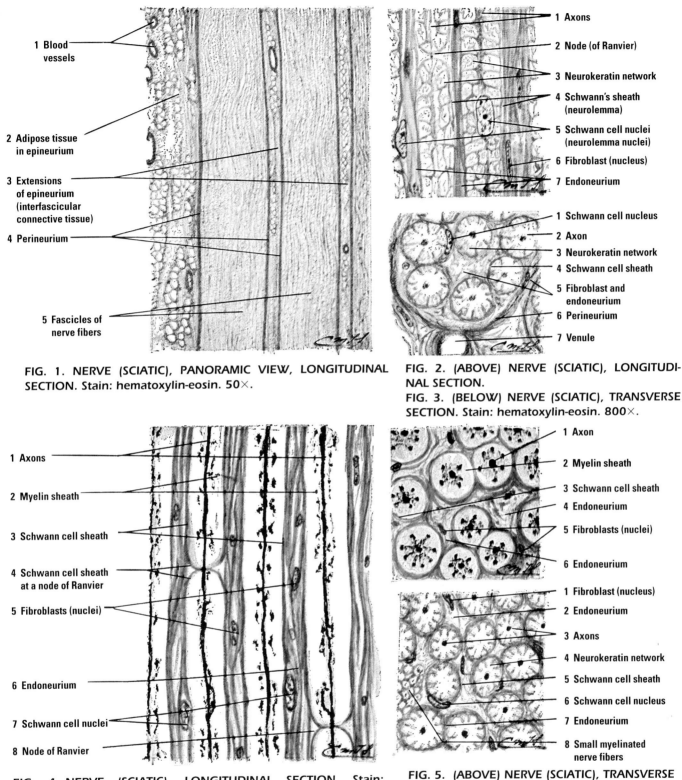

1 Blood vessels

2 Adipose tissue in epineurium

3 Extensions of epineurium (interfascicular connective tissue)

4 Perineurium

5 Fascicles of nerve fibers

1 Axons

2 Node (of Ranvier)

3 Neurokeratin network

4 Schwann's sheath (neurolemma)

5 Schwann cell nuclei (neurolemma nuclei)

6 Fibroblast (nucleus)

7 Endoneurium

1 Schwann cell nucleus

2 Axon

3 Neurokeratin network

4 Schwann cell sheath

5 Fibroblast and endoneurium

6 Perineurium

7 Venule

FIG. 1. NERVE (SCIATIC), PANORAMIC VIEW, LONGITUDINAL SECTION. Stain: hematoxylin-eosin. 50×.

FIG. 2. (ABOVE) NERVE (SCIATIC), LONGITUDINAL SECTION.

FIG. 3. (BELOW) NERVE (SCIATIC), TRANSVERSE SECTION. Stain: hematoxylin-eosin. 800×.

1 Axons

2 Myelin sheath

3 Schwann cell sheath

4 Schwann cell sheath at a node of Ranvier

5 Fibroblasts (nuclei)

6 Endoneurium

7 Schwann cell nuclei

8 Node of Ranvier

1 Axon

2 Myelin sheath

3 Schwann cell sheath

4 Endoneurium

5 Fibroblasts (nuclei)

6 Endoneurium

1 Fibroblast (nucleus)

2 Endoneurium

3 Axons

4 Neurokeratin network

5 Schwann cell sheath

6 Schwann cell nucleus

7 Endoneurium

8 Small myelinated nerve fibers

FIG. 4. NERVE (SCIATIC), LONGITUDINAL SECTION. Stain: Protargol and aniline blue. 800×.

FIG. 5. (ABOVE) NERVE (SCIATIC), TRANSVERSE SECTION.

FIG. 6. (BELOW) NERVE (BRANCH OF THE VAGUS), TRANSVERSE SECTION. Stain: Mallory-azan. 800×.

PLATE 32

■ **FIG. 1**
DORSAL ROOT GANGLION (PANORAMIC VIEW, LONGITUDINAL SECTION)

A **connective tissue layer (1)**, rich in adipose cells, nerves, and blood vessels **(13)**, surrounds the nervous tissue of a dorsal root ganglion. This layer merges with the external connective tissue capsule of the ganglion, the **epineurium (2)**, which is continuous with the **epineuria of the dorsal root (3)** and **spinal nerve (10)**. The perineurium and the endoneurium of the ganglion are not distinguishable at this magnification.

The round **pseudounipolar neurons (8)** of varying size constitute the majority of the **ganglion (8)**; these neurons are conspicuous because of their size and staining. Their vesicular nuclei with dark-staining nucleoli are better visible at higher magnification in Figure 2. Numerous fascicles of **nerve fibers (9)** are visible between the ganglion cells and course either in the **dorsal root (4)** or the **spinal nerve (11)**. These nerve fibers represent, respectively, the central processes and peripheral processes formed by bifurcation of a single axon process which emerges from each ganglion cell.

The **ventral root (7)**, surrounded by its **epineurium (6)**, joins the nerve fibers that emerge from the **ganglion (12)** and form the **spinal nerve (11)**.

■ **FIG. 2**
SECTION OF A DORSAL ROOT GANGLION

With a higher magnification, the **pseudounipolar neurons (2, 3)** appear variable in size. The characteristic vesicular **nucleus** with its prominent, dark-staining **nucleolus (2)** is conspicuous and the cytoplasm is filled with **Nissl bodies (3)**. Some cells exhibit small clumps of **lipofuscin pigment (5)**. Each cell has an axon hillock; however, it is not visible in this illustration.

Within the perineuronal space and in close association with the ganglion cells are the much smaller **satellite cells (6)**. These cells have spherical nuclei, are of neuroectodermal origin, and form a loose inner layer of the capsule around the ganglion cells. An outer **capsule (7)** of more flattened **fibroblasts (8)** and connective tissue fibers is continuous with the endoneurium. In different plane of sections, these two layers are not always clearly distinguishable; often the two cell types appear intermingled, as seen around the neuron with the **lipofuscin pigment (5)**.

Between ganglion cells are numerous **fibroblasts (4)**, randomly arranged in the connective tissue, or in rows in the endoneurium between **nerve fibers (1, 8)**. With hematoxylin-eosin stain, small axons and connective tissue fibers are not clearly defined. Large **myelinated fibers (1)** are recognizable when sectioned longitudinally.

■ **FIG. 3**
SECTION OF A SYMPATHETIC TRUNK GANGLION

Similar to the dorsal root ganglion cells, the cells of the sympathetic trunk ganglion exhibit a characteristic nucleus, a dark-staining nucleolus (sometimes multiple nucleoli), and Nissl bodies in their cytoplasm.

In contrast to cells in the dorsal root ganglion, however, these cells are multipolar neurons and are smaller and more uniform in size. As a result, the cell outlines are often irregular and remnants of their processes may be visible **(6)**. Their **nuclei (6)** are often eccentric and binucleated cells are not uncommon. Most of these neurons contain lipofuscin pigment in their cytoplasm.

The **satellite cells (2, 5)** are usually less numerous than around the cells in the dorsal root ganglion and the connective tissue capsule may or may not be well defined **(3)**. Present in the **intercellular area (4)** are fibroblasts, supportive connective tissue, blood vessels, and unmyelinated and myelinated axons. Nerve fibers aggregate into **bundles (1, 7)**, which course through the sympathetic trunk. These nerve fibers represent the preganglionic fibers, postganglionic visceral efferent fibers, and visceral afferent fibers.

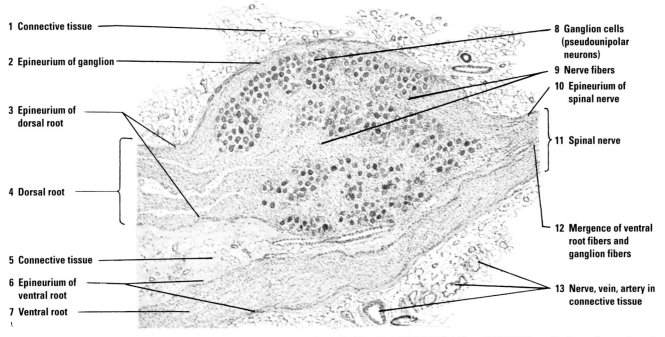

1 Connective tissue

2 Epineurium of ganglion

3 Epineurium of dorsal root

4 Dorsal root

5 Connective tissue

6 Epineurium of ventral root

7 Ventral root

8 Ganglion cells (pseudounipolar neurons)

9 Nerve fibers

10 Epineurium of spinal nerve

11 Spinal nerve

12 Mergence of ventral root fibers and ganglion fibers

13 Nerve, vein, artery in connective tissue

FIG. 1. DORSAL ROOT GANGLION: PANORAMIC VIEW (LONGITUDINAL SECTION). Stain: hematoxylin-eosin. 25×.

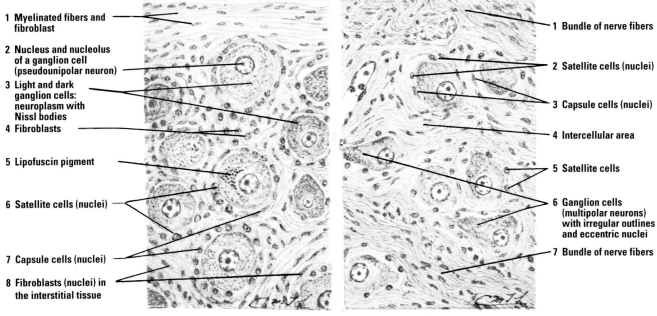

1 Myelinated fibers and fibroblast

2 Nucleus and nucleolus of a ganglion cell (pseudounipolar neuron)

3 Light and dark ganglion cells: neuroplasm with Nissl bodies

4 Fibroblasts

5 Lipofuscin pigment

6 Satellite cells (nuclei)

7 Capsule cells (nuclei)

8 Fibroblasts (nuclei) in the interstitial tissue

1 Bundle of nerve fibers

2 Satellite cells (nuclei)

3 Capsule cells (nuclei)

4 Intercellular area

5 Satellite cells

6 Ganglion cells (multipolar neurons) with irregular outlines and eccentric nuclei

7 Bundle of nerve fibers

FIG. 2. SECTION OF A DORSAL ROOT GANGLION. Stain: hematoxylin-eosin. 400×.

FIG. 3. SECTION OF A SYMPATHETIC TRUNK GANGLION. Stain: hematoxylin-eosin. 400×.

PLATE 33

■ **FIG. 1**
SPINAL CORD: CERVICAL REGION (TRANSVERSE SECTION)

To illustrate the white matter and the gray matter of the spinal cord, a cross section of the cord was prepared with silver impregnation technique. After staining, the dark brown, outer **white matter (3)** and the light-staining, inner **gray matter (4, 14)** are clearly visible. The white matter (3) consists primarily of ascending and descending myelinated nerve fibers or axons. By contrast, the gray matter contains the cell bodies of neurons, interneurons, and their axons. The gray matter also exhibits a symmetrical H-shape, whose two sides are connected across the midline of the spinal cord by the **gray commissure (15)** in whose center is located the **central canal (16)** of the spinal cord.

The **anterior horns (6)** of the gray matter extend toward the front of the cord and are more prominent than the **posterior horns (2, 13)**. The anterior horns contain the cell bodies of the large **motor neurons (7, 17)**. Some **axons (8)** from the motor neurons of the anterior horns cross the white matter and exit from the spinal cord as components of the **anterior roots (9, 21)** of the peripheral nerves. The posterior horns (2, 13) are the sensory areas and contain cell bodies of smaller neurons.

The spinal cord is surrounded by connective tissue meninges, consisting of an outer dura mater, a middle **arachnoid (5)**, and an inner **pia mater (18)**. The spinal cord is also partially divided into right and left halves by a narrow, posterior (dorsal) groove, the **posterior median sulcus (10)**, and a deep, anterior (ventral) cleft, the **anterior median fissure (19)**. In this illustration, pia mater (18) is best seen in the **anterior median fissure (19)**.

Between the posterior median sulcus (10) and the posterior horns (2, 13) of the gray matter are the prominent dorsal columns of the white matter. In the cervical region of the spinal cord, each dorsal column is subdivided into two fascicles, the posteromedial column, the **fasciculus gracilis (11)** and the posterolateral column, the **fasciculus cuneatus (1, 12)**.

■ **FIG. 2**
SPINAL CORD: ANTERIOR GRAY HORN AND ADJACENT ANTERIOR WHITE MATTER

A small section of the white matter and the gray matter of the anterior horn of the spinal cord are illustrated at a higher magnification. The gray matter of the anterior horn contains large, **multipolar motor neurons (2, 3)**. These are characterized by numerous **dendrites (5, 6)** that extend in different directions from the parikaryon (cell bodies). In some sections of the neurons, the **nucleus (8)** is visible with its prominent **nucleolus (8)**. In other neurons, the plane of section has missed the nucleus and the parikaryon appears empty **(2)**. Located in the vicinity of the motor neurons are the small, light-staining, supportive cells, the **neuroglia (7)**.

The white matter contains closely packed groups of myelinated axons. In cross sections, the **axons (1)** appear dark-stained and surrounded by a clear spaces, which are the remnants of the myelin sheaths. The axons of the white matter represent the ascending and descending tracts of the spinal cord. On the other hand, the **axons (4)** of the anterior horn motor neurons aggregate into groups, pass through the white matter, and exit from the spinal cord as the anterior (ventral) root fibers (See Fig. 1).

SPINAL CORD: CERVICAL REGION (TRANSVERSE SECTION)

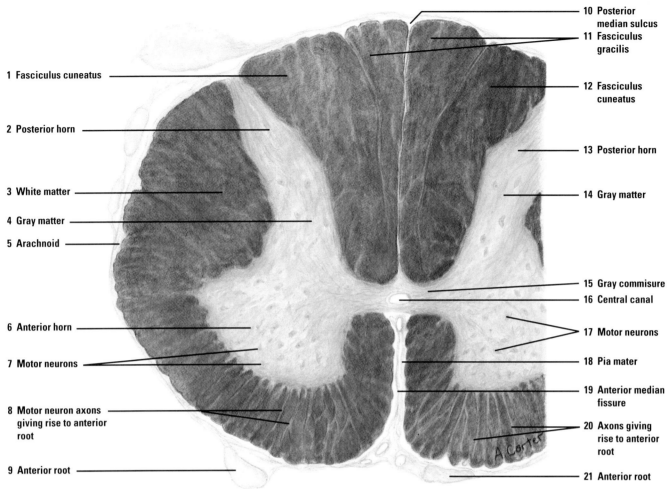

1 Fasciculus cuneatus

2 Posterior horn

3 White matter

4 Gray matter

5 Arachnoid

6 Anterior horn

7 Motor neurons

8 Motor neuron axons giving rise to anterior root

9 Anterior root

10 Posterior median sulcus

11 Fasciculus gracilis

12 Fasciculus cuneatus

13 Posterior horn

14 Gray matter

15 Gray commisure

16 Central canal

17 Motor neurons

18 Pia mater

19 Anterior median fissure

20 Axons giving rise to anterior root

21 Anterior root

FIG. 1. Spinal Cord.

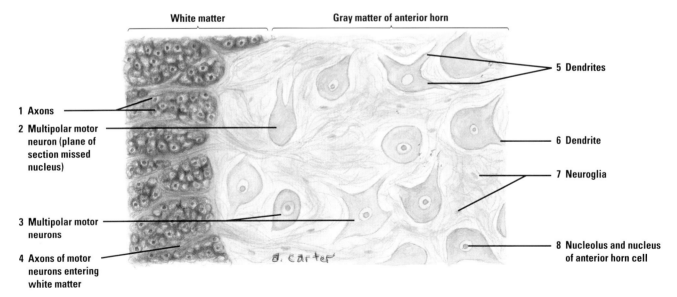

White matter

Gray matter of anterior horn

1 Axons

2 Multipolar motor neuron (plane of section missed nucleus)

3 Multipolar motor neurons

4 Axons of motor neurons entering white matter

5 Dendrites

6 Dendrite

7 Neuroglia

8 Nucleolus and nucleus of anterior horn cell

FIG. 2. ANTERIOR GRAY HORN AND ADJACENT WHITE MATTER. Silver impregnation: Cajal's method. 160 ×.

PLATE 34

■ **FIG. 1**
SPINAL CORD: MIDTHORACIC REGION (PANORAMIC VIEW, TRANSVERSE SECTION)

A transverse section of a spinal cord in the midthoracic region is illustrated with routine hematoxylin-eosin stain. This section of the spinal cord differs from the cervical region illustrated in Plate 33. The **posterior gray horns (5)** are slender. At the ventromedial basal portion of the posterior gray horn is seen the prominent **nucleus dorsalis (of Clarke) (22)**. The **anterior gray horns (24)** are also small, and the number of motor neurons is reduced to only a few cells in both the medial and lateral regions (24). The **lateral gray columns (23)** are well developed in the thoracic region of the spinal cord and contain the neurons of the sympathetic division of the autonomic nervous system. The remaining structures in the midthoracic region of the spinal cord correspond to the cervical cord region illustrated in Plate 33, differing only in appearance mainly because of the type of stain used in section preparation.

The meninges are also illustrated in this section of the spinal cord. The fibrous **pia mater (9)** is the innermost layer of the meninges. It adheres closely to the external glial limiting membrane of the spinal cord, which is not clearly seen in the figure. The pia mater (9) contains both the small and larger **blood vessels (1, 15)** that supply the cord. Fine trabeculae in the **subarachnoid space (10)** connect the pia mater with the **arachnoid (11)**. In life, the subarachnoid space is filled with cerebrospinal fluid. External to the arachnoid is a thick, fibrous **dura mater (13)**, separated from the arachnoid by the **subdural space (12)**. In this preparation, the subdural space is unusually large due to the artifactual retraction of the arachnoid.

■ **FIG. 2**
SPINAL CORD: ANTERIOR GRAY HORN AND ADJACENT ANTERIOR WHITE MATTER

A higher magnification of a small section of the spinal cord illustrates the appearance of gray matter, white matter, neurons, neuroglia, and axons stained with hematoxylin and eosin. The cells in the anterior gray horn of the thoracic region of the spinal cord are **multipolar motor neurons (2, 6)**. Their cytoplasm is characterized by a prominent vesicular **nucleus (7)**, a distinct **nucleolus (7)**, and coarse clumps of basophilic material called the **Nissl substance (3)**. The Nissl substance extends into the **dendrites (5)** but not the axons. One such neuron exhibits the root of an axon from the **axon hillock (4)**, which is devoid of the Nissl substance.

The non-neural **neuroglia (8)** cells, seen only as basophilic nuclei, are small in comparison to the prominent multipolar neurons (2, 4). The neuroglia occupy the spaces between the neurons. The anterior white matter of the spinal cord contains myelinated axons of various sizes. Because of the histologic preparation of this section, the myelin sheaths appear as clear spaces around the dark-staining **axons (1)**.

In certain neurons (2), the plane of section did not include the nucleus, and the cytoplasm appears enucleated (without nucleus).

SPINAL CORD: MID-THORACIC REGION (TRANSVERSE SECTION)

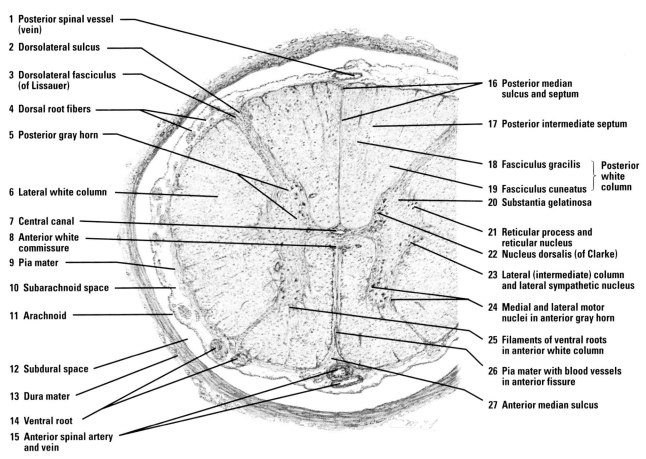

1 Posterior spinal vessel (vein)
2 Dorsolateral sulcus
3 Dorsolateral fasciculus (of Lissauer)
4 Dorsal root fibers
5 Posterior gray horn
6 Lateral white column
7 Central canal
8 Anterior white commissure
9 Pia mater
10 Subarachnoid space
11 Arachnoid
12 Subdural space
13 Dura mater
14 Ventral root
15 Anterior spinal artery and vein

16 Posterior median sulcus and septum
17 Posterior intermediate septum
18 Fasciculus gracilis } Posterior white column
19 Fasciculus cuneatus } Posterior white column
20 Substantia gelatinosa
21 Reticular process and reticular nucleus
22 Nucleus dorsalis (of Clarke)
23 Lateral (intermediate) column and lateral sympathetic nucleus
24 Medial and lateral motor nuclei in anterior gray horn
25 Filaments of ventral roots in anterior white column
26 Pia mater with blood vessels in anterior fissure
27 Anterior median sulcus

FIG. 1. PANORAMIC VIEW. Stain: hematoxylin-eosin. 18×.

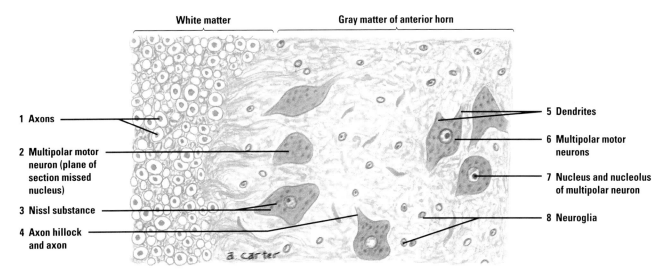

White matter

Gray matter of anterior horn

1 Axons
2 Multipolar motor neuron (plane of section missed nucleus)
3 Nissl substance
4 Axon hillock and axon

5 Dendrites
6 Multipolar motor neurons
7 Nucleus and nucleolus of multipolar neuron
8 Neuroglia

FIG. 2. ANTERIOR GRAY HORN AND ADJACENT WHITE MATTER. Hematoxylin and eosin. 160 ×.

89

PLATE 35

■ FIG. 1
CEREBELLUM (SECTIONAL VIEW, TRANSVERSE SECTION)

The cerebellum consists of an outer cortex of **gray matter (3)** and an inner **white matter (4, 10).** The white matter (4, 10) consists of myelinated nerve fibers or axons. These fibers are the afferent and efferent fibers of the cerebellar cortex. Their ramification (10) forms the core of the numerous cerebellar folds.

The gray matter constitutes the cortex, and three distinct cell layers can be distinguished in the cortex: an **outer molecular layer (6)** with relatively few cells and horizontally directed fibers, an **inner granular layer (7)** with numerous small cells with intensely stained nuclei, and a central layer of **Purkinje cells (8).** The Purkinje cells are pyriform in shape with ramified dendrites that extend into the molecular layer.

■ FIG. 2
CEREBELLUM: CORTEX

The **Purkinje cells (9)** are typically arranged in a single row at the junction of the **molecular (8)** and **granular cell (10)** layers. Their large "flask-shaped" bodies give off one or more thick **dendrites (3),** which extend through the molecular layer to the surface, giving off complex branchings along their course. The thin **axon (5)** leaves the base of the Purkinje cell, passes through the granular layer, and becomes myelinated as it enters the **white matter (12).**

The molecular layer contains scattered outer **stellate cells (8)** whose unmyelinated axons normally course in a horizontal direction. Descending collaterals of more deeply placed **basket cells (4)** arborize around the Purkinje cells (9) in a "basketlike" arrangement. Axons of the **granule cells (6)** in the granular layer extend into the molecular layer and also course horizontally **(2)** as unmyelinated fibers.

In the granular layer are found numerous small granule cells (6, 10) with dark-staining nuclei (an exception to the usual vesicular nucleus of nerve cells) and little cytoplasm. Also present in the granular layer are scattered larger **stellate cells** or **Golgi type II cells (7)** with typical vesicular nuclei and more cytoplasm. Throughout the granular layer are small, irregularly dispersed, clear spaces called the **"glomeruli" (11).** In these regions, the cells are absent and synaptic complexes occur.

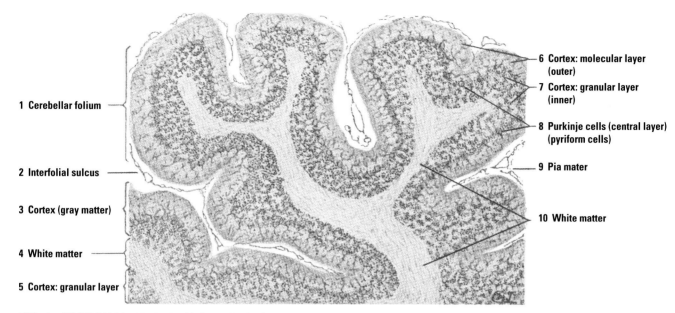

1 Cerebellar folium

2 Interfolial sulcus

3 Cortex (gray matter)

4 White matter

5 Cortex: granular layer

6 Cortex: molecular layer (outer)

7 Cortex: granular layer (inner)

8 Purkinje cells (central layer) (pyriform cells)

9 Pia mater

10 White matter

FIG. 1. SECTIONAL VIEW, TRANSVERSE SECTION. Silver impregnation: Cajal's method. 45×.

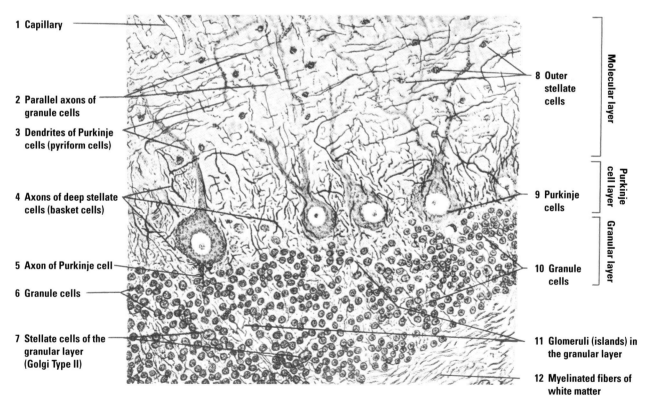

1 Capillary

2 Parallel axons of granule cells

3 Dendrites of Purkinje cells (pyriform cells)

4 Axons of deep stellate cells (basket cells)

5 Axon of Purkinje cell

6 Granule cells

7 Stellate cells of the granular layer (Golgi Type II)

8 Outer stellate cells

9 Purkinje cells

10 Granule cells

11 Glomeruli (islands) in the granular layer

12 Myelinated fibers of white matter

Molecular layer

Purkinje cell layer

Granular layer

FIG. 2. CORTEX. Silver impregnation: Cajal's method. 300×.

PLATE 36

■ **FIG. 1**
CEREBRAL CORTEX: SECTION PERPENDICULAR TO THE CORTICAL SURFACE

The silver nitrate stain used for this section of cerebral cortex demonstrates the neurofibrils.

The different cell types that constitute the cerebral cortex are distributed in layers, with one or more cell types predominant in each layer. Horizontal fibers associated with each layer give the cortex a laminated appearance. Fibers exhibiting a **radial arrangement (14)** are also present.

Although there are variations in arrangement of cells in different parts of the cerebral cortex, six distinct layers are recognized. These layers are labeled on the left side of the figure.

Starting at the periphery of the cortex, the outermost layer is the **molecular layer (1)**. Its peripheral portion is composed predominantly of horizontally directed neuronal processes, both dendrites and axons. Deep in the molecular layer lie the infrequent, stellate or spindle-shaped **horizontal cells of Cajal (10);** their axons contribute to the horizontal fibers. Overlying and covering the molecular cell layer is the delicate connective tissue of the brain, the **pia mater (8).**

In the next four layers, the predominant cells are the characteristic pyramidal cells of the cerebral cortex; these cells exhibit variable sizes. The figure illustrates that the **pyramidal cells (11, 13)** get progressively larger in layers 2, 3, 4, and 5. Their **dendrites (13)** are directed toward the periphery of the cortex and their axon extends from the cell base. In the **internal granular layer (4),** numerous smaller and larger **stellate cells (12)** form numerous complex connections with the pyramidal cells.

The **multiform layer (6)** lacks the pyramidal cells; however, the fusiform cells predominate and the granule cells, stellate cells, and cells of Martinotti are intermixed. All of these cells vary in size. Axons of the cells of Martinotti are directed peripherally, whereas the axons from other cells enter the **white matter (16).**

■ **FIG. 2**
CEREBRAL CORTEX: CENTRAL AREA OF THE CORTEX

Higher magnification of the cerebral cortex illustrates the large **pyramidal cells (1, 8). Neurofibrils (1, 8)** in the cell bodies have a characteristic network arrangement, whereas neurofibrils in the **dendrites (6)** and the **axons (7)** exhibit a more parallel arrangement. The typical large vesicular **nucleus (3)** with its prominent **nucleolus (3,** lower leader) is outlined. The most prominent cell process is the apical **dendrite (6),** which is directed toward the surface of the cortex. Several collaterals **(5)** are given off along its course through the cortex. Smaller dendrites (6, middle leader) arise from other parts of the cell body. The **axon (7)** arises from the base of the cell body and passes into the white matter.

The intercellular area is occupied by **nerve fibers (2)** of various cells in the cortex, small **astrocytes (4),** and blood vessels.

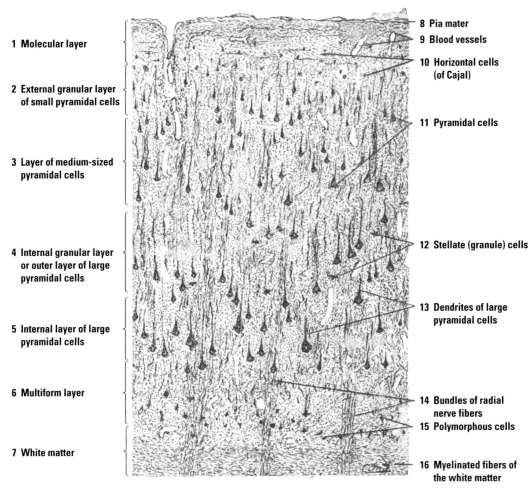

1 Molecular layer

2 External granular layer of small pyramidal cells

3 Layer of medium-sized pyramidal cells

4 Internal granular layer or outer layer of large pyramidal cells

5 Internal layer of large pyramidal cells

6 Multiform layer

7 White matter

8 Pia mater
9 Blood vessels
10 Horizontal cells (of Cajal)
11 Pyramidal cells
12 Stellate (granule) cells
13 Dendrites of large pyramidal cells
14 Bundles of radial nerve fibers
15 Polymorphous cells
16 Myelinated fibers of the white matter

FIG. 1. SECTION PERPENDICULAR TO THE CORTICAL SURFACE. Reduced silver nitrate method of Cajal. 80×.

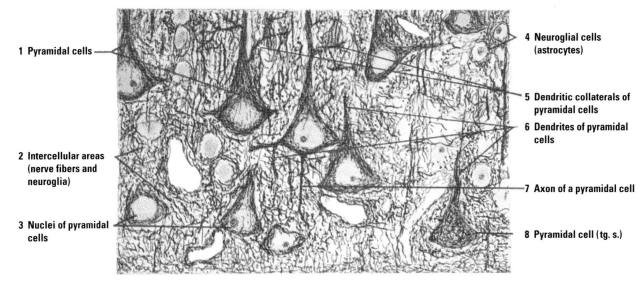

1 Pyramidal cells

2 Intercellular areas (nerve fibers and neuroglia)

3 Nuclei of pyramidal cells

4 Neuroglial cells (astrocytes)
5 Dendritic collaterals of pyramidal cells
6 Dendrites of pyramidal cells
7 Axon of a pyramidal cell
8 Pyramidal cell (tg. s.)

FIG. 2. CENTRAL AREA OF THE CORTEX. Reduced silver nitrate method of Cajal. 300×.

ORGANS

THE CARDIOVASCULAR SYSTEM

The circulatory system consists of a closed system of vessels whose main function is to transport blood to all cells, tissues, and organs of the body. The two components of the circulatory system are the cardiovascular system and lymph vascular system.

The cardiovascular system consists of the heart and the blood vessels. The blood vessels deliver nutrients, oxygen, and hormones to, and remove metabolic waste products from, all of the cells in the body. This exchange occurs at the level of the capillaries. The blood from the capillaries is then collected into the venules and veins, and is returned to the heart.

The Arteries

The rhythmic contraction of the heart forces the blood out of its chambers. The major function of the arterial system is the distribution of this blood to the capillary beds of the body. The three major categories of vessels in the arterial system are elastic arteries, muscular arteries, and arterioles. There is a gradual structural and functional transition from one type of vessel to the next.

The elastic arteries include the aorta and its major branches. The main function of the elastic arteries is to transport the blood from the heart and move it along the vascular path. The presence of increased amounts of elastic fibers in their walls allows the elastic arteries to expand during heart contraction (systole) and ejection of the blood into their lumina. During heart relaxation (diastole), the expanded elastic walls recoil. This effect forces the blood to move forward through the vascular channels and maintains the necessary arterial pressure. Also, as a result of the elastic fibers in the walls, the elastic arteries maintain a less variable blood pressure and a more even blood flow during the heart cycle.

The muscular or medium-sized arteries are branches of the elastic arteries and constitute the great majority of the arteries in the body. Their major function is to distribute blood to all organs of the body. As a result of the increased amount of smooth muscles in their walls, the muscular arteries control the blood flow and blood pressure through vasoconstriction or vasodilation of their lumina.

The arterioles are the smallest arterial vessels. Their walls consist of one to five layers of smooth muscle. By constricting or dilating their lumen, they regulate the flow of blood into the capillary beds. The terminal arterioles give rise to capillaries.

The Capillaries

The capillaries are the smallest blood vessels in the body. The average diameter of their lumina is about 8 μm, which almost equals the size of the erythrocytes. There are three types of capillaries in the body: continuous capillaries, fenestrated capillaries, and sinusoids.

The continuous capillaries are the most common type and are found in the connective tissue, all muscle tissue, the central nervous system, and other organs. In the continuous capillaries, the endothelial cells are joined and form an uninterrupted inner lining.

In contrast, the endothelial cells of the fenestrated capillaries contain circular openings or pores. The main function of the fenestrated capillaries is to allow a more rapid exchange of molecular substances between blood and the tissues than would normally occur in continuous capillaries. The fenestrated capillaries are primarily found in the endocrine organs, the small intestine, and the glomerulus of the kidneys.

The sinusoids exhibit irregular, tortuous paths through their organs and have much wider diameters than the ordinary capillaries. Endothelial cell junctions are rare, and wide gaps exist between endothelial cells. Also, the basement membrane is incomplete or absent in the sinusoids. As a result of these gaps, plasma as well as formed elements can pass through the sinusoids. Sinusoids are found in the liver, spleen, and bone marrow.

The Veins

There is a gradual transition from the capillaries to venules; venules usually accompany arterioles. The returning blood initially flows into postcapillary venules and then gradually into veins of increasing size. The veins exhibit increased structural variation and are arbitrarily classified as small, medium, and large. Veins are generally more numerous and have thinner walls and larger diameters than the arteries.

The blood pressure in the veins is lower than in the arteries. As a result, blood flow in the veins is passive. Venous blood flow in the head and trunk is primarily caused by negative pressure in the thorax and abdominal cavities due to the respiratory movements. The blood return from the extremities is aided by the contractions of muscles.

Small and medium-sized veins, particularly in the extremities, have valves; these prevent the backflow of blood. When the blood flows toward the heart, the valves are forced flat against the wall of the vein. As the blood starts to flow backwards, however, the valve flaps become distended with blood and prevent backflow. Thus, venous blood that is situated between the valves in the extremities is forced to flow toward the heart under the force of muscular contractions. The valves are absent in the veins of the central nervous system, large veins, and veins of the viscera.

The Lymph Vascular System

The lymph vascular system consists of the lymph capillaries and lymph vessels. In contrast to the blood capillaries, the lymph capillaries start as blind channels in the connective tissues. The larger lymphatic vessels have a similar structure to that of the veins except that their walls are thinner. Lymph movement is also similar to the movement of blood in the veins; however, there are more valves in the lymph vascular system.

The main function of the lymph vascular system is the passive collection of excess tissue fluid, the lymph, from the intercellular spaces of the connective tissue and returning it into the blood vascular system; lymph is an ultrafiltrate of the blood plasma. The lymph vessels also carry fatty acids absorbed in the small intestine and antibodies (immunoglobulins), produced in the lymph nodes, to the blood stream.

Vasa Vasorum

The walls of larger vessels are too thick to receive nourishment by direct diffusion from the lumen. As a result, the walls of these vessels have their own small vessels called vasa vasorum (vessels of the vessel).

PLATE 37

■ **FIG. 1**
BLOOD AND LYMPHATIC VESSELS

■ **FIG. 2**
LARGE VEIN: PORTAL VEIN (TRANSVERSE SECTION)

PLATE 37

■ **FIG. 1**
BLOOD AND LYMPHATIC VESSELS

This plate illustrates various types of blood and lymphatic vessels, surrounded by loose connective and **adipose tissue (13, 28)**. Most vessels have been cut in a transverse or oblique plane of section.

A **small artery (4)**, with its basic wall structure, is shown at the top center of the plate. In contrast to the vein, an artery has a relatively thick wall and a small lumen. In cross section, the wall of an artery exhibits the following layers:

a. tunica intima, composed of an inner layer of **endothelium (16)**, a **subendothelial (17)** layer of connective tissue, and an **internal elastic lamina (membrane) (19)**, which marks the boundary between the tunica intima and tunica media.

b. **tunica media (4)**, composed predominantly of circular smooth muscle fibers. A loose network of fine elastic fibers is interspersed among the smooth muscle cells.

c. **tunica adventitia (6)**, composed of connective tissue, which contains **small nerves (14)** and blood vessels **(15)**. The blood vessels in the adventitia are collectively called **vasa vasorum (15)**, or "blood vessels of blood vessel."

When arteries acquire about 25 or more layers of smooth muscle in tunica media, they are called muscular or distributing arteries. Elastic fibers become more numerous, but are still present as thin fibers and networks.

A **medium-sized vein (22)** is illustrated at the lower center of the plate. It has a relatively thin wall and a large lumen. In cross section, the wall of the vein exhibits the following layers:

a. **tunica intima**, composed of **endothelium (24)** and an extremely thin layer of fine collagenous and elastic fibers, which blend with the connective tissue of the tunica media.

b. **tunica media (25)**, consisting of a thin layer of circularly arranged smooth muscle loosely embedded in connective tissue. This layer is much thinner in veins than in arteries.

c. **tunica adventitia (26)**, consisting of a wide layer of connective tissue. This layer in veins is much thicker than the tunica media.

Arterioles (1, 5, 8) are also illustrated in the figure. The smallest arteriole (1) has a thin internal elastic lamina and one layer of smooth muscle cells in the tunica media. One **arteriole (8)** with a branching **capillary (9)** is sectioned longitudinally. Also illustrated are smaller **veins (18, 27)**, **venules (3, 10)**, **capillaries (9, 11, 20)** and small **nerves (2, 23)**.

A **lymphatic vessel (12)** can be recognized by the thinness of its walls and the flaps of a valve in the lumen. Many veins in the extremities have similar valves.

■ **FIG. 2**
LARGE VEIN: PORTAL VEIN (TRANSVERSE SECTION)

In large veins, the outstanding feature is the thick, muscular adventitia, in which the smooth muscle fibers exhibit a longitudinal orientation. In the illustrated transverse section of the portal vein, the typical arrangement in its wall is observed: the **smooth muscle fibers (1)** are segregated into bundles and seen mainly in cross section, with varying amounts of connective tissue of the tunica **adventitia (2)** dispersed among them. **Vasa vasorum (3, 7)** are present in the intervening connective tissue.

In contrast to the thick tunica adventitia, the **tunica media (6)** is a thinner layer of circularly arranged smooth muscle fibers and a more loosely arranged connective tissue. In other large veins, the tunica media may be extremely thin and compact. As seen in other vessels, the tunica intima is part of the **endothelium (4)** and supported by a small amount of connective tissue. In addition, large veins usually exhibit an **internal elastic lamina (5)**, which is not as well developed as in the arteries.

BLOOD AND LYMPHATIC VESSELS AND LARGE VEIN

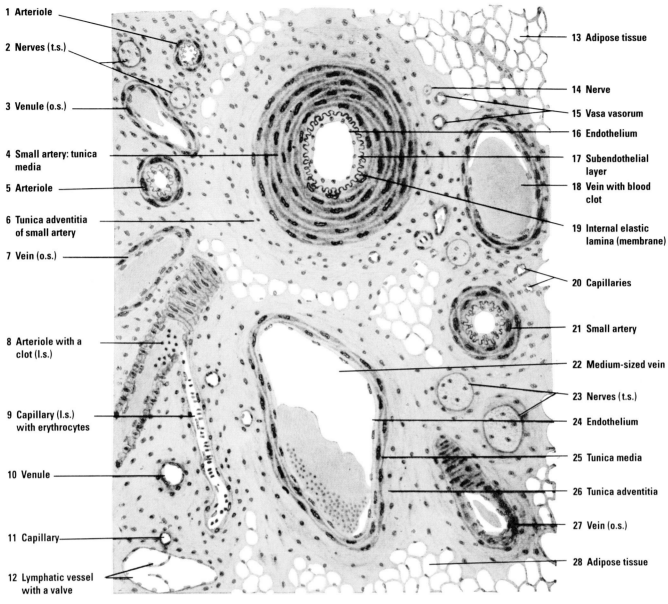

1 Arteriole

2 Nerves (t.s.)

3 Venule (o.s.)

4 Small artery: tunica media

5 Arteriole

6 Tunica adventitia of small artery

7 Vein (o.s.)

8 Arteriole with a clot (l.s.)

9 Capillary (l.s.) with erythrocytes

10 Venule

11 Capillary

12 Lymphatic vessel with a valve

13 Adipose tissue

14 Nerve

15 Vasa vasorum

16 Endothelium

17 Subendothelial layer

18 Vein with blood clot

19 Internal elastic lamina (membrane)

20 Capillaries

21 Small artery

22 Medium-sized vein

23 Nerves (t.s.)

24 Endothelium

25 Tunica media

26 Tunica adventitia

27 Vein (o.s.)

28 Adipose tissue

FIG. 1. BLOOD AND LYMPHATIC VESSELS. Stain: hematoxylin. 160×.

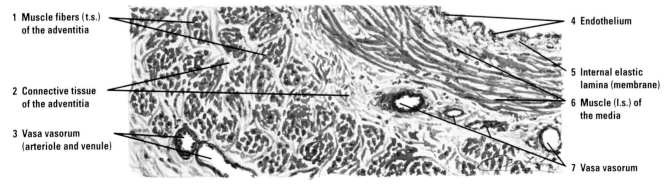

1 Muscle fibers (t.s.) of the adventitia

2 Connective tissue of the adventitia

3 Vasa vasorum (arteriole and venule)

4 Endothelium

5 Internal elastic lamina (membrane)

6 Muscle (l.s.) of the media

7 Vasa vasorum

FIG. 2. LARGE VEIN: PORTAL VEIN (TRANSVERSE SECTION). Stain: hematoxylin-eosin. 200×.

101

PLATE 38

■ FIG. 1
NEUROVASCULAR BUNDLE (TRANSVERSE SECTION)

In the center of the figure is a large, **elastic artery (18)** with a thick **tunica media (16)** consisting primarily of concentric layers of elastic lamina (membrane), between which are found thin layers of smooth muscle. The tunica intima consists of **endothelium (19)** whose round nuclei appear to project into the lumen of the artery, and a thin layer of subendothelial connective tissue (19) containing fine collagenous and elastic fibers. The first visible elastic membrane is the **internal elastic lamina (17).** The **tunica adventitia (15)** is a thin layer of connective tissue with vasa vasorum and the vasomotor nerves.

Several **arterioles (3, 9, 26)** are illustrated, distinguished by their thin muscular walls and relatively narrow lumina; also, numerous **capillaries (21)** are visible in the vicinity of the artery.

The **veins (4, 7, 22)** exhibit a highly variable morphology; however, each vein has a thin wall and a large lumen. Some veins can contain a blood clot or hemolyzed blood (7, 22).

Various-sized **nerves (2, 8, 10, 25)** accompany the blood vessels. Each nerve is surrounded by the connective tissue perineurium and is composed primarily of unmyelinated axons. Also illustrated in the figure is a **sympathetic ganglion (1)** surrounded by a connective tissue capsule. It contains multipolar neurons, axons, and small blood vessels.

The figure also shows part of a small **lymph node (5)**, its hilus, and several **efferent lymphatic vessels (6)**. The larger **lymph node (11)** shows its **capsule (14)**, the **subcapsular sinus (13), cortex (12)**, and **medulla (11)**.

■ FIG. 2
LARGE ARTERY: AORTA (TRANSVERSE SECTION)

The structure of the illustrated artery is similar to that of the vessel illustrated in Figure 1; however, it has been stained with orcein, which stains **elastic fibers (2)** dark brown. Other tissues in the wall of the aorta remain colorless or are only lightly stained. The size and arrangement of elastic lamina in the tunica media are clearly demonstrated. **Smooth muscle cells (3)** and fine elastic fibers between the laminae remain unstained.

The extent of **tunica intima (4)** is indicated but

remains unstained. The first elastic membrane is the **internal elastic lamina (membrane) (5)**. At times, smaller laminae appear in the subendothelial connective tissue, and a gradual transition is made to larger laminae of the tunica media.

The **tunica adventitia (1)**, also unstained, is a narrow zone of collagenous fibers. In the aorta and pulmonary arteries, tunica media occupies most of the wall of the vessel, whereas tunica adventitia is reduced to the proportionately small area, as illustrated in the figure.

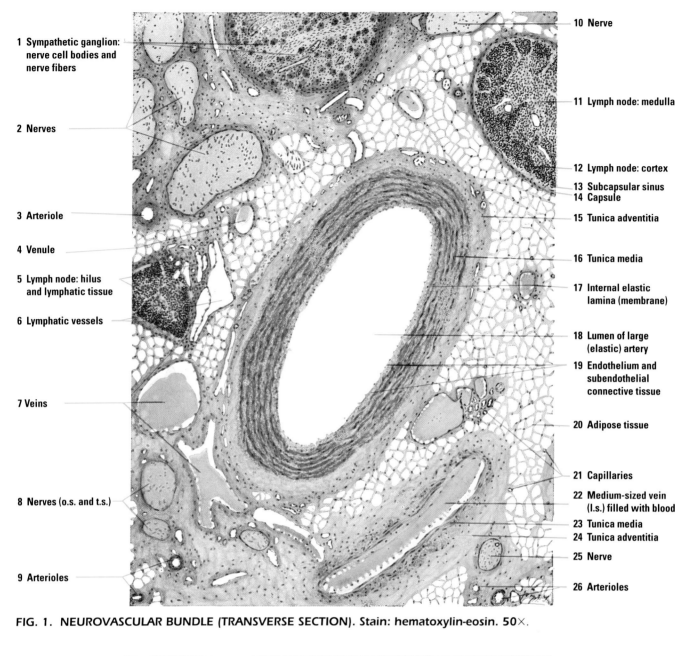

1 Sympathetic ganglion: nerve cell bodies and nerve fibers

2 Nerves

3 Arteriole

4 Venule

5 Lymph node: hilus and lymphatic tissue

6 Lymphatic vessels

7 Veins

8 Nerves (o.s. and t.s.)

9 Arterioles

10 Nerve

11 Lymph node: medulla

12 Lymph node: cortex

13 Subcapsular sinus
14 Capsule

15 Tunica adventitia

16 Tunica media

17 Internal elastic lamina (membrane)

18 Lumen of large (elastic) artery

19 Endothelium and subendothelial connective tissue

20 Adipose tissue

21 Capillaries

22 Medium-sized vein (l.s.) filled with blood

23 Tunica media
24 Tunica adventitia

25 Nerve

26 Arterioles

FIG. 1. NEUROVASCULAR BUNDLE (TRANSVERSE SECTION). Stain: hematoxylin-eosin. 50×.

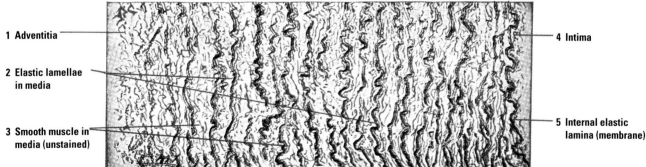

1 Adventitia

2 Elastic lamellae in media

3 Smooth muscle in media (unstained)

4 Intima

5 Internal elastic lamina (membrane)

FIG. 2. LARGE ARTERY: AORTA (TRANSVERSE SECTION). Orcein stain: aorta. Elastic fibers selectively stained dark brown. Approx. 300×.

PLATE 39

HEART: LEFT ATRIUM AND VENTRICLE, (PANORAMIC VIEW, LONGITUDINAL SECTION)

This figure illustrates a longitudinal section of the left side of the heart, showing a portion of the **atrium (1)**, the **atrioventricular (mitral) valve (4)**, and the **ventricle (6)**. In this plane of section, the cardiac musculature is seen in various planes.

In the atrial wall, the **endocardium (1)** consists of endothelium, a thick subendothelial layer of connective tissue, and a thick **myocardium (2)** of loosely arranged musculature. The **epicardium (13)** covers the heart and is lined externally by a single layer of mesothelium. A **subepicardial layer (14)** contains connective tissue and fat, which vary in amount in different regions of the heart. This layer also extends into the coronary (atrioventricular) and interventricular sulcus of the heart.

In the ventricle, the **endocardium (6)** is thin in comparison with that in the atrium, (1) whereas the **myocardium (7)** is thick and more compact. The **epicardium** and **subepicardial (16)** connective tissue are continuous with those in the atrium.

Between the atrium and ventricle is seen the **annulus fibrosus (3)**, which consists of dense fibrous connective tissue. The leaflet of the **atrioventricular valve (mitral) (4)** is formed by a double membrane of the **endocardium (4a)** and a core of dense **connective tissue (4b)**, which is continuous with the annulus fibrosus (3). On the ventral surface of the valve is seen the insertion of a section of **chorda tendina (5)** into the valve.

The inner surface of the ventricular wall exhibits the characteristic prominence of myocardium and endocardium: the **apex of papillary muscle (18)** and **trabeculae carneae (17)**.

The **Purkinje fibers (8)** or impulse-conducting fibers are located in the loose subendocardial tissue. They are distinguished by their larger size and lighter-staining properties. The small area within the rectangle **(9)** is illustrated in greater detail and higher magnification in Plate 40, Figure 2.

The larger blood vessels, such as the **coronary artery (10)**, course in the **subepicardial connective tissue (14)**. Below the coronary artery is a section through the **coronary sinus (11)**. Entering the coronary sinus is a **coronary vein (12)** with its valve. Smaller coronary **vessels (15)** are seen in the subepicardial connective tissue (14) and in the **perimyseal septa (15)** that extend into the myocardium (7).

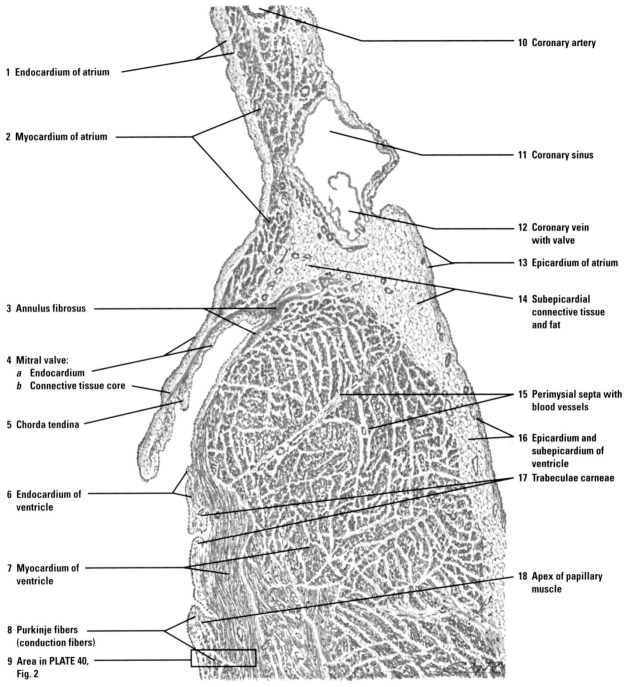

1 Endocardium of atrium

2 Myocardium of atrium

3 Annulus fibrosus

4 Mitral valve:
   a Endocardium
   b Connective tissue core

5 Chorda tendina

6 Endocardium of
   ventricle

7 Myocardium of
   ventricle

8 Purkinje fibers
   (conduction fibers)

9 Area in PLATE 40,
   Fig. 2

10 Coronary artery

11 Coronary sinus

12 Coronary vein
   with valve

13 Epicardium of atrium

14 Subepicardial
   connective tissue
   and fat

15 Perimysial septa with
   blood vessels

16 Epicardium and
   subepicardium of
   ventricle

17 Trabeculae carneae

18 Apex of papillary
   muscle

Stain: hematoxylin-eosin. 6×.

PLATE 40

■ FIG. 1
HEART: PULMONARY TRUNK, PULMONARY VALVE, RIGHT VENTRICLE
(PANORAMIC VIEW, LONGITUDINAL SECTION)

A portion of the right ventricle and a section of the **pulmonary trunk (6)** are illustrated. The endothelium of the tunica intima is visible on the right surface. Tunica media constitutes the thickest portion of its wall; however, its thick, elastic laminae are not apparent at this magnification. A thin adventitia merges into the surrounding **subepicardial connective tissue (2),** which is filled with fat in this specimen.

The **pulmonary trunk (8)** arises from the **annulus fibrosus (9).** One cusp of its **semilunar (pulmonary) valve (7)** is illustrated. Like the mitral valve, (illustrated in Plate 39), it is covered with endocardium. The connective tissue from the annulus fibrosus extends into the base of the **pulmonary valve (10)** and forms its central core.

The thick **myocardium (4)** of the right ventricle is lined internally by **endocardium (11).** The endocardium (11) extends over the pulmonary valve (7) and the annulus fibrosus (9), and blends in with tunica intima of the pulmonary trunk (8).

The external surface of the **pulmonary trunk (6)** is lined by the **subepicardial connective tissue** and **fat (2),** which, in turn, is covered by **epicardium (1).** Both of these layers cover the external surface of the ventricle. **Coronary vessels (3, 5)** are seen in the subepicardium (2).

■ FIG. 2
PURKINJE FIBERS (IMPULSE-CONDUCTING FIBERS)

The area outlined by a rectangle **(9)** in Plate 39 is illustrated here at higher magnification to show the impulse-conducting fibers. Located under the **endocardium (1)** are groups of **Purkinje fibers (2, 4).** These fibers are different from typical **cardiac (myocardial) muscle fibers (5)** because of their larger size and less intense staining. Some Purkinje fibers are sectioned transversely (2) and others longitudinally (4). In transverse section, the Purkinje fibers exhibit fewer myofi-brils, distributed peripherally, leaving a perinuclear zone of comparatively clear sarcoplasm. A nucleus is seen in some transverse sections; in others, a central area of clear sarcoplasm is seen, with the plane of section bypassing the nucleus.

Purkinje fibers merge with cardiac fibers at a **transitional fiber (3);** the upper part of the fiber corresponds to a Purkinje fiber and the lower part to an ordinary cardiac muscle fiber.

■ FIG. 3
PURKINJE FIBERS (IMPULSE-CONDUCTING FIBERS) (MALLORY-AZAN STAIN)

This figure illustrates a cardiac region with Purkinje fibers that are stained with Mallory-Azan; for this preparation, the same magnification as in Figure 2 was used. The characteristic features of **Purkinje fibers (2)** are demonstrated in both the longitudinal and transverse sections.

With a hematoxylin-eosin preparation, the connective tissue does not stain well. In this preparation, the blue-stained collagenous fibers accentuate the **subendocardial connective tissue (3)** around the Purkinje fibers (2). A **capillary (1)** with red blood cells is seen near these fibers.

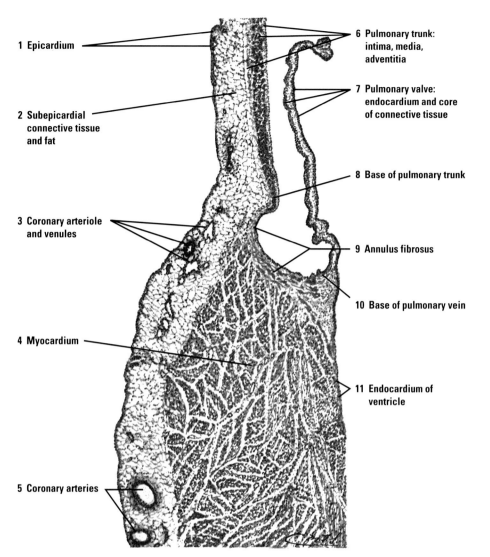

1 Epicardium

2 Subepicardial connective tissue and fat

3 Coronary arteriole and venules

4 Myocardium

5 Coronary arteries

6 Pulmonary trunk: intima, media, adventitia

7 Pulmonary valve: endocardium and core of connective tissue

8 Base of pulmonary trunk

9 Annulus fibrosus

10 Base of pulmonary vein

11 Endocardium of ventricle

FIG. 1. PULMONARY TRUNK, PULMONARY VALVE, RIGHT VENTRICLE (PANORAMIC VIEW, LONGITUDINAL SECTION).Stain: hematoxylin-eosin. 9×.

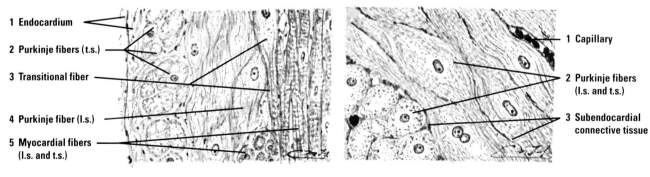

1 Endocardium

2 Purkinje fibers (t.s.)

3 Transitional fiber

4 Purkinje fiber (l.s.)

5 Myocardial fibers (l.s. and t.s.)

1 Capillary

2 Purkinje fibers (l.s. and t.s.)

3 Subendocardial connective tissue

FIG. 2. PURKINJE FIBERS (IMPULSE-CONDUCTING FIBERS). Stain: hematoxylin-eosin. 400×.

FIG. 3. PURKINJE FIBERS (IMPULSE-CONDUCTING FIBERS). Stain: Mallory-azan. 400×.

THE LYMPHOID SYSTEM

The lymphoid system includes all cells, tissues, and organs that contain aggregates of lymphocytes. The lymphocytes are distributed throughout the body as individual aggregates of cells in the loose connective tissue, distinct lymphatic nodules, or encapsulated individual lymphoid organs. The major lymphoid organs are the thymus gland, tonsils, spleen, and lymph nodes. Because the bone marrow produces lymphocytes, it can also be considered a lymphoid organ.

The lymphoid cells, tissue, and organs are the important components of the immune system. Their primary functions are the protection of the internal environment of the body against foreign substances or antigens. This crucial protective function of the immune system is performed by the lymphocytes because these cells have the ability to recognize and react specifically with antigens by producing antibodies. The antibodies are specialized to react with the antigens and initiate a complex immune process that protects the body from damage by eventually destroying the foreign substance. There are numerous types of lymphocytes in different organs of the body. Morphologically, these lymphocytes appear similar, but functionally they differ greatly.

The lymphoid tissue consists mainly of two types of lymphocytes: T lymphocytes and B lymphocytes. These are two functionally distinct types of lymphocytes found in the blood, lymph, and lymphoid tissues. Both types of lymphocytes, however, originate from precursor hemopoietic stem cells in the bone marrow. Whether the developing lymphocytes become B lymphocytes or T lymphocytes depends on where in the body they mature and become immunocompetent.

The B lymphocytes are believed to mature and become immunocompetent in the spleen and fetal liver, and possibly the bone marrow. After their maturation, the B lymphocytes are carried by the blood to the lymphoid tissue, where they reside, primarily in the lymph nodes and spleen. When the immunocompetent B lymphocytes encounter a specific antigen, they proliferate and develop into plasma cells. The plasma cells then synthesize and secrete specific antibodies against the particular antigen into the blood and lymph.

The T lymphocytes arise from lymphocytes that are carried to the thymus gland, where they undergo maturation before migrating to other lymphoid organs. Production of mature T lymphocytes by the thymus gland takes place early in the life of the individual.

After their stay in the thymus gland, the T lymphocytes are then distributed throughout the body in the blood stream, and populate the lymph nodes, spleen, and different lymphoid tissues.

The Lymphoid Organs

The Thymus Gland

The thymus gland is an important component of the immune system. During the fetal life and early childhood, this gland is large. It reaches its largest size during puberty, but is most functional in early life. As the individual ages, the thymus gland gradually atrophies and degenerates into connective tissue and adipose tissue.

Although all of its functions are not completely understood, the thymus gland performs an important role in developing the immune system of the organism. Undifferentiated lymphocytes migrate to the thymus gland, proliferate, and then differentiate into immunocompetent T lymphocytes. The T lymphocytes then leave the thymus gland by way of the blood stream and populate other lymphoid organs and tissues. The thymus gland also secretes a group of hormones, among which is thymosin, believed necessary for maturation of T lymphocytes and production of lymphocytes in other lymphoid organs.

If the thymus gland is removed in the newborn individual, the lymphoid organs will not become populated by the immunocompetent T lymphocytes. As a result of this deficiency, the individual does not acquire the necessary immunologic competence to fight invading pathogens and may die early from the complications of an infection.

The Lymph Nodes

The lymph nodes are distributed throughout the body and along the paths of the lymphatic vessels. They also have an important role in the defense mechanism of the body. The nodes are most prominent in the inguinal and axillary regions of the body. They serve an important function by filtering the lymph, removing from it particulate matter and bacteria.

109

Associated directly with lymph filtration is the phagocytic function of the lymph nodes. Within the mesh of the reticular fiber network in each node are fixed or free macrophages. By filtering and phagocytizing bacteria from the lymph, the lymph nodes assist in localizing and preventing the spread of infection.

The lymph nodes also have an important role in the formation of antibodies and in immunologic defense of the body in response to regional antigens. The antibodies are produced by the plasma cells that are concentrated in the lymph nodes.

The lymph nodes also produce and recirculate the B and T lymphocytes. As these lymphocytes enter the lymph node, the B lymphocytes aggregate in the lymphoid nodules in the cortex and the T lymphocytes concentrate in the paracortical regions.

The Spleen

The spleen is the largest lymphoid organ. One of its main functions is filtering the blood. As a result, the sinuses of the spleen are filled with blood cells. The dense reticular network of spleen's interior functions as an effective filter for antigens, microorganisms, platelets, and worn-out red blood cells. The trapped materi-al in the reticular meshwork is then removed from the blood by the macrophages and phagocytic reticular cells. The macrophages in the spleen also remove iron from the hemoglobin of the worn-out red blood cells and return it to the bone marrow for re-use during the production of new red blood cells. The heme from the breakdown of hemoglobin is then excreted in bile by the liver cells.

In fetal life, the spleen has an important function as a hemopoietic organ. It produces such blood cells as granulocytes and erythrocytes. This hemopoietic capability, however, ceases after the birth of an individual.

The spleen also serves as an important reservoir for blood. Because it has a sponge-like structure, increased amounts of blood volume can be stored in its interior. When the need arises, the stored blood is returned from the spleen to the general circulation.

This organ also performs an important function in defense mechanisms of the body because it contains large quantities of both B lymphocytes and T lymphocytes, as well as macrophages. The presence of antigens stimulates the proliferation of B lymphocytes, which then give rise to plasma cells. The plasma cells then produce large quantities of antibodies.

Although the spleen performs various important functions in the body, it is not essential to life.

PLATE 41

LYMPH NODE (PANORAMIC VIEW)

PLATE 41

LYMPH NODE (PANORAMIC VIEW)

The lymph node consists of lymphocyte aggregations intermeshed with lymphatic sinuses, supported by a reticular fiber framework, and surrounded by a **connective tissue capsule (2).** The lymph node has a **cortex (5)** and a **medulla (6).**

The cortex (5) of the lymph node contains lymphocytes that are aggregated into **lymphatic nodules (5, 16).** In many of the **cortical nodules (16),** the centers are lightly stained. These lighter-stained areas represent the **germinal centers (18),** which are the active sites of lymphocyte proliferation.

In the medulla (6) of the lymph node, the lymphocytes are arranged as irregular cords of lymphatic tissue, the **medullary cords (14).** The **medullary sinuses (13)** course between these cords.

The capsule (2) of the node is surrounded by **connective tissue and pericapsular fat (1).** From the capsule, **connective tissue trabeculae (7)** extend into the node, initially between the cortical nodules (7, upper leader) and then ramifying throughout the **medulla (15)** between medullary cords and sinuses. The trabeculae contain the major **blood vessels (15)** of the lymph node.

Afferent lymphatic vessels (4) course in the connective tissue of the lymph node and, at intervals, pierce the capsule to enter the **subcapsular sinus (9, 17).** From here, the trabecular sinuses (cortical sinuses) extend along the trabeculae to pass into medullary sinuses (13).

At the upper right section are the **hilus (12)** of the lymph node and the **efferent lymphatic vessels (11)** which drain the lymph from the node. Also found here are nerves, small arteries, and veins, which supply and drain the node.

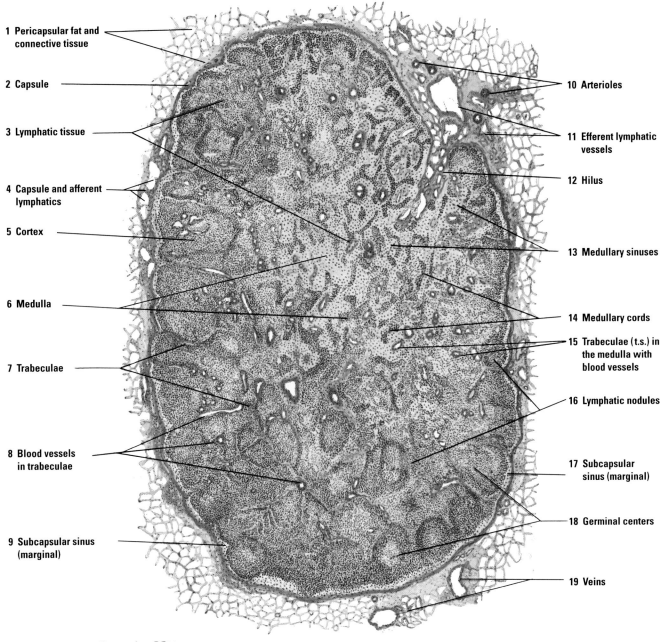

1 Pericapsular fat and connective tissue

2 Capsule

3 Lymphatic tissue

4 Capsule and afferent lymphatics

5 Cortex

6 Medulla

7 Trabeculae

8 Blood vessels in trabeculae

9 Subcapsular sinus (marginal)

10 Arterioles

11 Efferent lymphatic vessels

12 Hilus

13 Medullary sinuses

14 Medullary cords

15 Trabeculae (t.s.) in the medulla with blood vessels

16 Lymphatic nodules

17 Subcapsular sinus (marginal)

18 Germinal centers

19 Veins

Stain: hematoxylin-eosin. 32×.

PLATE 42

PLATE 42

■ FIG. 1
LYMPH NODE (SECTIONAL VIEW)

A small section of a cortical region of the lymph node is illustrated at a higher magnification.

The lymph node **capsule (5)** is surrounded by loose **connective tissue (1)** containing **blood vessels (2, 3, 4)** and afferent **lymphatic vessels (13);** the latter are lined with endothelium and contain **valves (14).** Arising from the inner surface of the capsule (5), connective tissue **trabeculae (15)** extend through the cortex and medulla. Associated with these connective tissue partitions are **trabecular blood vessels (18).**

The **cortex (7)** of the lymph node is separated from the connective tissue capsule (5) by the **subcapsular (marginal) sinus (6).** The cortex consists of lymphatic nodules situated adjacent to each other but incompletely separated by internodular trabeculae (15) and **trabecular (cortical) sinuses (16).** In this figure, one complete **lymphatic nodule** (7, lower leader; 8, 17, lower leader) and portions of two other nodules (7, upper leader; 17, upper leader) are illustrated. The deeper portion of the cortex, the **paracortical region (19),** is the thymus-dependent zone and is occupied by T lymphocytes. This is a transition area from the nodules to the medullary cords. The medulla consists of anastomosing cords of lymphatic tissue, the **medullary cords (12, 20),** interspersed with **medullary sinuses (11, 21)** which drain into the efferent lymphatic vessels located at the hilus.

Reticular connective tissue forms the stroma of the cortical nodules, the medullary cords, and all sinuses. Relatively few lymphocytes are seen in the sinuses (6, 11, 16, 21); thus, it is possible to distinguish the reticular framework (21) of the node. In the lymphatic nodules (7) and the medullary cords (12, 20), lymphocytes are so abundant that the reticulum is obscured unless it is specially stained, as shown in Figure 2. Most of the lymphocytes are small and contain large, deep-staining nuclei with condensed chromatin. The cells exhibit either a small amount or no cytoplasm at all.

Lymphatic nodules often exhibit **germinal centers (8),** which stain less intensely than the surrounding peripheral portion of the nodule (7). In the germinal center (8), the cells are more loosely aggregated and the developing lymphocytes have larger, lighter nuclei with more cytoplasm than the small lymphocytes (see Plate 43, Fig. 1).

■ FIG. 2
LYMPH NODE: RETICULAR FIBERS OF THE STROMA

A section of a lymph node has been stained with the Bielschowsky-Foot silver method to illustrate the intricate arrangement of the **reticular fibers (7).**

The various zones illustrated in Figure 1 are readily recognized: the **cortex (1), subcapsular (marginal) sinus (2), medullary cords (5),** and **medullary sinuses (6).** All of these regions contain a stroma of delicate reticular fibers **(4, 7),** which form the fine meshwork of the lymph node.

LYMPH NODE

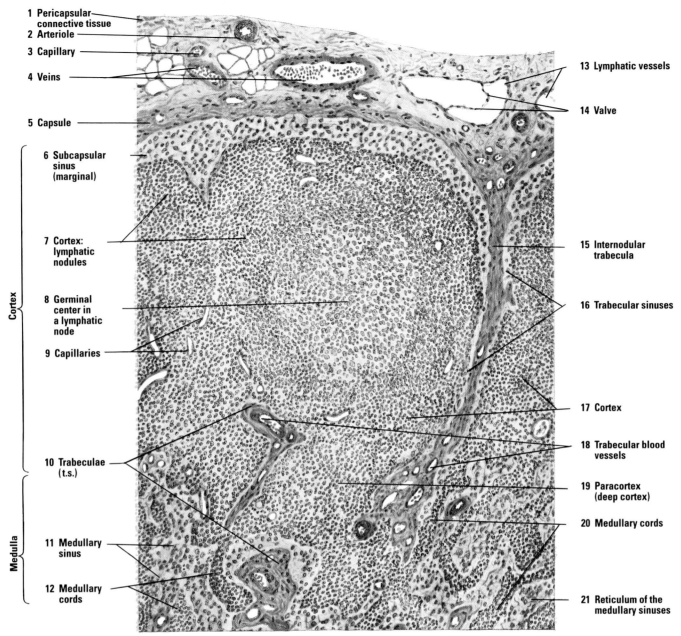

1 Pericapsular connective tissue
2 Arteriole
3 Capillary
4 Veins
5 Capsule

6 Subcapsular sinus (marginal)

7 Cortex: lymphatic nodules

8 Germinal center in a lymphatic node

9 Capillaries

10 Trabeculae (t.s.)

11 Medullary sinus

12 Medullary cords

Cortex

Medulla

13 Lymphatic vessels

14 Valve

15 Internodular trabecula

16 Trabecular sinuses

17 Cortex

18 Trabecular blood vessels

19 Paracortex (deep cortex)

20 Medullary cords

21 Reticulum of the medullary sinuses

FIG. 1. SECTIONAL VIEW. Stain: hematoxylin-eosin. 150×.

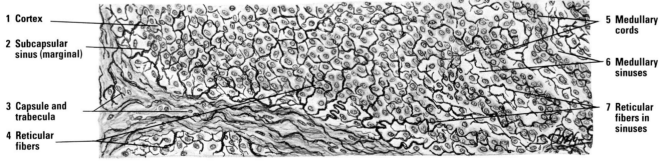

1 Cortex
2 Subcapsular sinus (marginal)
3 Capsule and trabecula
4 Reticular fibers

5 Medullary cords
6 Medullary sinuses
7 Reticular fibers in sinuses

FIG. 2. RETICULAR FIBERS OF THE STROMA. Stain: Bielschowsky-Foot silver method. 240×.

115

PLATE 43

■ **FIG. 1**
LYMPH NODE: PROLIFERATION OF LYMPHOCYTES

This figure illustrates, at a higher magnification than that in Plate 42, a portion of the lymph node **capsule (1)**, the **subcapsular (marginal) sinus (2)**, a lymphatic nodule with its **peripheral zone (5)**, and a **germinal center (6)** containing developing lymphocytes.

The reticular connective tissue of the node is seen in the subcapsular sinus (2), where **reticular cells (9)** and their processes and associated delicate fibers are distinguishable. **Small lymphocytes (11, upper leader)** and free **macrophages (3, 10)** are also visible in the subcapsular sinus. **Endothelial cells (4, limiting cells)** form an incomplete cover over the surface of the node. Occasional **reticular cells (15)** and free macrophages (3, 7, 10) may be seen in different regions of the node.

The peripheral zone (5) of the lymphatic nodule is dense because of the accumulations of **small lymphocytes (11, lower leader)**, which are characterized by dark-staining nuclei, condensed chromatin, and little or no cytoplasm.

The **germinal center (6)** contains a majority of cells that are **medium-sized lymphocytes (12)**. These are characterized by larger, lighter nuclei and more cytoplasm than seen in the small lymphocytes; the nuclei exhibit variations in size and density of chromatin. The largest lymphocytes, with less condensed chromatin, are derived from **lymphoblasts (14)**. With successive **mitosis (8)**, chromatin condenses and cell size decreases, resulting in the formation of small lymphocytes.

The lymphoblasts (14) are seen in small numbers in the germinal center (6). These are large, round cells with a broad band of cytoplasm and a large vesicular nucleus with one or more nucleoli. **Mitotic divisions of lymphoblasts (13)** produce other lymphoblasts and medium-sized lymphocytes.

Plate 45 illustrates developing lymphocytes and related cells that are either formed or found in lymphatic tissues.

■ **FIG. 2**
PALATINE TONSIL

The surface of the palatine tonsil is covered with **stratified squamous epithelium (1)**, which also lines the deep invaginations or **tonsillar crypts (3, 10)**. In the underlying connective tissue are numerous **lymphatic nodules (2)** distributed along the crypts. The lymphatic nodules are embedded in reticular connective tissue stroma and diffuse lymphatic tissue. The nodules frequently merge with each other **(8)** and usually exhibit a **germinal center (7)**.

The fibroelastic connective tissue underlies the tonsil and forms its **capsule (11)**. The **septa (trabeculae) (5, 9)** arise from the capsule (11) and pass upward as a core of connective tissue between the lymphatic nodules that form the walls of the crypts. **Skeletal muscle fibers (6, 12)** form an underlying layer of the tonsil.

LYMPH NODE AND PALATINE TONSIL

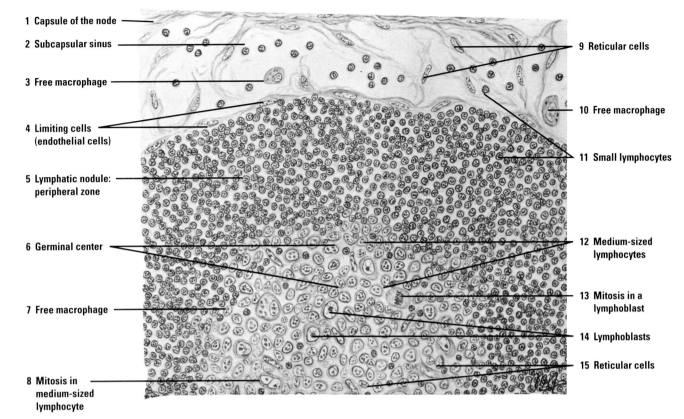

1 Capsule of the node

2 Subcapsular sinus

3 Free macrophage

4 Limiting cells (endothelial cells)

5 Lymphatic nodule: peripheral zone

6 Germinal center

7 Free macrophage

8 Mitosis in medium-sized lymphocyte

9 Reticular cells

10 Free macrophage

11 Small lymphocytes

12 Medium-sized lymphocytes

13 Mitosis in a lymphoblast

14 Lymphoblasts

15 Reticular cells

FIG. 1. LYMPH NODE: PROLIFERATION OF LYMPHOCYTES. Stain: hematoxylin-eosin. 450×.

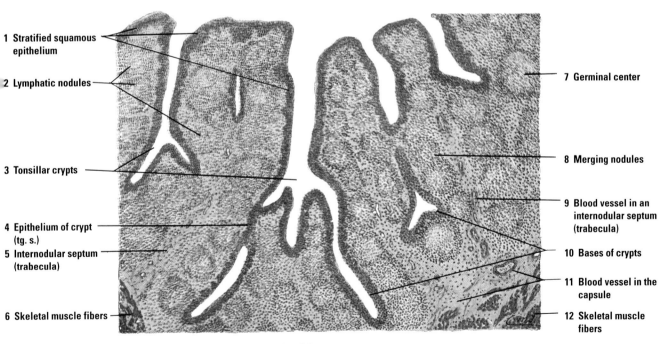

1 Stratified squamous epithelium

2 Lymphatic nodules

3 Tonsillar crypts

4 Epithelium of crypt (tg. s.)

5 Internodular septum (trabecula)

6 Skeletal muscle fibers

7 Germinal center

8 Merging nodules

9 Blood vessel in an internodular septum (trabecula)

10 Bases of crypts

11 Blood vessel in the capsule

12 Skeletal muscle fibers

FIG. 2. PALATINE TONSIL. Stain: hematoxylin-eosin. 32×.

117

PLATE 44

■ FIG. 1
THYMUS GLAND (PANORAMIC VIEW)

The thymus gland is a lobulated lymphoid organ. It is enclosed by a connective tissue **capsule (1)** from which arise numerous **trabeculae (2, 10).** The trabeculae extend into and subdivide the thymus gland into incomplete **lobules (8).** Each lobule (8) consists of a dark-staining outer **cortex (3, 13)** and a light-staining inner **medulla (4, 12).** Because the lobules are incomplete, the medulla exhibits continuity between neighboring lobules (4, 12). Numerous **blood vessels (5, 14)** pass into the thymus gland by way of the connective tissue of the capsule (1) and the trabeculae (2, 10).

The cortex (3, 13) of each lobule contains numerous densely packed lymphocytes without forming lymphatic nodules. In contrast, the medulla (4, 12) contains fewer lymphocytes but more epithelial reticular cells. The medulla also contains numerous **thymic (Hassall's) corpuscles (6, 9),** which are highly characteristic features of the thymus gland.

The histology of the thymus gland varies with the age of the individual. The gland attains its greatest development shortly after birth; however, by puberty, it begins to involute. The lymphocyte production declines and the thymic (Hassall's) corpuscles (6, 9) become larger. In addition, the parenchyma of the gland is gradually replaced by loose **connective tissue (10)** and **adipose cells (7, 11).** The thymus gland depicted in this illustration exhibits the changes associated with age involution.

■ FIG. 2
THYMUS GLAND (SECTIONAL VIEW)

A small section of the cortex and medulla of a thymus gland lobule is illustrated at a higher magnification. The thymic lymphocytes in the **cortex (1, 5)** exhibit dense aggregations. In the **medulla (3),** there are fewer lymphocytes but more **epithelial reticular cells (7).**

The **thymic (Hassall's) corpuscles (8)** are oval structures consisting of round or spherical aggregations of flattened epithelial cells. The corpuscles also exhibit calcification or **degeneration centers (9),** which stain as highly eosinophilic. The functional significance of these corpuscles is unknown.

Blood vessels (6) and **adipose cells (4)** are seen in both the lobules and the connective tissue **trabecula (2).**

THYMUS

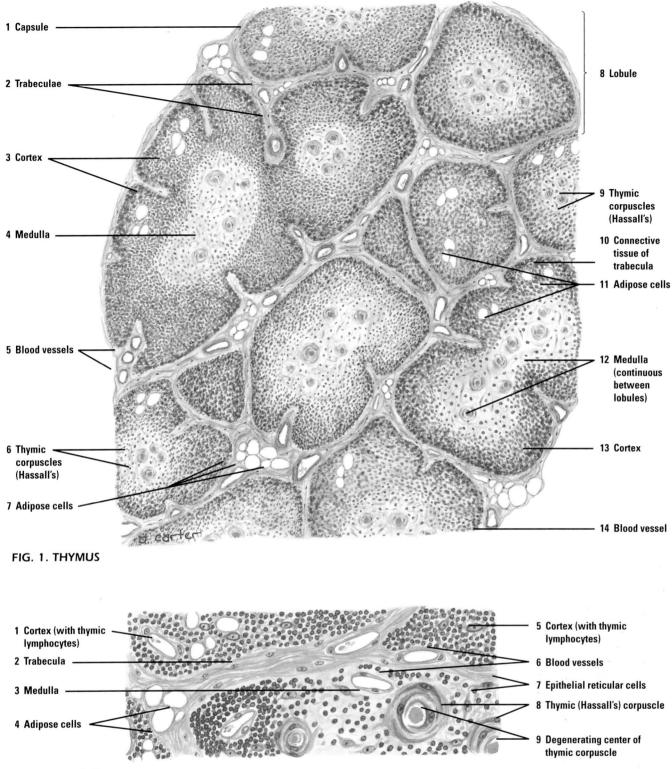

1 Capsule

2 Trabeculae

3 Cortex

4 Medulla

5 Blood vessels

6 Thymic corpuscles (Hassall's)

7 Adipose cells

8 Lobule

9 Thymic corpuscles (Hassall's)

10 Connective tissue of trabecula

11 Adipose cells

12 Medulla (continuous between lobules)

13 Cortex

14 Blood vessel

FIG. 1. THYMUS

1 Cortex (with thymic lymphocytes)

2 Trabecula

3 Medulla

4 Adipose cells

5 Cortex (with thymic lymphocytes)

6 Blood vessels

7 Epithelial reticular cells

8 Thymic (Hassall's) corpuscle

9 Degenerating center of thymic corpuscle

FIG. 2. THYMUS

119

PLATE 45

■ FIG. 1
SPLEEN (PANORAMIC VIEW)

The spleen is enclosed by a dense connective tissue **capsule (1),** from which extend connective tissue **trabeculae (3)** deep into the interior of the spleen. The main trabeculae enter the spleen at the hilus, branch throughout the organ, and carry with them trabecular **arteries (4)** and **veins (11).** **Trabeculae (12)** that are cut in transverse section have a round or nodular appearance.

The spleen is characterized by **lymphatic nodules (2, 8);** these constitute the white pulp of the organ. The lymphatic nodules contain **germinal centers (7),** which progressively decrease in number as the individual ages. Passing through each lymphatic nodule is a **central artery (6, 9),** which is usually displaced to one side, thus losing the central position. Central arteries (6, 9) are branches of trabecular arteries (4) which become ensheathed with lymphatic tissue as they leave the trabeculae. This sheath also forms the lymphatic nodules (2, 8), which then constitute the white pulp (2) of the spleen.

Surrounding the lymphatic nodules (2, 8) and intermeshed with the trabeculae is a diffuse cellular meshwork, which collectively forms the **red or splenic pulp (5, 10);** it exhibits a red color in fresh preparations. Red pulp contains **venous sinuses (10)** and **splenic cords (5)** (of Billroth); these appear as diffuse strands of lymphatic tissue between the venous sinuses. The cords form a spongy meshwork of reticular connective tissue, which is usually obscured by the density of other tissue.

The spleen does not exhibit a cortex and a medulla, as seen in lymph nodes; however, lymphatic nodules (2) are found throughout the spleen. The spleen contains venous sinuses, in contrast to lymphatic sinuses seen in lymph nodes, but the spleen does not have subcapsular or trabecular sinuses. The capsule and trabeculae in the spleen are thicker than those in the lymph nodes and contain some smooth muscle cells.

■ FIG. 2
SPLEEN: RED AND WHITE PULP

A higher magnification of the spleen illustrates a small area of red and white pulp and structural associations.

The **lymphatic (splenic) nodule (8)** represents the white pulp. Each nodule consists of a peripheral zone, the periarterial lymphatic sheath, densely packed small **lymphocytes (8),** a **germinal center (9),** which may not always be present, and an eccentric **central artery (10).** The cells found in the periarterial lymphatic sheath are mainly T lymphocytes. In the more lightly stained germinal center (9) are found the B lymphocytes, mainly medium-sized lymphocytes, some small lymphocytes, and lymphoblasts.

The red pulp contains the **splenic cords (6)** (of Billroth) and **venous sinuses (2, 7)** that course between the cords. The splenic cords (6) are thin aggregations of lymphatic tissue containing small lymphocytes, associated cells, and various blood cells. Venous sinuses (2, 7) are dilated vessels lined with modified endothelium; their elongated cells appear cuboidal in transverse sections.

Also present in the red pulp are **pulp arteries (11);** these are the branches of the central artery as it leaves the lymphatic nodule. Branches of these sheathed arteries are not illustrated; however, one vessel is seen in Figure 1:13. Capillaries and pulp veins (venules) are also present.

Trabeculae (1, 4) with **trabecular arteries (1)** and **veins (4, 5)** are also illustrated. These vessels have a tunica intima and tunica media but no apparent adventitia; connective tissue of the trabeculae surrounds the tunica media.

■ FIG. 3
SPLEEN: DEVELOPMENT OF LYMPHOCYTES AND RELATED CELLS

The illustrated cells may be found in lymph nodes, spleen, thymus, and/or other lymphatic tissues.

The large, phagocytic **macrophage (1),** 25 to 35 μm in diameter, exhibits an eccentric nucleus, cytoplasmic vacuoles (caused by dissolved lipid inclusions), fragments of ingested material, and a larger, unidentified inclusion.

The **lymphoblast (2),** 15 to 20 μm in diameter, has intensely basophilic cytoplasm, a round nucleus with dilated chromatin filaments, and two or more nucleoli. In the **medium-sized lymphocytes (3)** (prelymphocytes, 12 to 15 μm in diameter), the cytoplasm appears less basophilic and the nuclear chromatin more condensed, and the nucleoli are indistinct or absent. The **small lymphocytes (4),** 6 to 12 μm in diameter, exhibit a cytoplasm that is reduced to a small rim. The cytoplasm is slightly basophilic and may contain azurophilic granules. Nuclear chromatin is in small clusters and deeply stained.

In the **plasmablast (5),** 16 to 20 μm in diameter, the nuclear chromatin forms a heavier reticulum than in the lymphoblast. The **proplasmacyte (6),** 12 to 18 μm in diameter, exhibits a more basophilic cytoplasm than the prolymphocyte, a more eccentric nucleus, and heavier chromatin clumps. The **plasma cell (7)** (mature plasmacyte) is oval and exhibits a basophilic cytoplasm except for a pale area near the eccentric nucleus. The "cartwheel" arrangement of chromatin is a distinctive feature of plasma cells.

A **monoblast (8),** 18 to 20 μm in diameter, resembles a lymphoblast. The **monocyte (9),** 15 to 18 μm in diameter, has a distinct bean-shaped or indented nucleus with chromatin in filaments and strands. The abundant cytoplasm may exhibit fine **azurophilic granules (10).**

SPLEEN

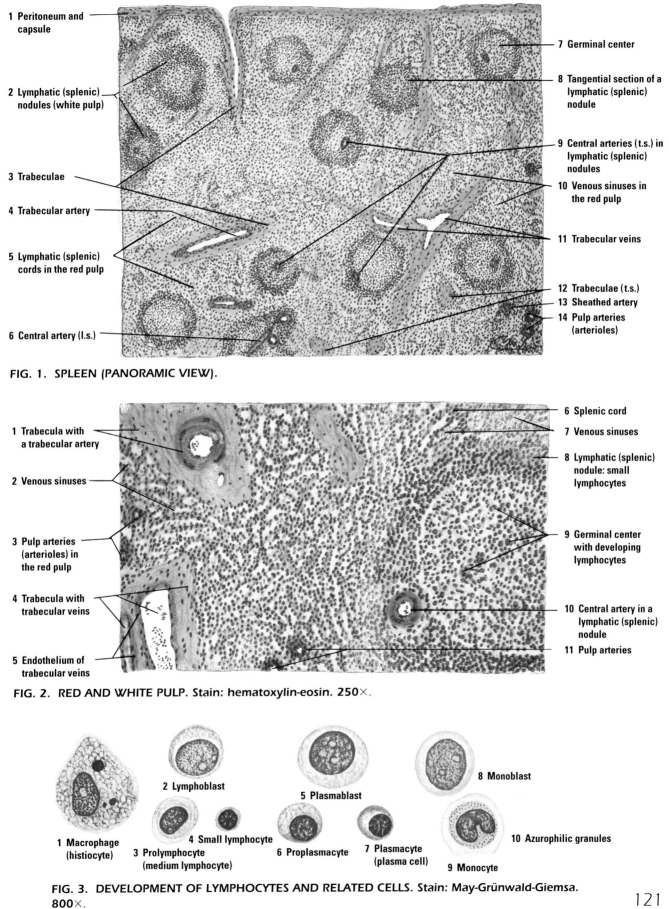

1 Peritoneum and capsule

2 Lymphatic (splenic) nodules (white pulp)

3 Trabeculae

4 Trabecular artery

5 Lymphatic (splenic) cords in the red pulp

6 Central artery (l.s.)

7 Germinal center

8 Tangential section of a lymphatic (splenic) nodule

9 Central arteries (t.s.) in lymphatic (splenic) nodules

10 Venous sinuses in the red pulp

11 Trabecular veins

12 Trabeculae (t.s.)

13 Sheathed artery

14 Pulp arteries (arterioles)

FIG. 1. SPLEEN (PANORAMIC VIEW).

1 Trabecula with a trabecular artery

2 Venous sinuses

3 Pulp arteries (arterioles) in the red pulp

4 Trabecula with trabecular veins

5 Endothelium of trabecular veins

6 Splenic cord

7 Venous sinuses

8 Lymphatic (splenic) nodule: small lymphocytes

9 Germinal center with developing lymphocytes

10 Central artery in a lymphatic (splenic) nodule

11 Pulp arteries

FIG. 2. RED AND WHITE PULP. Stain: hematoxylin-eosin. 250×.

1 Macrophage (histiocyte)

2 Lymphoblast

3 Prolymphocyte (medium lymphocyte)

4 Small lymphocyte

5 Plasmablast

6 Proplasmacyte

7 Plasmacyte (plasma cell)

8 Monoblast

9 Monocyte

10 Azurophilic granules

FIG. 3. DEVELOPMENT OF LYMPHOCYTES AND RELATED CELLS. Stain: May-Grünwald-Giemsa. 800×.

121

The skin and its derivatives or appendages form the integumentary system. In humans, the skin derivatives are the nails, hair, and several types of sweat glands and sebaceous glands. The skin is also called the integument and is composed of two distinct regions, the epidermis and dermis. The epidermis is the superficial, nonvascular layer that consists of cornified stratified squamous epithelium. The deeper, thicker, and vascular layer of the skin is the dermis, which lies under the epidermis. The dermis consists of connective tissue and contains blood vessels, nerves, and skin derivatives.

The histology of the skin is similar in different regions of the body; however, the thickness of the epidermis varies. In the regions of the palms and soles, where there is an increased amount of wear, tear, and abrasion, the epidermis is thick. This is thick skin. The rest of the body is covered by thin skin, in which the cell layers in the epidermis are thinner and simpler than in the thick skin.

The skin is the outer covering of the body and comes in direct contact with the external environment. As a result, the skin performs numerous important functions: protection, temperature regulation, sensory perception, excretion, and formation of vitamin D.

Protection The cornified, stratified layers of the skin epidermis protect the body from mechanical abrasion and form a physical barrier to pathogenic microorganisms that may otherwise enter the body. The epidermis is impermeable to water and also prevents the loss of body fluids through dehydration.

Temperature Regulation The skin participates in regulating the temperature of the body. In hot climates, heat is lost from the body by evaporation of sweat from the skin surface. In addition, there is increased dilation of blood vessels for maximum blood flow to the skin; this mechanism also increases the dissipation of heat from the body to the exterior. On the other hand, in cold climates, body heat is conserved by constriction of blood vessels and decreased blood flow to the skin.

Sensory Perception The skin is a large sense organ. It provides the main source of general sensations of the external environment of the body. Located in the skin are numerous sensory nerve endings that receive stimuli for temperature (heat and cold), touch, pain, and pressure.

Excretion Through the sweat glands, water, sodium salts, and nitrogenous wastes are excreted to the surface of the skin.

Formation of Vitamin D When the skin is exposed to the ultraviolet rays of the sun, vitamin D is formed from precursors synthesized in the epidermis.

Skin Derivatives or Appendages

The nails, glands, and hairs are derivatives of the skin. These derivatives develop directly from the surface epithelium of the epidermis and grow into and reside deep in the connective tissue of the dermis. Often the glands extend deeper into the hypodermis, which is the connective tissue situated below the dermis.

Hairs are the hard, cornified cylindrical structures that arise from the hair follicles. One portion of the hair projects through the skin to the exterior surface; the other portion is embedded in the dermis. Hair growth takes place in the expanded portion of the base of the hair follicle called the hair bulb. The base of the hair bulb is indented by a connective tissue papilla. This papilla is highly vascularized and serves an important function by bringing the essential nourishments to the hair follicle.

Associated with each hair follicle are one or more sebaceous glands that produce an oily secretion called sebum. Extending from the connective tissue around the hair follicle to the papillary layer of the dermis is a bundle of smooth muscle called the arrector pili. The sebaceous glands are located between the arrector pili muscle and the hair follicle. The arrector pili muscle is controlled by the autonomic nervous system and contracts during conditions such as fear, strong emotions, or cold. The contraction of this muscle bundle erects the hair shaft, depresses the skin where it inserts, and produces a small bump on the surface of the skin often called a "goose-bump." In addition, contraction of the arrector pili muscle forces the sebum from the sebaceous glands onto the hair follicle and the skin. The main functions of sebum are to oil and keep the skin smooth, prevent it from drying, and provide some antibacterial protection to the skin.

The sweat glands are widely distributed in the skin. They are subdivided into two types, the eccrine sweat glands and apocrine sweat glands. The eccrine type are simple, coiled tubular glands. Their secretory portion is found deep in the connective tissue of the dermis, from which a coiled excretory duct leads to the surface of the skin. The eccrine sweat glands contain two types of cells: clear cells without secretory granules and dark cells containing secretory granules. Surrounding the glandular cells are myoepithelial cells, whose contraction forces the secretion from the sweat glands. The eccrine sweat glands are most numerous in the skin of the palms and soles. The sweat consists primarily of water and some sodium salts, ammonia, uric acid, and urea. The main function of the sweat is to assist the body in temperature regulation.

The apocrine sweat glands have a limited distribution in the skin and are primarily limited to the axillary, anal, and areolar breast regions of the body. These glands are larger than the eccrine sweat glands and their ducts open into the hair follicle. The apocrine sweat glands produce a viscous secretion, which acquires a distinct odor following bacterial decomposition.

PLATE 46

■ **FIG. 1**
THIN SKIN (CAJAL'S TRICHROME STAIN)

■ **FIG. 2**
THICK SKIN, PALM, SUPERFICIAL LAYERS

PLATE 46

■ FIG. 1
THIN SKIN (CAJAL'S TRICHROME STAIN)

The skin is composed of two principal layers: epidermis and dermis. The epidermis is the most superficial and cellular layer. The dermis is located directly below the epidermis and consists of connective tissue components. This illustration depicts a section of skin from the general body surface where wear and tear are minimal. In this type of skin, the **epidermis (1)** consists of stratified squamous epithelium. This type of skin is thin and is in contrast to thick skin, which is found on the palms and soles.

The single layer of low columnar cells at the base of the epidermis is the **stratum basale or germinativum (7).** Located directly above this layer are a few rows of polygonal cells that form the **stratum spinosum (6).** Above these cells are usually found one or two layers of granular cells; these blend with the elongated, cornified cells of the **stratum corneum (5).**

The narrow zone of dense irregular connective tissue below the epidermis is the **papillary layer (2)** of the dermis. It projects into the base of the epidermis and forms the **dermal papillae (8).** The deeper **reticular layer (3)** of the dermis consists of dense, irregular connective tissue; this layer comprises the bulk of the dermis. A small portion of **hypodermis (4),** the superficial region of the underlying subcutaneous tissue, is also illustrated.

Most of the skin appendages are located in the dermis. Illustrated in the figure are parts of hair follicles and a sweat gland, which is illustrated in greater detail on Plate 47. The lower portion of the hair follicle is in longitudinal section and exhibits the **papilla** and **hair bulb (13)** at its base; these structures are located deep in the dermis. The section of the upper portion of another **hair follicle (9)** exhibits the smooth muscle, **arrector pili muscle (10),** and a **sebaceous gland (11).** An **oblique section** of the **hair follicle (14)** is illustrated deep in the subcutaneous tissue.

The dermis contains numerous examples of the cross sections of a coiled portion of the **sweat gland (12).** The sections with light-staining epithelium are from the **secretory (12a)** portion of the gland, whereas the darker-staining sections are from the **duct (12b)** portion.

Cajal's trichrome stain illustrates the variations in collagenous fiber density and distinguishes between the muscle and connective tissue. Aniline dyes stain the nuclei and cytoplasm. The nuclei are stained bright red by basic fuchsin. Indigo carmine in picric acid solution is used to stain cytoplasm orange. Collagenous fibers stain deep blue.

■ FIG. 2
THICK SKIN, PALM, SUPERFICIAL LAYERS

A section of palm skin is illustrated in which both the epidermis and dermis are much thicker than in the thin skin illustrated in Figure 1. The thicker epidermis also has a more complex structure and five distinct cell layers. The outermost layer, the **stratum corneum (1),** is a wide layer of flattened, dead cells that are constantly desquamated or shed **(10)** from the surface. Beneath the stratum corneum (1) is a narrow, lightly stained **stratum lucidum (2).** At higher magnification are occasionally seen outlines of flattened cells and eleidin droplets in this layer. Located under the stratum lucidum is the **stratum granulosum (3),** whose cells contain dark-staining **keratohyalin granules (7),** better seen at a higher magnification in the insert. Below this layer is the thick **stratum spinosum (4),** composed of several layers of polyhedral-shaped cells. The deepest cell layer is the basal layer, the **stratum basale (5),** consist-

ing of columnar cells which rest on the basement membrane.

Cells of **stratum spinosum (4, 8)** appear to be connected by spinous processes or **intercellular bridges (9** in the insert), which represent the desmosomes (macula adherens). **Mitotic activity (12)** is normally seen in the deeper layers of stratum spinosum (4) and stratum basale (5).

Ducts of sweat glands penetrate the epidermis between two dermal papillae, lose their epithelial wall, and spiral through the **epidermis (11)** to the skin surface as small channels with a thin cuticular lining.

Dermal papillae (6) are prominent in thick skin. Some of the dermal papillae contain **tactile corpuscles (13)** (Meissner's corpuscles); other papillae have capillary loops.

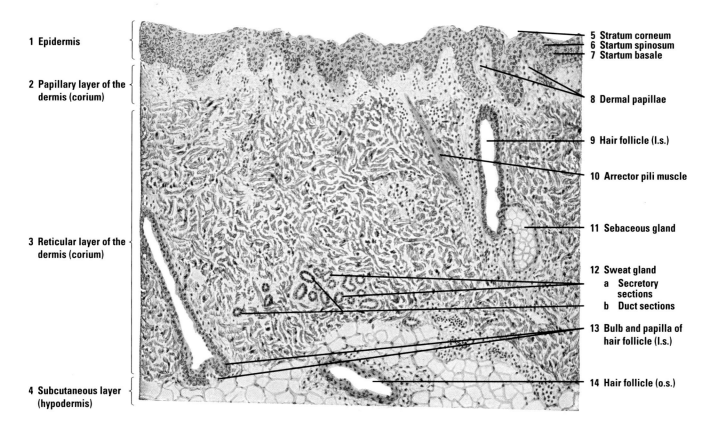

1 Epidermis

2 Papillary layer of the
dermis (corium)

3 Reticular layer of the
dermis (corium)

4 Subcutaneous layer
(hypodermis)

5 Stratum corneum
6 Startum spinosum
7 Startum basale

8 Dermal papillae

9 Hair follicle (l.s.)

10 Arrector pili muscle

11 Sebaceous gland

12 Sweat gland
a Secretory
sections
b Duct sections

13 Bulb and papilla of
hair follicle (l.s.)

14 Hair follicle (o.s.)

FIG. 1. THIN SKIN. STAIN: Cajal's trichrome. Cytoplasm: orange; nuclei: bright red; collagenous fibers: deep blue.
About 50×.

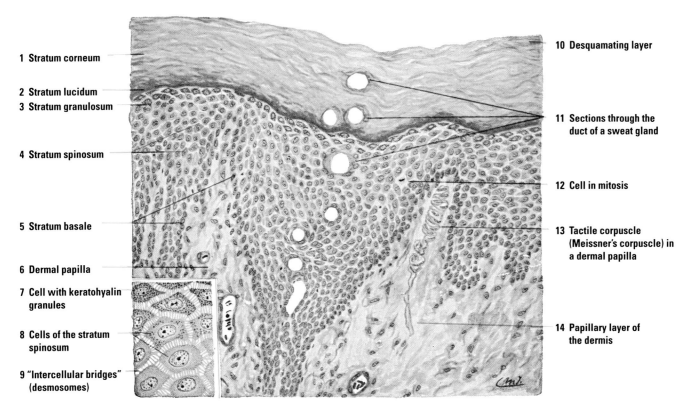

1 Stratum corneum

2 Stratum lucidum
3 Stratum granulosum

4 Stratum spinosum

5 Stratum basale

6 Dermal papilla

7 Cell with keratohyalin
granules

8 Cells of the stratum
spinosum

9 "Intercellular bridges"
(desmosomes)

10 Desquamating layer

11 Sections through the
duct of a sweat gland

12 Cell in mitosis

13 Tactile corpuscle
(Meissner's corpuscle) in
a dermal papilla

14 Papillary layer of
the dermis

FIG. 2. THICK SKIN, PALM: SUPERFICIAL LAYERS. STAIN: hematoxylin-eosin. 200×.

127

PLATE 47

SWEAT GLAND

The sweat gland is a simple, highly coiled tubular gland that extends deep into the dermis or the upper portion of the hypodermis. To illustrate this, the sweat gland is shown in both cross-sectional (left side) and diagrammatic views (right side).

The coiled portion of the sweat gland located deep in the dermis represents its **secretory (8)** region. The **secretory cells (3, 4)** in this region are large, columnar, and stain light eosinophilic. Surrounding the secretory cells are thin, spindle-shaped **myoepithelial cells (5);** these are located between the base of the secretory cells (3, 4) and the basement membrane (not illustrated).

Leaving the secretory region of the sweat gland is a thinner, darker-staining **excretory duct (2, 7).** The cells of the excretory duct are smaller than the cells of the secretory acini. Also, the duct is smaller in diameter and is lined by two layers of deep-staining cuboidal cells. There are no myoepithelial cells around the excretory duct. As the excretory duct ascends through the dermis, it straightens out and penetrates the cell layers of the **epidermis (1, 6),** where it loses its epithelial wall. In the epidermis (1, 6), the duct follows a spiral course through the cells to the surface of the skin.

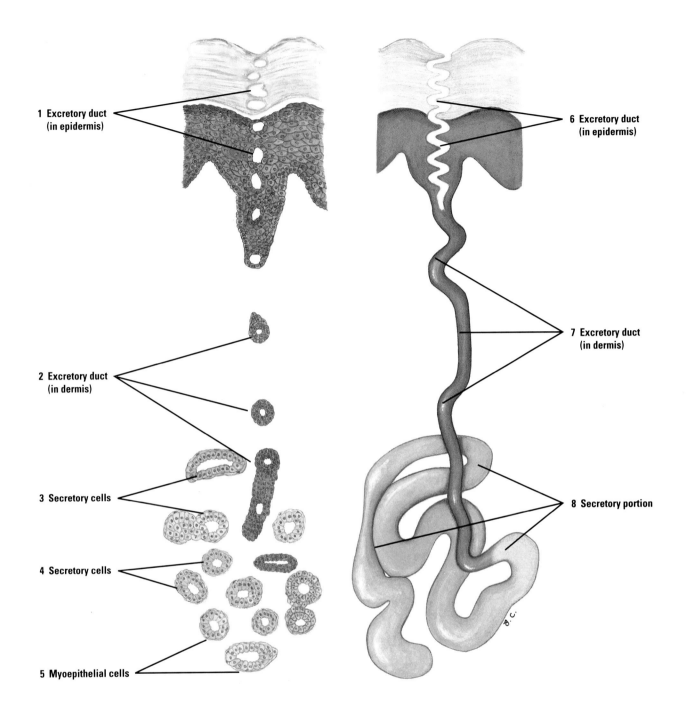

1 Excretory duct
(in epidermis)

2 Excretory duct
(in dermis)

3 Secretory cells

4 Secretory cells

5 Myoepithelial cells

6 Excretory duct
(in epidermis)

7 Excretory duct
(in dermis)

8 Secretory portion

129

PLATE 48

■ FIG. 1
SKIN: SCALP

This low magnification of a section of the skin illustrates the different cell layers in the skin: the **stratum corneum (1)** with cornified superficial cells, **stratum spinosum (2),** and stratum basale.

The **dermal papillae (3)** form typical indentations in the **epidermis (14)** of the skin. The thin papillary layer of the dermis, located immediately under the epidermis, is not visible at this magnification. The thick **reticular layer (4)** of the dermis extends from just below the epidermis to the **subcutaneous layer (23),** which contains increased amounts of adipose tissue. Beneath this layer is found the **skeletal muscle (13).**

Hair follicles in the skin of the scalp are numerous, close together, and placed at an angle to the surface of the skin. A complete **hair follicle (17, 21)** in longitudinal section is illustrated in the center of the plate. Parts of other **hair follicles, (5, 8, 18, 20)** sectioned in different planes, are also illustrated. The hair follicles consist of the following structures: cuticle, **internal root sheath (18), external root sheath (20), connective tissue sheath (19), hair bulb (10),** and a **connective tissue papilla (11).** The hair passes upward through the follicle (17, 21) to the surface of the skin.

The **sebaceous glands (6, 15)** are aggregated clusters of clear cells connected to a duct that opens into the hair follicle (see Fig. 2).

The **arrector pili muscles (7)** are smooth muscles that are aligned at an oblique angle to the hair follicle. These muscles bind to the papillary layer of the dermis and to the connective tissue sheath (19) of the hair follicle. The contraction of arrector pili muscle moves the hair shaft to a more vertical position.

The basal portions of the sweat glands lie deep in the dermis or in the subcutaneous layer (see also Plate 47). Sections of the sweat gland that exhibit lightly stained columnar epithelium represent the **secretory portions (12)** of the gland. These are distinct from sections of the **sweat gland duct (9),** which exhibit two layers of smaller, darker-stained epithelial cells (stratified cuboidal). Each sweat gland duct (9) is coiled in the deep dermis, then straightens out in the upper dermis **(16)** and follows a spiral course through the epidermis **(14).**

The **Pacinian corpuscles (22)** are located in the subcutaneous tissue. These corpuscles are important sensory receptors, such as pressure and possibly vibration. (See also Plate 49, Fig. 2.)

■ FIG. 2
SEBACEOUS GLAND AND ADJACENT HAIR FOLLICLE

This figure illustrates a sebaceous gland sectioned through the middle. The potential lumen is filled with secretory cells undergoing **cytolysis (3)** (holocrine secretion), a process whereby the cells degenerate to become the oily secretory product of the gland called sebum. The gland is lined with a stratified epithelium that has continuity with the **external root sheath (1)** of the hair follicle. Its epithelium is modified, and along the base of the gland is a single row of columnar or cuboidal cells, the **basal cells (5),** whose nuclei may be flattened. These cells rest on a basement membrane, which is surrounded by the connective tissue of the dermis. The basal cells (5) exhibit mitotic activity and fill the alveolus with larger, polyhedral cells which enlarge, accumulate secretory material, and become round **(4, 6).** The cells in the interior of the alveolus undergo cytolysis (3) and, together

with the secretory product sebum, pass through the short **duct (2)** of the gland into the lumen of the hair follicle. The sebaceous glands lie in the connective tissue of the dermis and in the angle between the hair follicles and the **arrector pili muscles (11).**

The various layers of the hair follicle at the level of the sebaceous gland may be identified. The follicle is surrounded by a **connective tissue sheath (7)** of the dermis. The **external root sheath (8)** is composed of several cell layers and is continuous with stratum spinosum of the dermis. The **internal root sheath (9)** is composed of a thin, pale epithelial stratum (Henle's layer) and a thin, granular epithelial stratum (Huxley's layer) (9). The latter is in direct contact with the cortex of the **hair (10),** which is illustrated as a pale yellow layer with cells.

■ FIG. 3
BULB OF HAIR FOLLICLE AND ADJACENT SWEAT GLAND

This figure illustrates the bulb of a hair follicle and its surrounding cell layers. A sheath of fibrous **connective tissue (7)** surrounds the bulb. The **external root sheath (1)** at this level of the bulb is a single layer of cells, which are columnar above the bulb and flat at the base of the bulb, where they cannot be distinguished from the matrix cells of the hair follicle. Above the bulb is the internal root sheath, composed of a thin, pale **epithelial stratum (Henle's layer) (2),** and a thin, **granular stratum (Huxley's layer) (3).** These two cell layers become indistinguishable as their cells merge with the cells of the bulb. Internal to these cell layers are the **cuticles (4), cortex (5),** and **medulla (6)** of the hair. In the bulb, these layers

merge into undifferentiated cells of the **hair matrix (12),** which cap the **connective tissue papilla (11)** of the hair follicle. Cell **mitosis (10)** can be seen in the matrix cells.

In the dermal connective tissue and adjacent to the hair follicle are sections through the basal portion of a coiled **sweat gland (8, 9).** The **secretory cells (9)** of the sweat gland are tall columnar and stain light. Along their bases may be seen the flattened nuclei of the contractile **myoepithelial cells (14).** The **excretory ducts (8)** of the sweat gland are smaller in diameter, are lined with a stratified cuboidal epithelium, and stain characteristically darker than the secretory cell.

INTEGUMENT

1 Stratum corneum
2 Stratum spinosum
3 Dermal papillae
4 Dermis: reticular layer
5 Hair follicles (tg. s.)
6 Sebaceous glands
7 Arrector pili muscles
8 Hair follicles (l.s.)
9 Ducts of sweat glands
10 Hair bulbs (bases of hair follicles)
11 Papillae of hair follicles
12 Secretory sections of sweat glands
13 Skeletal muscle

14 Epidermis traversed by duct of a sweat gland
15 Sebaceous gland
16 Duct of a sweat gland (l.s.)
17 Hair (cortex)
18 Internal root sheath of hair follicle
19 Connective tissue sheath of hair follicle
20 External root sheath of hair follicle
21 Medulla and matrix of hair
22 Pacinian corpuscles
23 Adipose tissue in subcutaneous layer
24 Vein
25 Arteriole

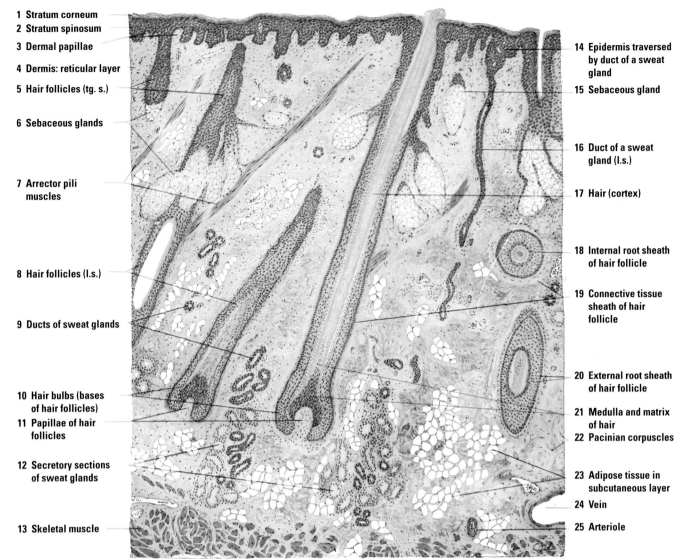

FIG. 1. SKIN (SCALP). STAIN: hematoxylin-eosin. 50×.

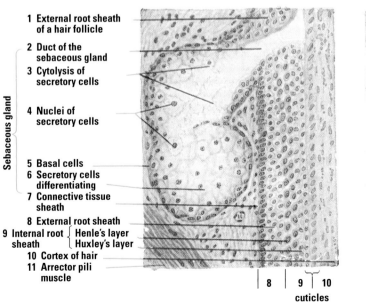

Sebaceous gland

1 External root sheath of a hair follicle
2 Duct of the sebaceous gland
3 Cytolysis of secretory cells
4 Nuclei of secretory cells
5 Basal cells
6 Secretory cells differentiating
7 Connective tissue sheath
8 External root sheath
9 Internal root sheath { Henle's layer / Huxley's layer
10 Cortex of hair
11 Arrector pili muscle

8 | 9 | 10
cuticles

FIG. 2. SEBACEOUS GLAND AND ADJACENT HAIR FOLLICLE.

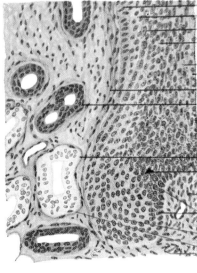

1 External root sheath
2 Henle's layer
3 Huxley's layer
4 Cuticles of hair and inner root sheath
5 Cortex of hair
6 Medulla of hair
7 Connective tissue sheath of hair follicle
8 Duct of sweat gland
9 Secretory section of sweat gland
10 Mitosis in matrix cells
11 Papilla of hair follicle
12 Matrix of hair
13 Matrix of follicle
14 Myoepithelial cell (nucleus)

FIG. 3. BULB OF HAIR FOLLICLE AND ADJACENT SWEAT GLAND.

STAIN: hematoxylin-eosin. 200×.

131

PLATE 49

■ FIG. 1
GLOMUS IN THE DERMIS OF THICK SKIN

Arteriovenous anastomoses are numerous in the thick skin of fingers and toes. Some anastomoses form direct connections; in others, the arterial portion of the anastomosis forms a specialized thick-walled structure called the **glomus (2)**. The vessel is coiled and, as a result, more than one lumen may be seen in a transverse section. The smooth muscle cells in the tunica media have hypertrophied and the specialized muscle cells with the epithelioid appearance are now called the **epithelioid cells (5)**. The tunica media wall, however, becomes thin again before the arteriole empties into a venule. The small artery (3, middle leader) may represent the terminal part of the glomus.

Small nerves and capillaries are present in the glomus and a **connective tissue sheath (6)** encloses the entire structure.

The dermis that surrounds the glomus contains **blood vessels (3), nerves (4),** and **ducts (1, 7)** of sweat glands. The PAS and hematoxylin (PASH) stains demonstrate the basement membrane of these ducts.

■ FIG. 2
PACINIAN CORPUSCLES IN THE DEEP DERMIS OF THICK SKIN

Pacinian corpuscles (1, 6) in the thick skin are located deep in the dermis and subcutaneous tissue. The corpuscles are important sensory receptors for pressure and possibly vibration. One corpuscle is illustrated in a transverse section (1) and another in an oblique section (6).

The Pacinian corpuscles are ovoid structures when seen in longitudinal or oblique sections (6) and contain an elongated central core, the **inner bulb (8).** This area usually appears empty in sections, but in life, the corpuscle contains a terminal myelinated nerve fiber. The inner bulb (8) is surrounded by **concentric lamellae (10)** of compact collagenous fibers, which become denser peripherally (inner and outer lamellae). Between the lamellae is a small amount of loose connective tissue with flat **fibroblasts (6).** A thin, dense connective tissue **sheath (9)** encloses the Pacinian corpuscle.

In a transverse section of the corpuscle (1), the layers of lamellae surrounding the inner bulb resemble a sliced onion.

In the dense irregular connective tissue of the **dermis (3), adipose cells (5), blood vessels (7), nerves (2, 11),** and a **sweat gland (4)** surround the Pacinian corpuscle.

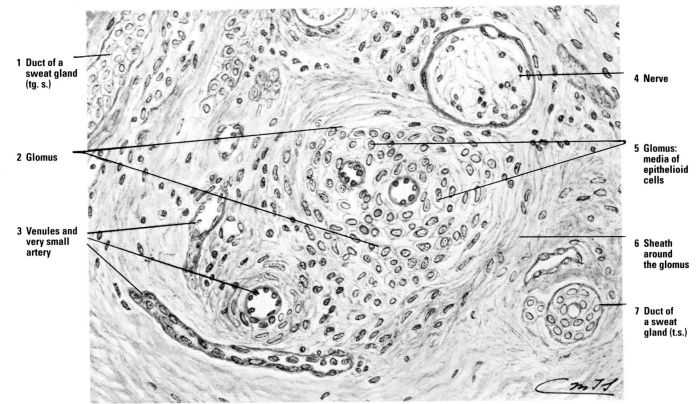

1 Duct of a sweat gland (tg. s.)

4 Nerve

2 Glomus

5 Glomus: media of epithelioid cells

3 Venules and very small artery

6 Sheath around the glomus

7 Duct of a sweat gland (t.s.)

FIG. 1. GLOMUS IN THE DERMIS OF THICK SKIN. STAIN: PASH. 350×.

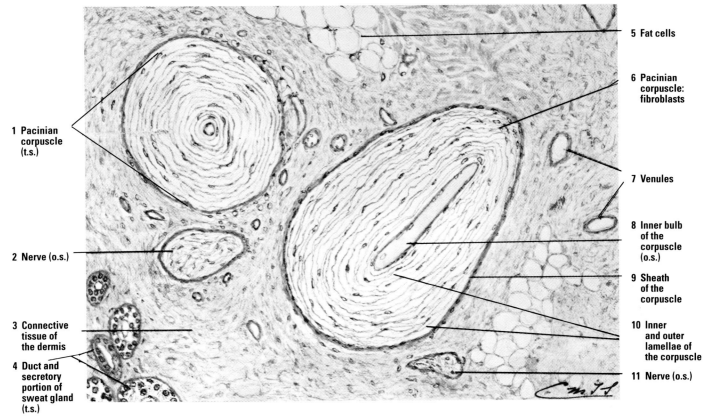

5 Fat cells

6 Pacinian corpuscle: fibroblasts

1 Pacinian corpuscle (t.s.)

7 Venules

8 Inner bulb of the corpuscle (o.s.)

2 Nerve (o.s.)

9 Sheath of the corpuscle

3 Connective tissue of the dermis

10 Inner and outer lamellae of the corpuscle

4 Duct and secretory portion of sweat gland (t.s.)

11 Nerve (o.s.)

FIG. 2. PACINIAN CORPUSCLES IN THE DEEP DERMIS OF THICK SKIN. STAIN: PASH. 350×.

THE DIGESTIVE SYSTEM: THE ACCESSORY DIGESTIVE ORGANS

The salivary glands are the accessory digestive organs that are associated with the oral cavity. These glands are located outside of the mouth and produce saliva. Saliva is delivered into the oral cavity by way of numerous excretory ducts.

The Oral Cavity and the Salivary Glands

The Tongue

The tongue consists of a core of interlacing bundles of skeletal muscle fibers covered by a mucous membrane. Its main functions during digestion are to perceive taste and to assist in chewing and swallowing food (bolus). The sensation of taste is detected by specialized cells located in numerous taste buds that are found in the stratified epithelium of the fungiform, circumvallate, and foliate papillae of the tongue; in humans, the foliate papillae are rudimentary. In addition to the tongue, where the taste buds are most numerous, the taste buds are also found in the mucous membrane of the soft palate, pharynx, and epiglottis.

Substances that stimulate the taste buds must first be dissolved in saliva, which is normally present in the oral cavity and during food intake. In addition, taste buds in the circumvallate papillae are continuously washed by watery secretions produced by the serous (von Ebner's) glands located in the connective tissue of the tongue. This secretory process allows different chemicals in the solution to enter the taste pore in the taste bud and stimulate the receptor cells.

There are four primary taste sensations to which the cells in the taste buds respond: sour, salt, bitter, and sweet. All other taste sensations are a combinations of these four. Certain regions of the tongue exhibit more sensitivity to certain taste sensations than others. The tip of the tongue is most sensitive to sweet and salt, the posterior portion to bitter, and the lateral edges to sour sensations.

The Salivary Glands

There are three major salivary glands, the parotid, submandibular, and sublingual. These glands produce a watery secretion called saliva. Saliva is a mixture of mucus, enzymes, and ionic secretions produced by the different salivary glands, although the major component of saliva is water. The sight, smell, thought, taste, or the actual presence of food in the mouth causes an autonomic increase of saliva secretion from the salivary glands and its release into the oral cavity.

Saliva performs numerous functions in the oral cavity. It moistens the food and lubricates the bolus to facilitate its swallowing and passage through the esophagus toward the stomach. Saliva also contains numerous electrolytes (calcium, potassium, sodium, chloride, bicarbonate ions, and others). The digestive enzyme amylase (ptyalin) is also found in the saliva. This enzyme is produced mainly by the serous acini of the salivary glands. The enzyme amylase initiates the breakdown of starch into smaller carbohydrates during the short time that the food is present in the oral cavity.

Saliva also controls bacterial flora in the mouth and protects the oral cavity against pathogens. The enzyme lysozyme, released also by the cells of the serous glands into the saliva, hydrolyzes the cell walls of bacteria and inhibits their growth in the oral cavity. Also, the immunoglobulins in saliva, primarily the IgA produced by the lymphocytes and plasma cells in the connective tissue, assist in immunologic defense against bacteria found in the mouth.

135

PLATE 50

LIP (LONGITUDINAL SECTION)

The core of the lip contains fibers of the striated muscle, **orbicularis oris (8).** Special stains would reveal the presence of intermixed dense fibroelastic connective tissue in the core. The right side illustrates the skin of the lip and the left side the mucosal lining of the mouth.

The skin of the lip is lined with **epidermis (9)** composed of stratified squamous, keratinized epithelium. Beneath the epidermis (9) is the **dermis (10)** with **sebaceous glands (11), hair follicles (12),** and **sweat glands (14);** all of these are epidermal derivatives. The dermis also contains the **arrector pili muscles (13, 15)** and a **neurovascular bundle (7)** on the lip periphery.

The mucosa is lined with a stratified squamous, nonkeratinized **epithelium (1).** The surface cells, without becoming cornified, slough off in the fluids of the mouth (see Plate 1, Fig. 1). Underlying the mucosal epithelium is the **lamina propria (2),** the counterpart of the dermis as related to the epidermis. In the submucosa are found tubuloacinar **labial glands (4),** which are predominantly mucous with occasional serous demilunes. Their secretion moistens the oral mucosa and their **small ducts (4, lower leader)** open into the oral cavity.

Transition of the skin epidermis to epithelium of oral mucosa illustrates a mucocutaneous junction. The "red line" or vermilion **border of the lip (6)** is illustrated. Epithelium (1) of the lip and oral mucosa is relatively smoother than that of the epidermis (9). The underlying papillae of the lip and oral mucosa are high, numerous, and abundantly supplied with capillaries. The color of the blood shows through the overlying cells, giving the lips a characteristic red color. The epithelium of the labial mucosa (1) is also thicker than the epidermis of the skin (9).

LIP (LONGITUDINAL SECTION)

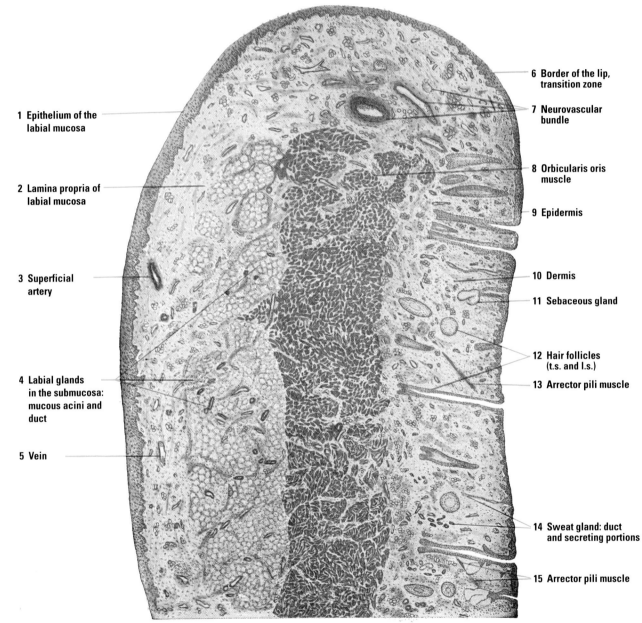

1 Epithelium of the labial mucosa

2 Lamina propria of labial mucosa

3 Superficial artery

4 Labial glands in the submucosa: mucous acini and duct

5 Vein

6 Border of the lip, transition zone

7 Neurovascular bundle

8 Orbicularis oris muscle

9 Epidermis

10 Dermis

11 Sebaceous gland

12 Hair follicles (t.s. and l.s.)

13 Arrector pili muscle

14 Sweat gland: duct and secreting portions

15 Arrector pili muscle

STAIN: hematoxylin-eosin. 20×.

PLATE 51

TONGUE: APEX (PANORAMIC VIEW, LONGITUDINAL SECTION)

The mucosa of the tongue consists of a **stratified squamous epithelium (1)** and a thin papillated **lamina propria (1),** which may contain diffuse lymphatic tissue. The dorsal surface of the tongue is characterized by mucosal projections called **papillae (4, 6, 7).** Most numerous are the slender **filiform papillae (6)** with cornified tips. Less numerous are the **fungiform papillae (4, 7),** which exhibit a broad, round surface of noncornified epithelium and a prominent core of **lamina propria (4).** All papillae are located on the dorsal surface of the tongue but are absent on the entire ventral (lower) surface **(18),** where the mucosa is smooth.

The core of the tongue consists of crisscrossing bundles of **skeletal muscle (3, 5).** As a result, the tongue muscle is typically seen in longitudinal, transverse, or oblique planes of section. In the connective tissue around the muscle bundles may be seen numerous **blood vessels (9, 10, 15, 16)** and **nerves (8, 17).**

In the lower half of the tongue near the apex and embedded in the muscle (3, 5) is illustrated a portion of the anterior lingual gland. This gland is of a mixed type and contains **serous (11), mucous (13),** and mixed acini with serous demilunes (not illustrated). The **interlobular ducts (12)** pass into the larger **excretory ducts (14),** which then open into the oral cavity on the ventral surface of the tongue.

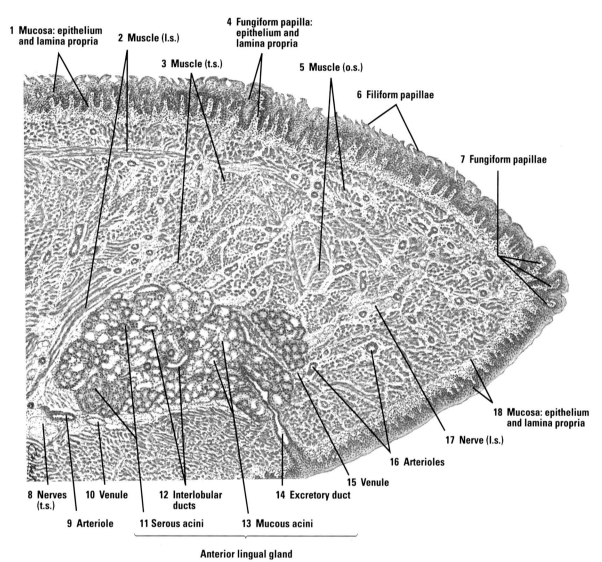

1 Mucosa: epithelium and lamina propria

2 Muscle (l.s.)

3 Muscle (t.s.)

4 Fungiform papilla: epithelium and lamina propria

5 Muscle (o.s.)

6 Filiform papillae

7 Fungiform papillae

8 Nerves (t.s.)

9 Arteriole

10 Venule

11 Serous acini

12 Interlobular ducts

13 Mucous acini

14 Excretory duct

15 Venule

16 Arterioles

17 Nerve (l.s.)

18 Mucosa: epithelium and lamina propria

Anterior lingual gland

STAIN: hematoxylin-eosin. 25×.

PLATE 52

■ **FIG. 1**
TONGUE: CIRCUMVALLATE PAPILLA (CROSS SECTION)

This illustration depicts a circumvallate papilla in cross section. The **lamina propria (2)** of the papilla exhibits numerous, **secondary papillae (3)** which project into the overlying **stratified squamous epithelium (8).** The underlying connective tissue contains an abundance of blood vessels (4). The upper part of the circumvallate papilla usually does not project above the level of the adjacent **lingual epithelium (1).** A deep trench or **furrow (9)** encircles the papilla.

Numerous oval **taste buds (5, 11)** are found in the epithelium of the lateral surfaces of the circumvallate papilla; some taste buds may also be present in the epithelium of the outer **wall of the furrow (10).**

Located in the lamina propria (2) and among the **skeletal muscle fibers (6, 14)** in the core of the tongue are the **tubuloacinar glands (of von Ebner) (12).** These glands are serous type and their **excretory ducts (7, 13)** open at the bottom of the circular furrow (9) in the circumvallate papilla.

■ **FIG. 2**
TONGUE: TASTE BUDS

Two oval **taste buds (3)** are illustrated at a high magnification. They are embedded within the stratified epithelium of the lingual **mucosa (1).** The taste buds (3) are distinguished from the surrounding epithelium by their oval shape and elongated cells (modified columnar) arranged perpendicularly to the surface of the epithelium.

The taste buds (3) contain several types of cells. Two types of cells in the taste buds are identified in the illustration. **Type I cells (6)** are elongated with darker cytoplasm and slender, dark nucleus. **Type II cells (5)** exhibit a lighter cytoplasm and a more oval, lighter nucleus. It is possible that these cells (Type II) are the neuroepithelial receptor cells for taste and Type I the supportive cells; however, it is difficult to assign a specific functional role to either type of cell with any degree of certainty. A third type of cell, the basal cell (not illustrated), is located at the periphery of the taste bud near the basement membrane. It is believed that this cell gives rise to the other two cell types.

The apical surfaces of both Type I and II cells exhibit long microvilli. These are **taste hairs (2)** and represent clusters of microvilli that protrude through the **taste pore (4)** into the furrow (Fig. 1:9) surrounding the circumvallate papilla.

TONGUE

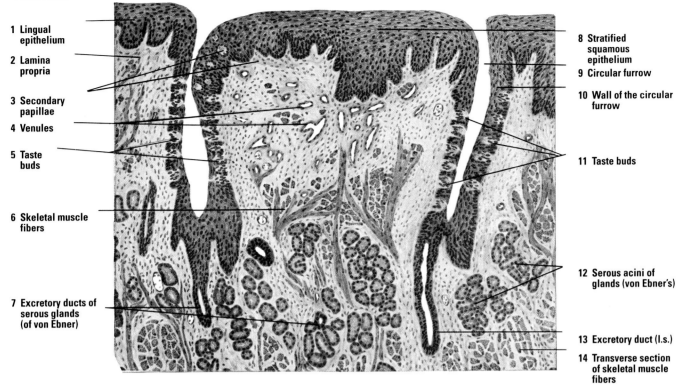

1 Lingual epithelium

2 Lamina propria

3 Secondary papillae

4 Venules

5 Taste buds

6 Skeletal muscle fibers

7 Excretory ducts of serous glands (of von Ebner)

8 Stratified squamous epithelium

9 Circular furrow

10 Wall of the circular furrow

11 Taste buds

12 Serous acini of glands (von Ebner's)

13 Excretory duct (l.s.)

14 Transverse section of skeletal muscle fibers

FIG. 1. CIRCUMVALLATE PAPILLA (CROSS SECTION). STAIN: hematoxylin-eosin. 115×.

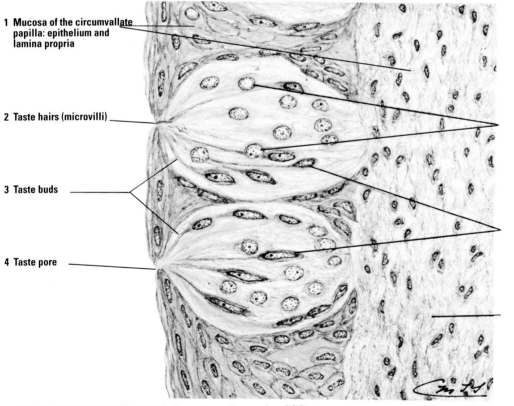

1 Mucosa of the circumvallate papilla: epithelium and lamina propria

2 Taste hairs (microvilli)

3 Taste buds

4 Taste pore

5 Type II cells: oval light nucleus, light cytoplasm

6 Type I cells: elongated darker nucleus, darker cytoplasm

7 Loose connective tissue of the lamina propria

FIG. 2. TASTE BUDS. STAIN: hematoxylin-eosin. 900×.

PLATE 53

■ FIG. 1
POSTERIOR TONGUE NEAR CIRCUMVALLATE PAPILLA (LONGITUDINAL SECTION)

The posterior region of the tongue is located behind the circumvallate papillae and near the lingual tonsils. Its dorsal surface typically exhibits large **mucosal ridges (1)** and round **elevations** or **folds (6)** that resemble large fungiform papillae. Lymphatic nodules of the lingual tonsils can be seen in such elevations; however, the typical filiform and fungiform papillae normally seen in the anterior region of the tongue are absent.

The lamina propria of the mucosa is wider but similar to that in the anterior two thirds of the tongue. Under the epithelium are seen diffuse **lymphatic tissue (2), adipose cells (3),** blood vessels, and **nerves (9).**

Numerous mucous **acini (4)** of the posterior lingual mucosal glands lie deep in the lamina propria and connective tissue between the **skeletal muscles (5, 10).** The **excretory ducts (7)** of the lingual glands open onto the dorsal surface of the tongue, usually between bases of the mucosal ridges and folds (1, 6); however, in this figure, the duct opens at the apex of a ridge. Anteriorly, these glands come in contact with the serous glands (van Ebner's) of the circumvallate papilla; posteriorly, the glands extend through the root of the tongue.

■ FIG. 2
LINGUAL TONSILS (TRANSVERSE SECTION)

This figure depicts a transverse section of the **lingual tonsils (2)** in the posterior tongue. The **lymphatic nodules (2)** are in the **lamina propria (7)** below the **stratified squamous surface epithelium (6).** The **crypts** of the **tonsils (3, 8)** form deep invaginations of the surface. The crypts are also lined with **stratified squamous epithelium (9)** and may extend deep into the lamina propria (7).

Deep in the lamina propria (7) and near the **adipose tissue (11)** are **mucous acini (5)** of the **posterior lingual glands (4).** Small **excretory ducts (4)** unite to form larger excretory ducts, most of which open into the crypts, although some open on the lingual surface (4, upper leader). Skeletal muscles, not shown, lie below the glands.

The lingual tonsils (2) are an aggregation of small, individual tonsils, each with its own crypt. They are situated in the lamina propria (7) at the root of the tongue. This arrangement may not be apparent in a small section of the tissue. The lingual tonsils are not a single encapsulated mass of lymphatic nodules as are the palatine tonsils.

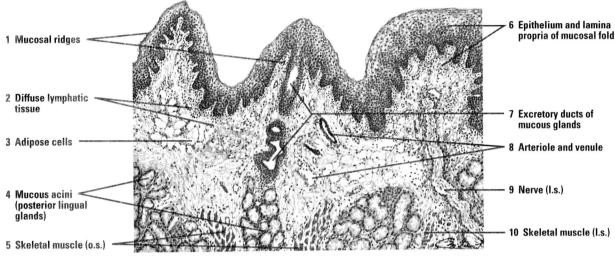

1 Mucosal ridges

2 Diffuse lymphatic tissue

3 Adipose cells

4 Mucous acini (posterior lingual glands)

5 Skeletal muscle (o.s.)

6 Epithelium and lamina propria of mucosal fold

7 Excretory ducts of mucous glands

8 Arteriole and venule

9 Nerve (l.s.)

10 Skeletal muscle (l.s.)

FIG. 1. POSTERIOR TONGUE NEAR CIRCUMVALLATE PAPILLA (LONGITUDINAL SECTION). STAIN: hematoxylin-eosin. 85×.

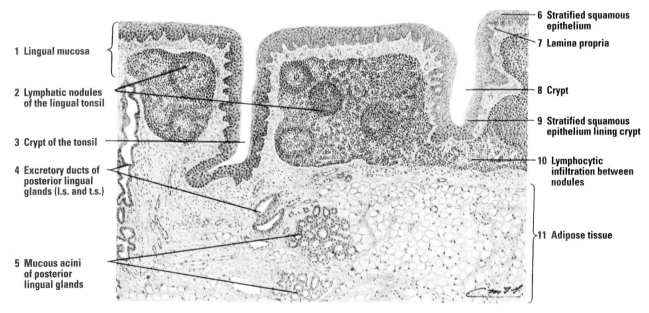
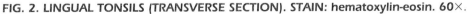

1 Lingual mucosa

2 Lymphatic nodules of the lingual tonsil

3 Crypt of the tonsil

4 Excretory ducts of posterior lingual glands (l.s. and t.s.)

5 Mucous acini of posterior lingual glands

6 Stratified squamous epithelium

7 Lamina propria

8 Crypt

9 Stratified squamous epithelium lining crypt

10 Lymphocytic infiltration between nodules

11 Adipose tissue

FIG. 2. LINGUAL TONSILS (TRANSVERSE SECTION). STAIN: hematoxylin-eosin. 60×.

143

PLATE 54

■ **FIG. 1**

DRIED TOOTH (PANORAMIC VIEW, LONGITUDINAL SECTION)

Dentin (3, 5) surrounds the **pulp cavity (4)** and its extension, the **root canal (6).** In life, the pulp cavity and root canal are filled with fine connective tissue, which contains fibroblasts, histiocytes, odontoblasts, blood vessels, and nerves. Dentin (3) exhibits wavy, parallel dentinal tubules. The earlier or primary dentin (3) is located at the periphery of the tooth; the later or secondary dentin (5) lies along the pulp cavity, where it is formed throughout life by odontoblasts. In the crown of a dried tooth and at the junction of dentin with **enamel (1)** are numerous irregular, air-filled spaces that appear black in the section. These are the **interglobular spaces (12)** which, in life, are filled with incompletely calcified dentin (interglobular dentin). Similar areas, but smaller and spaced closer together, are present in the root, close to the dentinal-cementum junction, where they form the **granular layer (of Tomes) (13).**

The dentin in the crown of the tooth is covered with a thick layer of enamel (1), composed of enamel rods or prisms held together by interprismatic cementing substance. The incremental **growth lines (of Retzius) (8)** represent the variations in the rate of enamel deposition. Light rays passing through a dried section of the tooth are refracted by twists that occur in the enamel rods as they course toward the surface of the tooth. These are the light **bands of Schreger (9).** At the dentinoenamel junction may be seen **enamel spindles (10)** and **enamel tufts (11);** these are illustrated at a higher magnification in Figure 2.

Cementum (7) covers the dentin of the root. In life, cementum contains **lacunae (14)** with cementocytes and canaliculi.

■ **FIG. 2**

DRIED TOOTH: LAYERS OF THE CROWN

A section of **enamel (1)** and **dentin (6)** are illustrated at a high magnification. The enamel consists of elongated **enamel rods** or **prisms (1).** In the enamel region, near the junction with dentin **(4),** are the **enamel spindles (2).** These are pointed or spindle-shaped processes of dentin

that penetrate the enamel. The **enamel tufts (3),** which are the poorly calcified, twisted enamel rods, extend from the **dentinoenamel junction (4)** into the enamel. Dentin (6) is clearly visible with its dentinal tubules (6) and black, air-filled **interglobular spaces (5).**

■ **FIG. 3**

DRIED TOOTH: LAYERS OF THE ROOT

Dentin (1) and **cementum (4)** are illustrated at a high magnification. Near the dentinoenamel junction is the **granular layer (of Tomes) (2).** Internal to this layer are the large, irregular **interglobular spaces (3)** which are

commonly seen in the crown of the tooth but may also be present in the root. **Cementum (4)** contains **lacunae (5)** with their canaliculi.

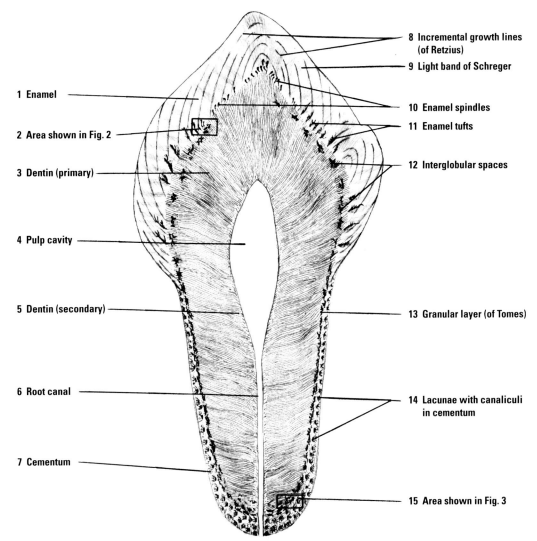

1 Enamel

2 Area shown in Fig. 2

3 Dentin (primary)

4 Pulp cavity

5 Dentin (secondary)

6 Root canal

7 Cementum

8 Incremental growth lines (of Retzius)

9 Light band of Schreger

10 Enamel spindles

11 Enamel tufts

12 Interglobular spaces

13 Granular layer (of Tomes)

14 Lacunae with canaliculi in cementum

15 Area shown in Fig. 3

FIG. 1. PANORAMIC VIEW, LONGITUDINAL SECTION.

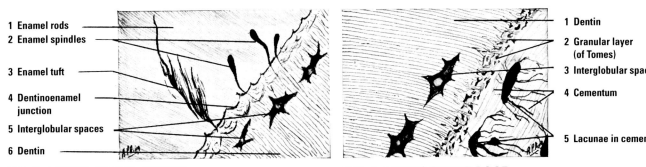

1 Enamel rods
2 Enamel spindles

3 Enamel tuft

4 Dentinoenamel junction

5 Interglobular spaces

6 Dentin

1 Dentin

2 Granular layer (of Tomes)

3 Interglobular space

4 Cementum

5 Lacunae in cementum

FIG. 2. LAYERS OF THE CROWN.
Area Corresponding to (2) in Fig. 1. 160×.

FIG. 3. LAYERS OF THE ROOT.
Area Corresponding to (15) In Fig. 1. 160×.

145

PLATE 55

■ **FIG. 1**
DEVELOPING TOOTH (PANORAMIC VIEW)

A developing deciduous tooth is shown embedded in a socket, the **dental alveolus (22)**, in the **bone** (4) of the jaw. A layer of **connective tissue (3)** surrounds the developing tooth and forms a compact layer around the tooth, the **dental sac (5)**. Enclosed within the sac is the enamel organ. It is composed of the **external enamel epithelium (18)**, the **stellate reticulum of enamel pulp (6, 19)**, the **intermediate stratum (20)**, and the **ameloblasts** or **inner enamel epithelium (7)**. All of these structures differentiate from the downgrowth of the gum epithelium. The ameloblasts secrete enamel around the **dentin (9, 16)**. The **enamel (8, 15)** appears as a narrow band of deep-staining pink material.

The **dental pulp (21)** originates from the primitive connective tissue and forms the core of the developing tooth. Blood vessels and nerves extend into and innervate the dental pulp from below. The mesenchymal cells in the dental papilla differentiate into **odontoblasts (11)** and form the outer margin of the dental pulp (21). The odontoblasts (11) secrete **predentin (10, 17)**, which is an uncalcified dentin. As predentin calcifies (10, 17), it forms a layer of dentin (9, 16) adjacent to enamel.

The **oral mucosa (1, 13)** covers the developing tooth. An epithelial downgrowth from the oral epithelium indicates the **germ of a permanent tooth (2)**. At the base of the tooth, the outer and inner enamel epithelium form the **epithelial root sheath (of Hertwig) (12)**.

■ **FIG. 2**
DEVELOPING TOOTH (SECTIONAL VIEW)

The left side of the figure shows a small area of dental pulp, **fibroblasts (1)**, and fine fibers, illustrated at a higher magnification. The **odontoblasts (2)** are located at the margin of the pulp and secrete the **uncalcified predentin (3)**, which later calcifies as **dentin (4)**. The odontoblasts (2) remain in the predentin and dentin as the **odontoblast processes (of Tomes) (3)**.

On the right side of the figure is a small area of **stellate reticulum (7)** of enamel. Seen here are the process- es of its modified epithelial cells, the **intermediate stratum (8)**, a transition region, and the tall columnar **ameloblasts (6)** that secrete the **enamel (5, 10)** in the form of enamel rods or prisms. During enamel formation, the apical ends of ameloblast become transformed into a terminal processes of Tomes. In advanced enamel formation, these processes appear as a separate layer of **enamel processes (of Tomes) (9)**.

DEVELOPING TOOTH

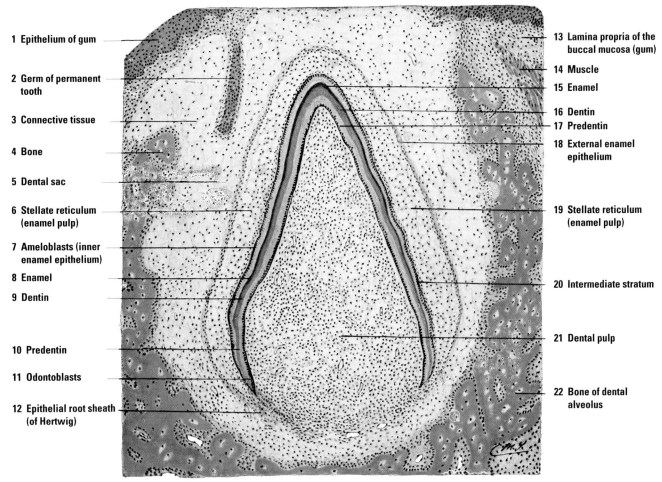

1 Epithelium of gum

2 Germ of permanent tooth

3 Connective tissue

4 Bone

5 Dental sac

6 Stellate reticulum (enamel pulp)

7 Ameloblasts (inner enamel epithelium)

8 Enamel

9 Dentin

10 Predentin

11 Odontoblasts

12 Epithelial root sheath (of Hertwig)

13 Lamina propria of the buccal mucosa (gum)

14 Muscle

15 Enamel

16 Dentin

17 Predentin

18 External enamel epithelium

19 Stellate reticulum (enamel pulp)

20 Intermediate stratum

21 Dental pulp

22 Bone of dental alveolus

FIG. 1. PANORAMIC VIEW. STAIN: hematoxylin-eosin. 50×.

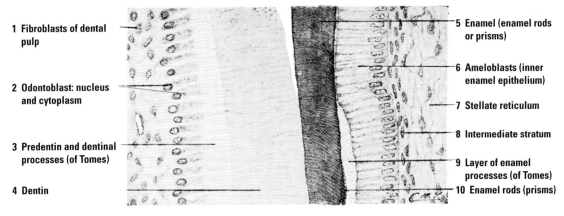

1 Fibroblasts of dental pulp

2 Odontoblast: nucleus and cytoplasm

3 Predentin and dentinal processes (of Tomes)

4 Dentin

5 Enamel (enamel rods or prisms)

6 Ameloblasts (inner enamel epithelium)

7 Stellate reticulum

8 Intermediate stratum

9 Layer of enamel processes (of Tomes)

10 Enamel rods (prisms)

FIG. 2. SECTIONAL VIEW. STAIN: hematoxylin-eosin. 300×.

147

PLATE 56

SALIVARY GLAND: PAROTID

The parotid salivary gland is a large serous gland, classified as a compound tubuloacinar gland (see Plate 6). In this illustration, a section of the parotid gland is depicted at lower magnification, while the specific features of the gland are presented at a higher magnification in separate boxes below.

The parotid gland is surrounded by a connective tissue capsule from which arise numerous **septa (2, 8)** that subdivide the gland into several lobes and lobules. Located in the connective tissue septa (2, 8) between the lobules are small **arterioles (12), venules (13), interlobular excretory ducts (1, 4, 9, IV)** and numerous **adipose cells (3).**

Each lobule consists of closely packed masses of secretory cells, the **serous acini (5, 10, 16, I).** These acini (I) consist of pyramid-shaped cells arranged around a small lumen. The spherical nuclei of these cells are located at the base of the slightly basophilic cytoplasm. In certain sections, the lumen is not always visible in all acini. At a higher magnification, small **secretory granules (15, I)** are visible in the cell apices. The number of secretory granules in these cells varies with the functional activity of the gland. The serous acini (5, 10, 16, I) are also surrounded by thin, contractile **myoepithelial cells (14, I),** located between the basement membrane and the serous cells; usually, only their nuclei are visible.

The secretory acini empty their product into narrow channels, the **intercalated ducts (6, 11, II).** These ducts have small lumina, are lined by a simple squamous or low cuboidal epithelium, and are often surrounded by myoepithelial cells (See Plate 57:23, III). The secretory product from the intercalated ducts drains into larger **striated ducts (7, III).** These ducts have larger lumina and are lined by simple columnar cells that exhibit **basal striations (17, III);** the striations are formed by deep infolding of the basal cell membrane.

The striated ducts empty their product into the **interlobular excretory ducts (1, 4, 9, IV)** that are located in the connective tissue septa (2, 8). Their lumina become progressively wider and the epithelium taller as the ducts increase in size. The ductal epithelium (IV) varies from columnar to pseudostratified or stratified columnar in large excretory (lobar) ducts that drain the lobes of the parotid gland.

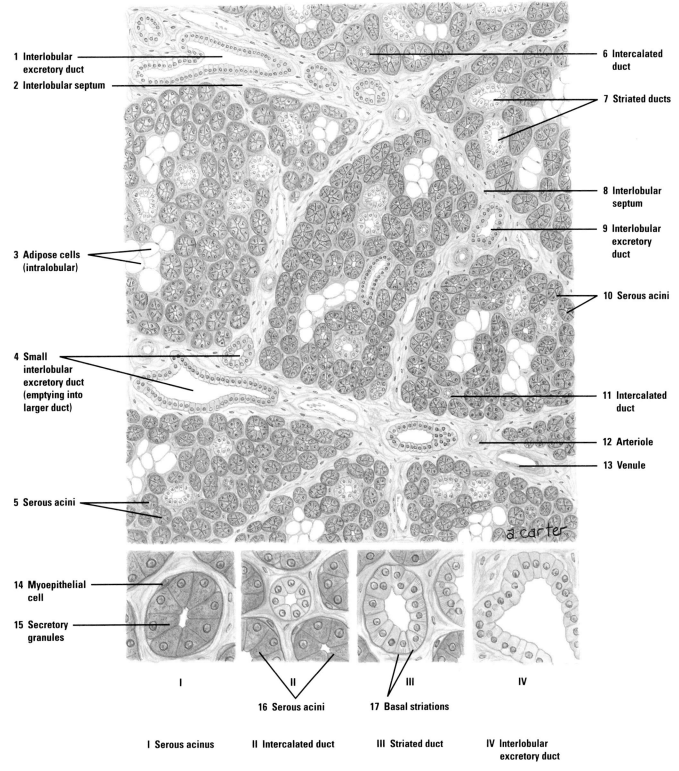

1 Interlobular excretory duct

2 Interlobular septum

3 Adipose cells (intralobular)

4 Small interlobular excretory duct (emptying into larger duct)

5 Serous acini

6 Intercalated duct

7 Striated ducts

8 Interlobular septum

9 Interlobular excretory duct

10 Serous acini

11 Intercalated duct

12 Arteriole

13 Venule

14 Myoepithelial cell

15 Secretory granules

16 Serous acini

17 Basal striations

I Serous acinus

II Intercalated duct

III Striated duct

IV Interlobular excretory duct

a. carter

FIG. 1. SALIVARY GLAND. Parotid. Stain: Hematoxylin-eosin.

149

PLATE 57

SALIVARY GLAND: SUBMANDIBULAR

Like the parotid salivary gland, the submandibular is also a compound tubuloacinar gland. The submandibular gland, however, is a mixed type, being composed predominantly of serous acini. The presence of serous and mucous acini distinguishes the submandibular gland from the parotid gland, which is a purely serous gland. This low-power illustration depicts portions of several lobules of the submandibular gland in which a few **mucous acini (6, 11, 14)** are intermixed with **serous acini (7, 18)**. The more detailed features of the gland are illustrated at higher magnification in separate boxes below.

The **serous acini (7, 18, I)** are similar to those observed in the parotid gland (Plate 56). These acini are characterized by smaller size, darker-stained pyramidal cells, spherical nucleus located basally, and **secretory granules (20)** in the cell apices, visible at higher magnification (I). The **mucous acini (6, 11, 14, II)** are larger than the serous acini (7, 18, I) and are more variable in their size and shape. The mucous cells are more columnar and exhibit pale or almost colorless cytoplasm after routine histologic staining. Their **nuclei (II)** are flattened and pressed against the base of the cell membrane. The mucous acini also have a somewhat larger and more apparent lumina.

The mixed acini (serous and mucous) are normally mucous acini surrounded or capped by one or more groups of serous cells, forming a crescent-shaped **serous demilune (8, 12)**. The thin, contractile **myoepithelial cells (21, 22, 23)** surround the serous (I), mucous (II), and intercalated duct cells (III).

The duct system of the submandibular gland is similar to that of the parotid gland. The intralobular **intercalated ducts (9, 13, 15, 19, III)** have small lumina and are shorter while the **striated ducts (5, 16, IV)** are longer than in the parotid gland. Illustrated is a **mucous acinus (14)** that opens into an **intercalated duct (15)**, which then opens into a larger **striated duct (16)**. Numerous **interlobular excretory ducts (3, 17)** of different sizes are located in the interlobular connective tissue **septa (4)**. These septa (4) penetrate and divide the gland into lobes and lobules. Also located in the connective tissue septa (4) are nerves and numerous, different-sized **arterioles (1)** and **venules (2)**. Numerous **adipose cells (10)** are seen scattered among the various acini and in the connective tissue septa.

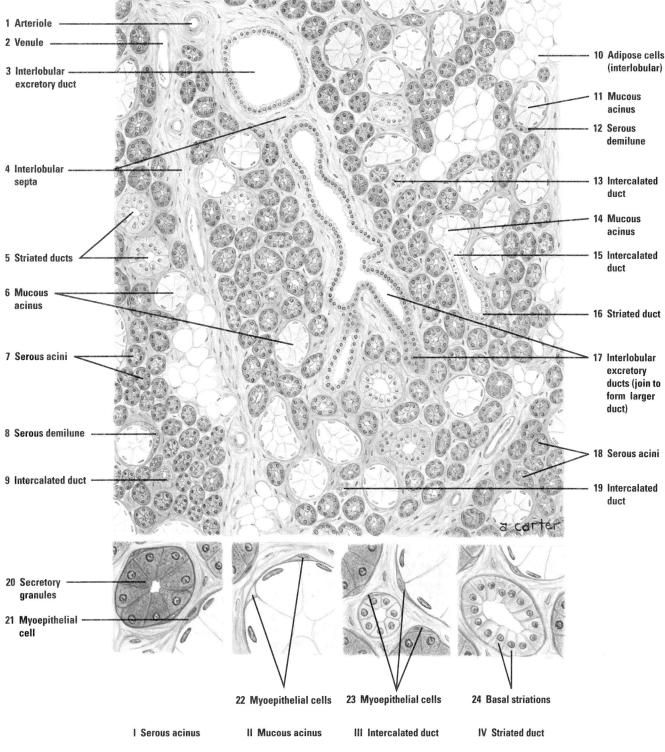

1 Arteriole

2 Venule

3 Interlobular excretory duct

4 Interlobular septa

5 Striated ducts

6 Mucous acinus

7 Serous acini

8 Serous demilune

9 Intercalated duct

10 Adipose cells (interlobular)

11 Mucous acinus

12 Serous demilune

13 Intercalated duct

14 Mucous acinus

15 Intercalated duct

16 Striated duct

17 Interlobular excretory ducts (join to form larger duct)

18 Serous acini

19 Intercalated duct

20 Secretory granules

21 Myoepithelial cell

22 Myoepithelial cells

23 Myoepithelial cells

24 Basal striations

I Serous acinus

II Mucous acinus

III Intercalated duct

IV Striated duct

a carter

FIG. 1. SALIVARY GLAND. Submandibular. Stain: Hematoxylin-eosin.

151

PLATE 58

SALIVARY GLAND: SUBLINGUAL

The sublingual gland is a compound mixed tubuloacinar gland. This gland resembles the submandibular gland because it is composed of both serous and mucous acini. Most of the secretory acini, however, are **mucous (5, 15, I, II)** and mucous acini capped with **serous demilunes (9, 14, 18, 19, II, III).** The light-stained mucous acini (5, 15, I, II) are conspicuous in this section. Purely serous acini are scarce; however, the composition of the gland is variable. In this low-magnification illustration, **serous acini (3, 16)** appear frequently, whereas in other sections of the sublingual gland such serous acini may be absent. At higher magnification, the **myoepithelial cells (17, I)** are seen around individual acini.

In comparison to other salivary glands, the duct system is somewhat different. Typical **intercalated ducts (2, 10, III)** are infrequent or are absent. In the sublingual gland, the intercalated ducts (2, 10, III) are short and are not readily observed in a given section. The nonstriated **intralobular excretory ducts (4, 6, IV)** are more prevalent in the sublingual glands. These ducts are equivalent to the striated ducts of the submandibular and parotid glands, but lack the extensive basal striations.

The interlobular connective tissue **septa (13)** are more abundant in the sublingual than in the parotid and submandibular glands. Numerous **arterioles (12), venules (8),** nerve fibers, and **interlobular excretory ducts (1, 11)** are seen in the septa. The epithelial lining of the interlobular excretory ducts (1, 11) varies from low columnar in the smaller ducts to pseudostratified or stratified columnar in the larger ducts.

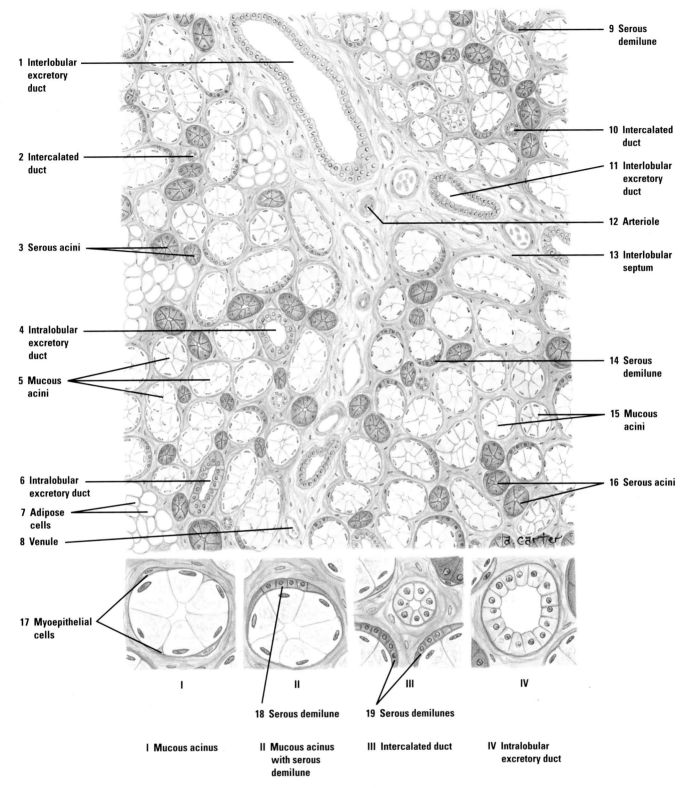

1 Interlobular excretory duct

2 Intercalated duct

3 Serous acini

4 Intralobular excretory duct

5 Mucous acini

6 Intralobular excretory duct

7 Adipose cells

8 Venule

9 Serous demilune

10 Intercalated duct

11 Interlobular excretory duct

12 Arteriole

13 Interlobular septum

14 Serous demilune

15 Mucous acini

16 Serous acini

17 Myoepithelial cells

18 Serous demilune

19 Serous demilunes

I Mucous acinus

II Mucous acinus with serous demilune

III Intercalated duct

IV Intralobular excretory duct

I   II   III   IV

a. carter

FIG. 1. SALIVARY GLAND. Sublingual. STAIN: hematoxylin-eosin.

153

THE DIGESTIVE SYSTEM: THE STOMACH

The stomach is a dilated, hollow organ of the digestive tract situated between the esophagus and the small intestine. Anatomically, the stomach is divided into the cardia, fundus, body or corpus, and pylorus. Histologically, the stomach has only three distinct regions because the fundus and body have identical histology. The cardia is the most superior region in the stomach and surrounds the entrance of the esophagus into the stomach. The fundus and body form the major portions of the stomach; their mucosa contains deep gastric glands that produce most of the gastric secretions. The pylorus is the most inferior region in the stomach and ends at the duodenum of the small intestine.

The luminal surface of the stomach is lined by a single layer of mucus-secreting, columnar epithelium, whose secretion forms a thick layer of mucus that protects the stomach surface from the corrosive action of the gastric juices. The surface epithelium of the stomach invaginates the lamina propria of the mucosa and forms numerous gastric pits, into which open the tubular gastric glands.

The main functions of the stomach are to receive, store, mix, and digest the food products. Some of these stomach functions are performed by mechanical and chemical actions, which reduce the ingested food material to a semiliquid mass called chyme. The mechanical reduction of food products in the stomach is produced by strong, muscular contractions of its thick wall in the form of peristalsis. This activity churns and mixes the food with gastric juices produced by the gastric glands when the food enters and distends the stomach wall. Nerve cells and nerve fibers located in the submucosal and myenteric nerve plexuses in the stomach wall regulate the peristaltic activity of the stomach musculature. The stomach also has some absorptive functions; however, these are limited to the absorption of water, alcohol, salts, and certain drugs.

The chemical reduction of food in the stomach is the result of the watery gastric secretions produced by different cells in the gastric glands, especially those in the fundus and body regions of the stomach. The main components of the gastric secretions are pepsin, hydrochloric acid, mucus, intrinsic factor, water, and different electrolytes.

Gastric Glands and the Cell Types

The gastric glands of the cardia and pylorus regions are located at the opposite ends of the stomach; however, their cell types are similar and predominantly mucus-secreting. The gastric glands found in the fundus and body of the stomach, however, are composed of three major types of cells. Located in the upper region of the gastric gland near the gastric pits are the mucous neck cells. The product of these cells, along with that of the cells in the surface epithelium, is mucus, which covers the stomach lining with its protective layer.

The large, polygonal, distinctive eosinophilic cells located in the upper half of the gastric glands between other gland cells are the parietal cells. These cells secrete hydrochloric acid, a major component of the gastric juice. It is also believed that, in humans, parietal cells produce gastric intrinsic factor, a glycoprotein that is necessary for vitamin B_{12} absorption in the small intestine. Vitamin B_{12} is necessary for red blood cell production in the red bone marrow and its deficiency reduces this important function.

The basophilic, cuboidal cells that are distributed predominantly in the lower region of the gastric glands are the chief or zymogenic cells. The cytoplasm of these cells exhibits numerous secretory granules that contain the enzyme pepsinogen, an inactive form of pepsin. Release of pepsinogen during gastric secretion into the acidic environment of the stomach converts pepsinogen into the highly active, proteolytic enzyme pepsin.

Enteroendocrine or APUD cells

In addition to the cells in the gastric glands just described, the mucosa of the digestive tract contains a wide distribution of enteroendocrine or APUD cells. These cells are poorly seen in histologic sections unless they are prepared with special silver staining techniques. The enteroendocrine (APUD) cells secrete polypeptides and proteins with hormonal activity that influence different functions of the digestive tract. Additional details, a description, and an illustration of the enteroendocrine (APUD) cells are found in Plate 69, Figure 2.

PLATE 59

UPPER ESOPHAGUS: WALL (TRANSVERSE SECTION)

The esophagus is a long, hollow tube whose wall is composed of the mucosa, submucosa, muscularis externa, and adventitia.

The **mucosa** (1,2,3) consists of an inner lining of nonkeratinized **stratified squamous epithelium (1);** an underlying thin layer of fine connective tissue, the **lamina propria (2);** and a layer of longitudinal smooth muscle fibers, the **muscularis mucosae (3),** illustrated in either cross or oblique sections. The connective tissue papillae in the lamina propria indent the epithelium. The lamina propria (2) contains small blood vessels, diffuse lymphatic tissue, and a small **lymphatic nodule (9).**

The **submucosa (4)** is a wide layer of moderately dense irregular connective tissue which often contains **adipose cells (14). The esophageal glands proper (11)** are present in the submucosa at intervals throughout the length of the esophagus. These are the tubuloacinar mucous glands, and their **ducts (12)** pass through the **muscularis mucosae (3, 10)** and the lamina propria (2), and open into the esophageal lumen. The ductal epithelium merges with stratified squamous surface epithelium of the esophagus (see Plate 60). Large **blood vessels (13)** are present in the connective tissue of the submucosa (4).

Located beneath the submucosa (4) is the **muscularis externa (5,6,7),** composed of two well-defined muscle layers. The inner muscle layer is **circular (5)** and, in this transverse section of the esophagus, sectioned longitudinally. The outer muscle layer is **longitudinal (7),** and the muscle fibers are seen mainly in transverse sections. A thin layer of **connective tissue (6)** lies between the two muscle layers.

The muscularis externa of the esophagus is highly variable in different species. In humans, the muscularis externa in the upper third of the esophagus consists primarily of striated skeletal muscles. In the middle third, both layers exhibit a mixture of smooth muscle, and in the lower third of the esophagus, only smooth muscle is found.

The **adventitia (8)** of the esophagus consists of a loose connective tissue layer that blends with the adventitia of the trachea and the surrounding structures. **Adipose tissue (16),** large **blood vessels (17, 18),** and **nerves (19)** forming the neurovascular bundles are present in the adventitia.

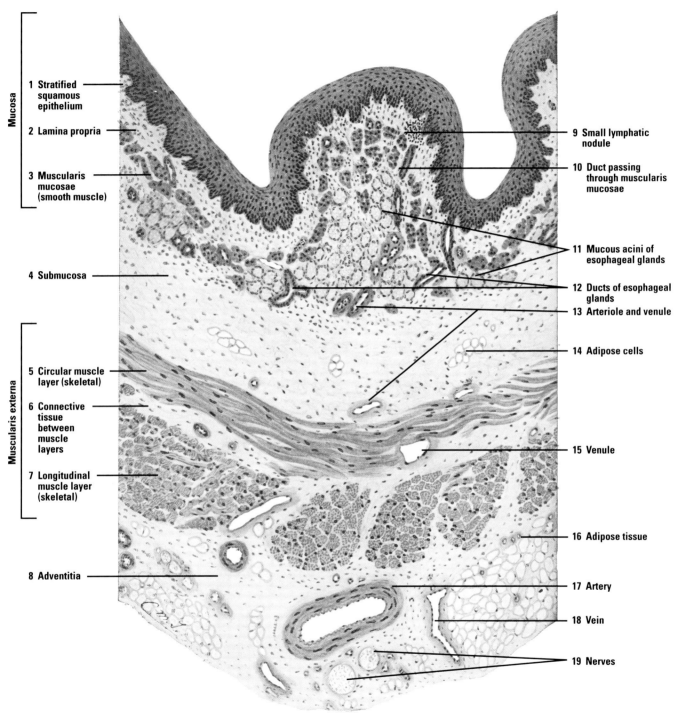

Mucosa

1 Stratified squamous epithelium

2 Lamina propria

3 Muscularis mucosae (smooth muscle)

4 Submucosa

Muscularis externa

5 Circular muscle layer (skeletal)

6 Connective tissue between muscle layers

7 Longitudinal muscle layer (skeletal)

8 Adventitia

9 Small lymphatic nodule

10 Duct passing through muscularis mucosae

11 Mucous acini of esophageal glands

12 Ducts of esophageal glands

13 Arteriole and venule

14 Adipose cells

15 Venule

16 Adipose tissue

17 Artery

18 Vein

19 Nerves

STAIN: hematoxylin-eosin. 50×.

PLATE 60

UPPER ESOPHAGUS: MUCOSA AND SUBMUCOSA (TRANSVERSE SECTION)

Higher magnification of the upper esophageal wall illustrates the **mucosa (1,2,3)** with the **stratified squamous epithelium (1)** and the **submucosa (4).** In the luminal epithelium, the **squamous cells (6)** form the outer layers, the numerous **polyhedral cells (7)** form the intermediate layers, and **low columnar cells (9)** form the basal layer. **Mitotic activity (8)** is seen in the deeper layers of the epithelium.

The **lamina propria (2,10)** contains **blood vessels (11)** and aggregates of **lymphocytes (12).** The smooth muscle of **muscularis mucosae (13)** is illustrated as bundles of muscle fibers sectioned in a transverse plane.

The submucosa (4) contains **mucous acini (15)** of the esophageal glands proper. Small **excretory ducts (16, lower leaders)** from these glands, lined with simple epithelium, join the larger excretory ducts (16, upper leader) that are lined with stratified epithelium. A large **duct,** sectioned tangentially **(14),** reveals that its epithelium is continuous with the stratified squamous epithelium of the esophageal lumen.

In the submucosa (4) are also seen **blood vessels (17,18), nerves (19),** and **adipose cells (20).** A section of skeletal muscle fibers from the inner circular layer of the **muscularis externa (5)** is illustrated in the lower left corner of the figure.

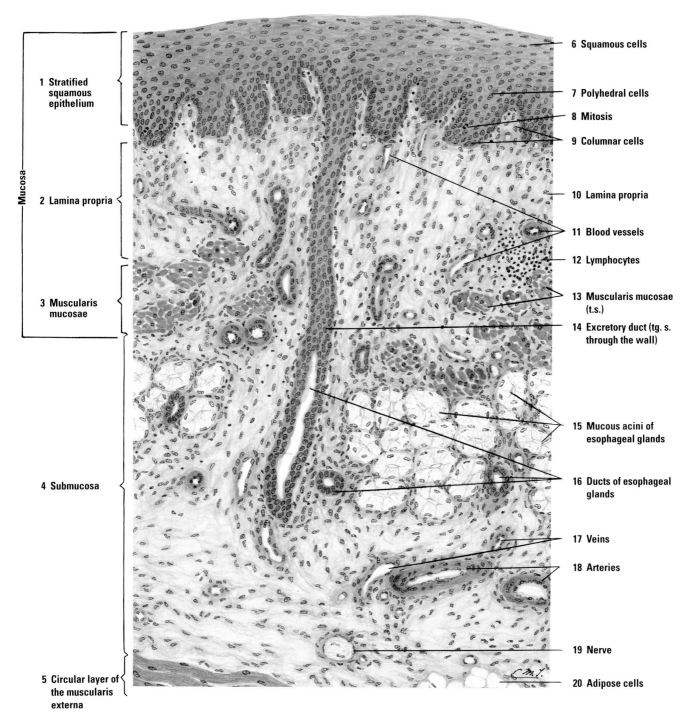

1 Stratified squamous epithelium

2 Lamina propria

3 Muscularis mucosae

4 Submucosa

5 Circular layer of the muscularis externa

Mucosa

6 Squamous cells

7 Polyhedral cells

8 Mitosis

9 Columnar cells

10 Lamina propria

11 Blood vessels

12 Lymphocytes

13 Muscularis mucosae (t.s.)

14 Excretory duct (tg. s. through the wall)

15 Mucous acini of esophageal glands

16 Ducts of esophageal glands

17 Veins

18 Arteries

19 Nerve

20 Adipose cells

STAIN: hematoxylin-eosin. 250×.

PLATE 61

■ **FIG. 1**
UPPER ESOPHAGUS

This section of the upper esophagus is similar to the illustration in Plate 59 except that it is stained with Heidenhain's modification of Mallory's trichrome (Mallory-azan). Azocarmine stains the nuclei an intense red. A mixture of aniline blue and orange G selectively stains other tissues. The collagen fibers of the **connective tissue (1, 4, 5, 7, 9)** stain bright blue, whereas the cytoplasm of **epithelium (6)** and **muscle cells (2, 3, 8)** stains orange to red.

The different layers of the esophagus are easily distinguishable. In the upper esophagus (as in Plate 60), the outermost layer is the **adventitia (1),** and the **muscularis externa (2, 3)** is skeletal muscle. Aniline blue stains the large amounts of connective tissue in the **submucosa (9)** and adventitia (1) and the smaller amounts between (4) and within muscle layers (5). The connective tissue of the **lamina propria (7)** appears distinct from the smooth muscle of the **muscularis mucosae (8).**

■ **FIG. 2**
LOWER ESOPHAGUS

This section of the terminal portion of the esophagus (in the peritoneal cavity near the stomach) is stained with Van Gieson's trichrome, which uses iron hematoxylin (Weigert's or Heidenhain's) as a nuclear stain and picrofuchsin to stain other components. As a result, cellular details are not well defined, but the **connective tissue (3, 5, 7)** and **smooth muscle (2, 4, 8)** are nicely differentiated. Nuclei are stained dark brown. Collagenous fibers (3, 5, 7) are stained red with acid fuchsin, whereas muscle (and other tissues) (2, 4, 6, 8, 9) are stained yellow with picric acid.

The layers in the wall of the lower esophagus are similar to those in the upper region, except for regional modifications. The outermost layer is the **serosa (1)** (visceral peritoneum). This is in contrast to the adventitia, which lines the esophagus in the thoracic region. The **muscularis externa (2, 4)** layers are entirely smooth muscle, although this is not apparent with this stain and this magnification. Distribution of the **mucous glands (9)** in the submucosa is variable, and in some regions, they may be absent; however, some are illustrated in this section.

The collagenous fibers in the **submucosa (5)** are abundant. The distribution of finer **connective tissue fibers (3, 8)** in lesser amounts is seen between and around **smooth muscle fibers (2, 3),** in serosa (1), and in the **lamina propria (7).**

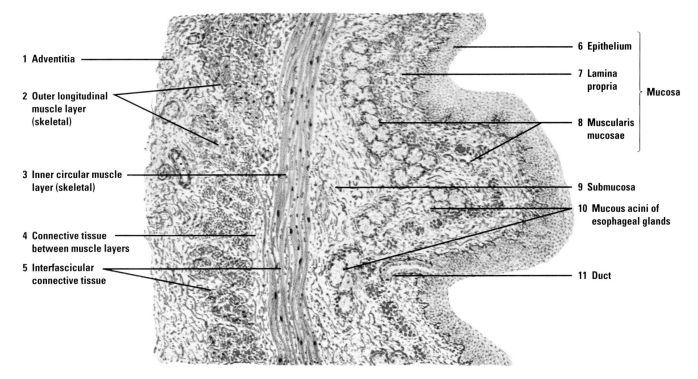

1 Adventitia

2 Outer longitudinal muscle layer (skeletal)

3 Inner circular muscle layer (skeletal)

4 Connective tissue between muscle layers

5 Interfascicular connective tissue

6 Epithelium

7 Lamina propria

} Mucosa

8 Muscularis mucosae

9 Submucosa

10 Mucous acini of esophageal glands

11 Duct

FIG. 1. UPPER ESOPHAGUS (TRANSVERSE SECTION). Stain: Mallory's trichrome. 40×. (Nuclei, red; connective tissue, blue; epithelium and muscle, orange to red.)

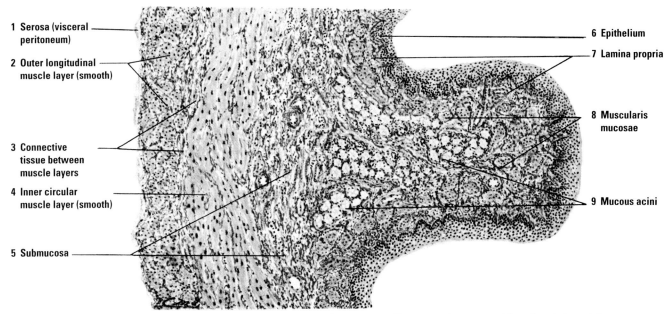

1 Serosa (visceral peritoneum)

2 Outer longitudinal muscle layer (smooth)

3 Connective tissue between muscle layers

4 Inner circular muscle layer (smooth)

5 Submucosa

6 Epithelium

7 Lamina propria

8 Muscularis mucosae

9 Mucous acini

FIG. 2. LOWER ESOPHAGUS (TRANSVERSE SECTION). Stain: Van Gieson's trichrome. 40×. (Nuclei, dark brown; connective tissue, red; epithelium and muscle, yellow.)

161

PLATE 62

ESOPHAGEAL-STOMACH JUNCTION

At the esophageal-stomach junction, the **esophageal glands proper (11)** may be seen in the **submucosa. Excretory ducts (13, 15)** from these glands course through the **muscularis mucosae (8)** and the **lamina propria (14)** to open into the lumen of the **esophagus.** The lamina propria (14) of the esophagus may also contain some **cardiac glands (12).**

At the esophageal-stomach junction, the **stratified squamous epithelium (10)** of the esophagus abruptly changes to simple columnar, mucus-secreting epithelium of the **stomach (18).** Consequently, the boundary between these two organs is sharply defined.

The **lamina propria** of the **esophagus (14)** is continuous with the lamina propria of the **stomach (16),** where it becomes a wide layer of glands and diffuse lymphatic tissue. The lamina propria of the stomach (16) is penetrated by numerous shallow **gastric pits (19),** into which empty the **glands (17, 20)** of the mucosa.

The upper region of the stomach contains two types of glands. The simple tubular **cardiac glands (17)** are primarily limited to the transition region, the cardia of the stomach. These glands are lined with a single type of cell, the mucus-secreting columnar cell. Below the cardiac region of the stomach, the glands are replaced by simple tubular **gastric glands (20),** some of which may exhibit basal branching.

The gastric glands (20) contain four different cell types: the **chief or zymogenic cells (21), parietal cells (23), mucous neck cells (22),** and several different types of endocrine cells (not illustrated), collectively called enteroendocrine cells (Plate 69).

The muscularis mucosae (8) of the stomach is also continuous with that of the esophagus. In the esophagus, the muscularis mucosae is usually a single layer of longitudinal smooth muscle fibers, whereas in the stomach, a second layer of smooth muscle the inner circular layer (8), is added.

The **submucosa (7)** and **muscularis externa (6)** layers of the esophagus are continuous in the stomach. Numerous **blood vessels (1, 2, 3, 4, 5, 9)** are found in the submucosa (7). From here, smaller blood vessels are distributed to other regions of the organ.

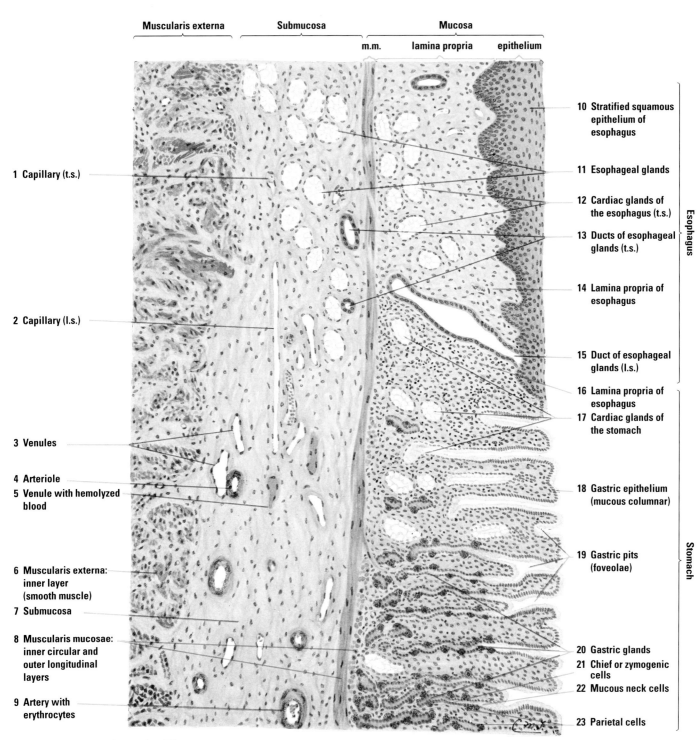

Muscularis externa   Submucosa   Mucosa

m.m.   lamina propria   epithelium

Esophagus

Stomach

1 Capillary (t.s.)

2 Capillary (l.s.)

3 Venules

4 Arteriole
5 Venule with hemolyzed blood

6 Muscularis externa: inner layer (smooth muscle)
7 Submucosa
8 Muscularis mucosae: inner circular and outer longitudinal layers
9 Artery with erythrocytes

10 Stratified squamous epithelium of esophagus

11 Esophageal glands

12 Cardiac glands of the esophagus (t.s.)

13 Ducts of esophageal glands (t.s.)

14 Lamina propria of esophagus

15 Duct of esophageal glands (l.s.)

16 Lamina propria of esophagus
17 Cardiac glands of the stomach

18 Gastric epithelium (mucous columnar)

19 Gastric pits (foveolae)

20 Gastric glands
21 Chief or zymogenic cells
22 Mucous neck cells

23 Parietal cells

STAIN: hematoxylin-eosin. 70×.

163

PLATE 63

STOMACH: FUNDUS OR BODY REGION (TRANSVERSE SECTION)

The human stomach is divided into three distinct histologic areas: the cardia, fundus or body, and pylorus. The fundus or body is the most extensive region in the stomach.

This low magnification figure illustrates a transverse section of the fundic stomach. The stomach wall exhibits four general regions that are characteristic of the entire digestive tract. The four regions are the **mucosa (1, 2, 3), submucosa (4), muscularis externa (5, 6, 7),** and **serosa (8).**

Mucosa (1, 2, 3): The mucosa of the stomach consists of three layers: the epithelium, lamina propria and muscularis mucosae. The luminal surface of the mucosa is lined by a layer of **simple columnar epithelium (1, 11).** This epithelium also extends into and lines the **gastric pits (10),** which are tubular infoldings of the surface epithelium **(11).** In the fundic region of the stomach, the gastric pits (10) are not deep and extend into the mucosa about one fourth of its thickness. Beneath the surface epithelium is a layer of loose connective tissue, the **lamina propria (2, 12),** which fills the narrow spaces between the gastric glands. The outer layer of mucosa is lined by a thin band of smooth muscle, the **muscularis mucosae (3, 15),** consisting of an inner circular and an outer longitudinal layer. Thin slips of muscle from the muscularis mucosae (3, 15) extend into lamina propria (2, 12) between the **gastric glands (13, 14)** toward the surface epithelium (1, 11) (See Plate 64:8).

The gastric glands (13, 14) are tightly packed in the lamina propria and occupy the entire thickness of the mucosa (1, 2, 3). These glands open in small groups into the bottom of the gastric pits (10). The surface epithelium of the entire gastric mucosa contains the same cell type, from the cardiac to the pyloric region; however, there are distinct regional differences in the type of cells that comprise the gastric glands. At lower magnification, two distinct types of cells can be identified in the gastric glands of the fundic stomach. The acidophilic **parietal cells (13)** are seen in the upper portions of the glands; the more basophilic **chief (zymo-**genic) **(14)** cells occupy the lower regions. The subglandular regions of the lamina propria may contain small accumulations of lymphatic tissue or **nodules (16).**

The mucosa of an empty stomach exhibits numerous folds called the **rugae (9).** These folds are temporary and are formed from the contractions of the smooth muscle layer, the muscularis mucosae (3, 15). As the stomach fills with solid or liquid material, the rugae disappear and the mucosa appears smooth.

Submucosa (4): The prominent layer directly beneath the muscularis mucosae (3, 15) is the submucosa (4). In an empty stomach, this layer can extend into the folds or the rugae (9). The submucosa (4) contains denser irregular connective tissue and more **collagenous fibers (17)** than the lamina propria (2, 12). In addition to the normal complement of connective tissue cells, the submucosa (4) contains numerous lymph vessels, **capillaries (22),** large **arterioles (18),** and **venules (19).** Isolated or small clusters of the parasympathetic ganglia of the **submucosal (Meissner's) nerve plexus (21)** are also seen in the deeper regions of the submucosa.

Muscularis Externa (5, 6, 7): In the stomach, the muscularis externa (5, 6, 7) consists of three layers of smooth muscle, each oriented in a different plane: an inner **oblique (5),** a middle **circular (6),** and an outer **longitudinal (7)** layer. The oblique layer is not complete and, as a result, this layer is not always seen in sections of stomach wall. In this illustration, the circular layer has been sectioned longitudinally and the longitudinal layer transversely. Located between the circular and longitudinal smooth muscle layers is a prominent **myenteric (Auerbach's) nerve plexus (23)** of parasympathetic ganglia and nerve fibers.

Serosa (8): The outermost layer of the stomach wall is the serosa (8). This is a thin layer of connective tissue that overlies the muscularis externa (5, 6, 7). Externally, this layer is covered by a simple squamous mesothelium of the **visceral peritoneum (8).** The connective tissue covered by the visceral peritoneum can contain numerous **adipose cells (24).**

STOMACH: FUNDUS OR BODY (TRANSVERSE SECTION)

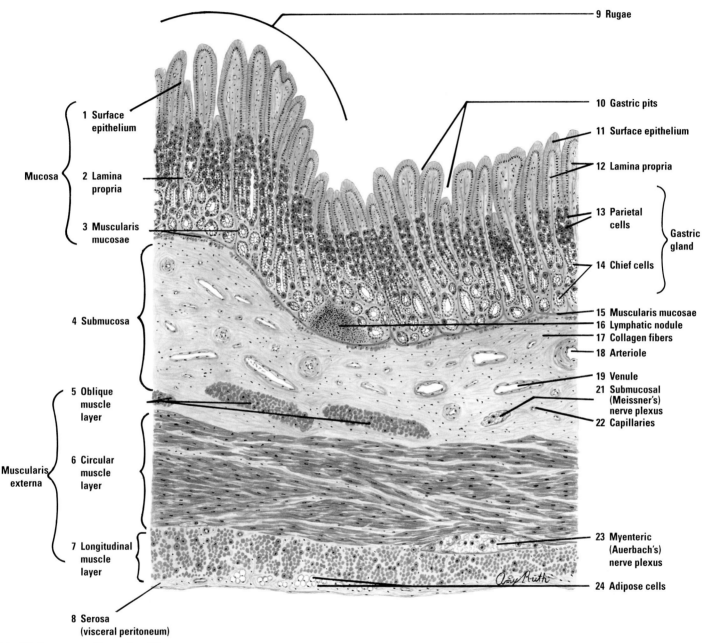

9 Rugae

1 Surface epithelium

10 Gastric pits

11 Surface epithelium

Mucosa

2 Lamina propria

12 Lamina propria

13 Parietal cells

Gastric gland

3 Muscularis mucosae

14 Chief cells

4 Submucosa

15 Muscularis mucosae

16 Lymphatic nodule

17 Collagen fibers

18 Arteriole

19 Venule

21 Submucosal (Meissner's) nerve plexus

5 Oblique muscle layer

22 Capillaries

Muscularis externa

6 Circular muscle layer

7 Longitudinal muscle layer

23 Myenteric (Auerbach's) nerve plexus

24 Adipose cells

8 Serosa (visceral peritoneum)

STAIN: hematoxylin-eosin. 57×.

165

PLATE 64

STOMACH: MUCOSA OF THE FUNDUS OR BODY (TRANSVERSE SECTION)

The mucosa and submucosa of the fundic region of the stomach are illustrated at a higher magnification. The extension of the simple columnar **surface epithelium (1, 13)** into the **gastric pits (11)** and the opening of the tubular **gastric glands (5)** into these pits are clearly seen. The loose irregular connective tissue of the **lamina propria (6)** fills the narrow spaces between the tightly packed gastric glands (5) and extends from the surface epithelium (1) to the **muscularis mucosae (9).**

The lamina propria (6) is better seen in the **mucosal ridges (2);** it consists primarily of fine reticular and collagenous fibers. Scattered throughout this connective tissue are the oval nuclei of the fibroblasts. Also seen in the lamina propria (6) are accumulations of lymphoid tissue in the form of **lymphatic nodules (17),** in addition to individual lymphocytes and other cell types normally encountered in the loose connective tissue.

The gastric glands (5) extend the entire length of the mucosa. In the deeper regions of the mucosa, the gastric glands may branch, as seen by the numerous transverse and oblique sections. Each gastric gland generally consists of three regions. At the junction of the gastric pit with the gastric gland is the **isthmus (14),** containing the surface epithelial cells (1, 13) and **parietal cells (4).** Lower in the gland is the **neck (15),** composed primarily of **mucous neck cells (3)** and also parietal cells (4). The base or **fundus (16)** is the deep portion of the gland, composed predominantly of **chief (zymogenic) cells (7)** with a few scattered parietal cells (4). In addition to these cells, the fundic glands contain undifferentiated cells and a variety of enteroendocrine cells (not illustrated) that belong to the APUD group. (The

characteristics of the APUD cells are discussed and illustrated in greater detail in Plate 69).

In the hematoxylin-eosin preparations, three types of cells can be easily identified in the fundic gastric glands. In this illustration, the parietal cells stain intensely and uniformly acidophilic (4). This staining characteristic distinguishes clearly the parietal cells from other cells in the fundic glands. In contrast, the chief cells (zymogenic) (7) are distinctly basophilic and are readily distinguishable from the surrounding acidophilic parietal cells. The mucous neck cells (3) are located just below the gastric pits (11) and are interspersed between the parietal cells in the neck region of the glands.

The muscularis mucosae (9) is well illustrated in this stomach section. It is composed of two thin strips of smooth muscle, the **inner circular layer (9a)** and **outer longitudinal layer (9b).** In this illustration, the circular layer is sectioned longitudinally and the outer layer is sectioned transversely. Extending into the lamina propria (6) from the muscularis mucosae (9) toward the surface epithelium (1, 13) are strands of **smooth muscle (8, 12).**

Directly below the muscularis mucosae is a prominent layer of denser connective tissue, the **submucosa (10).** In this section, abundant **collagen fibers (18)** and the nuclei of numerous **fibroblasts (19)** are readily seen. The submucosa layer also contains numerous vessels, including **arterioles (20), venules (21),** lymphatics, and capillaries. Some adipose cells may also be seen in this layer.

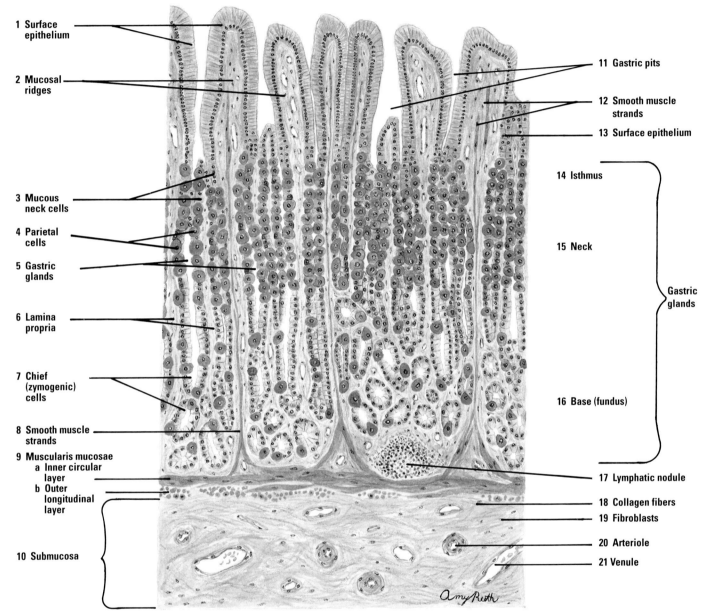

1 Surface epithelium
2 Mucosal ridges
3 Mucous neck cells
4 Parietal cells
5 Gastric glands
6 Lamina propria
7 Chief (zymogenic) cells
8 Smooth muscle strands
9 Muscularis mucosae
  a Inner circular layer
  b Outer longitudinal layer
10 Submucosa

11 Gastric pits
12 Smooth muscle strands
13 Surface epithelium
14 Isthmus
15 Neck
16 Base (fundus)

Gastric glands

17 Lymphatic nodule
18 Collagen fibers
19 Fibroblasts
20 Arteriole
21 Venule

STAIN: hematoxylin-eosin. 180×.

PLATE 65

■ FIG. 1
STOMACH: FUNDUS OR BODY, SUPERFICIAL REGION OF GASTRIC MUCOSA

Higher magnification of the stomach illustrates the characteristic features of different cells that compose the superficial region of the gastric mucosa of the fundus or body.

The tall columnar **surface epithelium (1)** exhibits basal oval nuclei and is lightly stained because of the presence of mucigen droplets in the cytoplasm. It is delimited from the adjacent fibroelastic connective tissue **lamina propria (3)** by a thin but distinct **basement membrane (2)**. The surface epithelium extends downward into the **gastric pits (4, 8)**.

The **gastric glands (5, 12)** lie in the **lamina propria (11)** below the **gastric pits (4, 9)**. The **necks (5, 10)** of the gastric glands are also lined with low columnar **mucous neck cells (6)** that have round, basal nuclei. The constricted necks of the gastric glands (10) open by a short transition region into the bottom of the gastric pit (8).

The prominent **parietal cells (7)** are interspersed among the mucous neck cells (6); their free surfaces are on the border of the **glandular lumen (12)**. The parietal cells (7) are most conspicuous in the gastric mucosa and are predominantly found in the upper half of the gastric glands. These cells are large and pyramidal in shape wtih round nucleus and highly acidophilic cytoplasm; some pyramidal cells may be binucleate.

Deeper in the gastric glands (5, 12), toward the lower half or third of the gland, the mucous cells are replaced by basophilic **chief or zymogenic cells (13)**, which border on the lumen of the gland. Parietal cells (7) are also seen here; however, they are displaced peripherally and lie against the basement membrane without reaching the lumen.

■ FIG. 2
DEEP REGION OF THE MUCOSA

The **gastric glands (1)** are branched tubular glands; the branching is normally seen at the base of the glands. A section through the deep region of the mucosa illustrates basal portions of the gastric glands **(1,10)** sectioned in various planes.

As in the higher region of the gland, the **chief or zymogenic cells (4, 9, 12)** border the glandular lumen. The **parietal cells (3, 8, 11)** are wedged against the basement membrane and are not in direct contact with the lumen. This is well demonstrated in several transverse sections of the glands (3, lower leader).

Also illustrated in this figure are the **lamina propria (2)** between the gastric glands (1,10) and a narrow zone of **subglandular lamina propria (5)**, which is not always distinguishable.

The two layers, inner circular and outer longitudinal, of **muscularis mucosae (13, 14)**, are also illustrated.

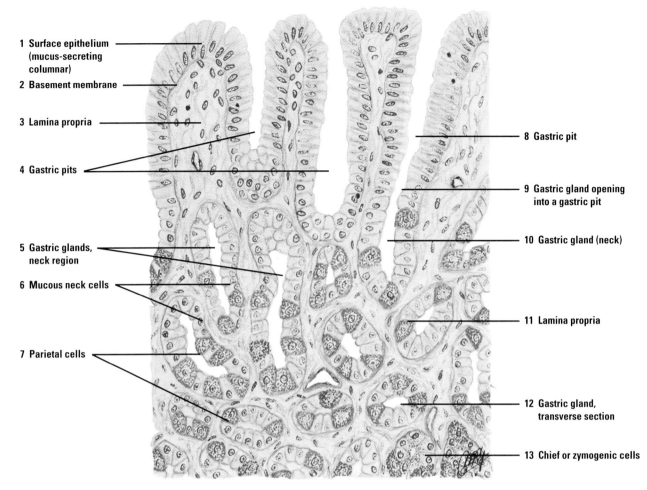

1 Surface epithelium (mucus-secreting columnar)

2 Basement membrane

3 Lamina propria

4 Gastric pits

5 Gastric glands, neck region

6 Mucous neck cells

7 Parietal cells

8 Gastric pit

9 Gastric gland opening into a gastric pit

10 Gastric gland (neck)

11 Lamina propria

12 Gastric gland, transverse section

13 Chief or zymogenic cells

FIG. 1. SUPERFICIAL REGION OF THE GASTRIC MUCOSA. Stain: hematoxylin-eosin. 350×.

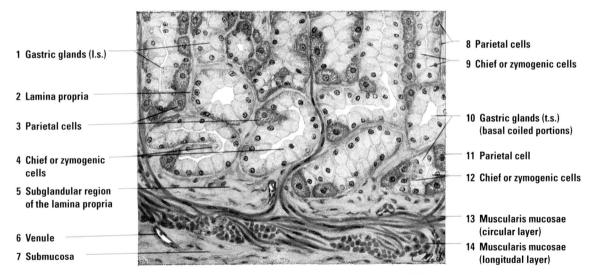

1 Gastric glands (l.s.)

2 Lamina propria

3 Parietal cells

4 Chief or zymogenic cells

5 Subglandular region of the lamina propria

6 Venule

7 Submucosa

8 Parietal cells

9 Chief or zymogenic cells

10 Gastric glands (t.s.) (basal coiled portions)

11 Parietal cell

12 Chief or zymogenic cells

13 Muscularis mucosae (circular layer)

14 Muscularis mucosae (longitudal layer)

FIG. 2. DEEP REGION OF THE MUCOSA. Stain: hematoxylin-eosin. 350×.

PLATE 66

STOMACH: MUCOSA OF THE PYLORIC REGION

In the pyloric region of the stomach, the **gastric pits (4, 12)** are deeper than those in the body or fundus regions of the stomach. The gastric pits (4, 12) extend into the mucosa to about one half or more of its thickness. The simple columnar mucous **epithelium (10)** that lines the surface of the stomach extends into and lines the gastric pits (4,12).

The pyloric **gastric glands (5, 6, 14)** are either branched or coiled tubular mucous glands. As in the cardia region of the stomach, only one type of cell is normally found in these glands. This is a tall columnar cell, with slightly granular cytoplasm, lightly stained because of mucigen content, and a flattened or oval nucleus at the base. The pyloric glands (5, 6, 14) open into the bottom of the gastric pits (4, lower leader). Enteroendocrine or APUD cells are also present in this region of the stomach and can usually be demonstrated with special staining techniques.

The remaining structures in this region are similar to those in the upper stomach. The **lamina propria (13)** contains diffuse lymphatic tissue, an occasional **lymphatic nodule (16)** may be seen in its deepest part. The lymphatic nodules may increase in size and penetrate through the **muscularis mucosae** (18) into the **submucosa** (20). **Smooth muscle fibers (7)** from the circular layer of the **muscularis mucosae (18)** pass upward into the lamina propria (13) between the pyloric glands (6) and into **mucosal ridges (2, 3).**

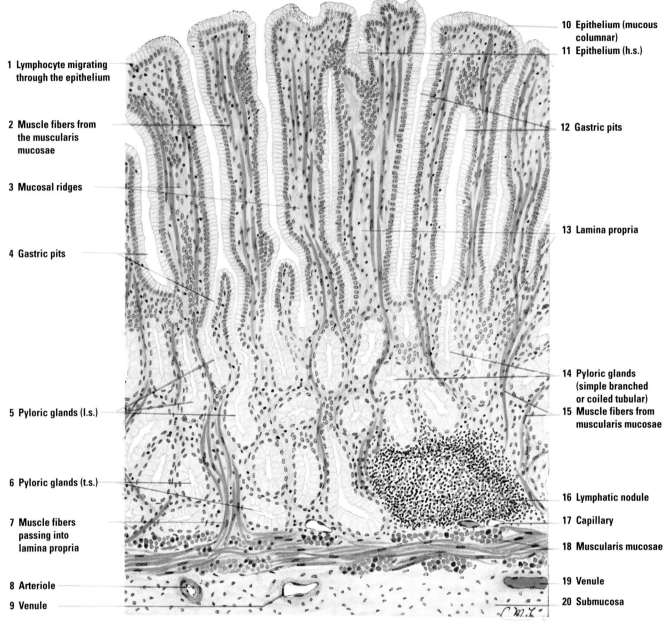

1 Lymphocyte migrating through the epithelium

2 Muscle fibers from the muscularis mucosae

3 Mucosal ridges

4 Gastric pits

5 Pyloric glands (l.s.)

6 Pyloric glands (t.s.)

7 Muscle fibers passing into lamina propria

8 Arteriole

9 Venule

10 Epithelium (mucous columnar)

11 Epithelium (h.s.)

12 Gastric pits

13 Lamina propria

14 Pyloric glands (simple branched or coiled tubular)

15 Muscle fibers from muscularis mucosae

16 Lymphatic nodule

17 Capillary

18 Muscularis mucosae

19 Venule

20 Submucosa

STAIN: hematoxylin-eosin. 100×.

PLATE 67

PYLORIC-DUODENAL JUNCTION (LONGITUDINAL SECTION)

The **pyloric region (1)** of the stomach is separated from the **duodenum (2)** by a **pyloric sphincter (7).** This sphincter is formed by thickened circular layer of the muscularis externa.

As the pylorus joins the duodenum, the **mucosal ridges (5),** which surround the **gastric pits (6),** become broader and more irregular. As a result, their shape becomes highly variable. Coiled tubular **pyloric (mucous) glands (4),** located in the lamina propria, open at the bottom of the gastric pits (6). **Lymphatic nodules (10)** are frequently seen in the transition region.

The **duodenum (2)** exhibits surface modification in the form of **villi (13).** Each villus (13) is a leaf-shaped surface projection with a pointed end. Between individual villi are **intervillous spaces (16)** that represent the continuation of the intestinal lumen. The mucus-secreting epithelium of the stomach (3) changes abruptly to intestinal epithelium (11). This epithelium consists of goblet cells and columnar cells with striated borders (microvilli), which are present throughout the length of the small intestine.

Short simple tubular **intestinal glands (crypts of Lieberkühn) (12)** are now seen in the lamina propria. These glands consist primarily of goblet cells and cells with striated borders (microvilli) from the surface epithelium. One or more **intestinal glands** are shown opening between the villi **(17).**

Duodenal (Brunner's) glands (14) occupy most of the submucosa in the upper duodenum. In this region, the **muscularis mucosae (15)** is disrupted and strands of its muscle are dispersed among the glands. Except for the esophageal (submucosal) glands proper, the duodenal glands (14) are the only submucosal glands in the digestive tract.

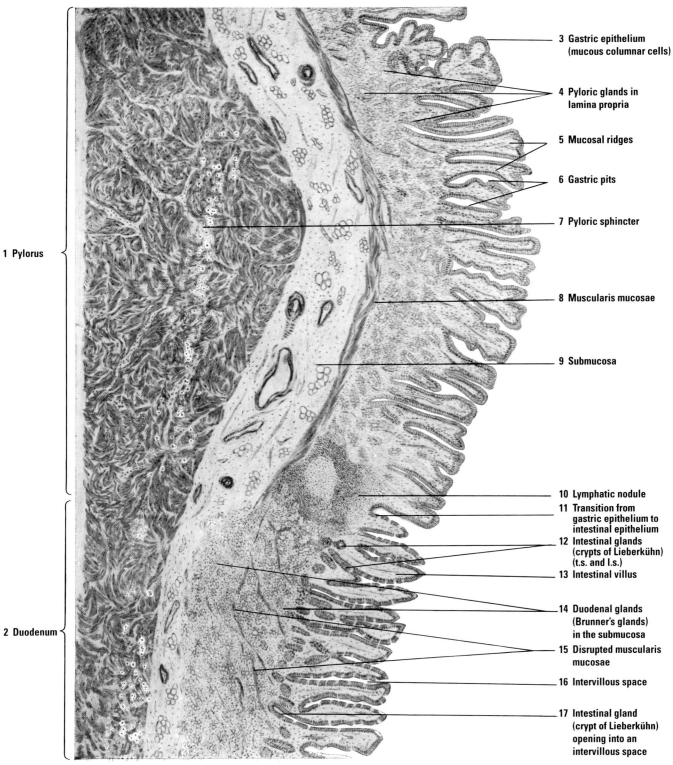

1 Pylorus

2 Duodenum

3 Gastric epithelium (mucous columnar cells)

4 Pyloric glands in lamina propria

5 Mucosal ridges

6 Gastric pits

7 Pyloric sphincter

8 Muscularis mucosae

9 Submucosa

10 Lymphatic nodule

11 Transition from gastric epithelium to intestinal epithelium

12 Intestinal glands (crypts of Lieberkühn) (t.s. and l.s.)

13 Intestinal villus

14 Duodenal glands (Brunner's glands) in the submucosa

15 Disrupted muscularis mucosae

16 Intervillous space

17 Intestinal gland (crypt of Lieberkühn) opening into an intervillous space

STAIN: hematoxylin-eosin. 25×.

THE DIGESTIVE SYSTEM: THE SMALL AND LARGE INTESTINES

The Small Intestine

The small intestine consists of three parts: the duodenum, jejunum, and ileum. It is a long tube that extends from the junction with the stomach to the junction with the large intestine or colon. The small intestine performs numerous important functions in the digestive processes, among which are: (1) completing the digestion of the food products (chyme), initiated in the stomach, by the chemicals and enzymes produced in the liver and pancreas and by cells in its own mucosa, (2) selective absorption of nutrients into the blood and lymph capillaries, (3) transportation of chyme and waste material of digestion to the large intestine, and (4) release of different hormones that regulate the digestive processes.

The mucosa of the small intestine shows certain specializations that increase its surface area for absorption. These mucosal specializations are the plicae circulares, villi, and microvilli. The plicae circulares are spiral folds with submucosal core that extend into the intestinal lumen; they are most prominent in the proximal portion of the small intestine, where most of the absorption takes place, and decrease in size toward the ileum. The villi are fingerlike projections that cover the surface of the intestine and also extend into the lumen. The villi are also more prominent in the proximal portion of the small intestine. The microvilli are the cytoplasmic extensions that cover the apices of the intestinal cells and are seen with light microscopy as striated (brush) border.

Although the epithelium that lines the stomach surface is of one type (mucus-secreting), the epithelium of small intestine exhibits numerous cell types. Most cells in the intestinal epithelium are the tall columnar absorptive cells with a prominent striated border (microvilli), which is covered by a thick glycocalyx coat. The outer glycocalyx coat protects the intestinal surface from digestion; it also contains numerous digestive enzymes. The intestinal cells absorb amino acids, glucose, and fatty acids, the end products of protein, carbohydrate, and fat digestion, respectively. Amino acids and glucose are transported through the intestinal cells to the blood capillaries. Most of the fatty acids, however, enter the blind-ending lymphatic vessels, called the lacteals, which are located in the lamina propria of the villi.

Interspersed among the columnar absorptive cells in the intestine are the goblet cells, which increase in number toward the distal region of the small intestine (ileum). The goblet cells secrete mucus that lubricates, coats, and protects the intestinal surface from the corrosive action of the digestive chemicals.

The small intestine also contains intestinal glands (crypts of Lieberkuhn). These glands are located in the intestinal mucosa and open into the intestinal lumen at the base of the villi. The surface epithelium of the villi also extends into and lines the intestinal glands. Located at the base of the intestinal glands are the Paneth cells, characterized by deep-staining eosinophilic granules. These cells are believed to produce lysozyme, an enzyme that digests the cell walls of some bacteria and controls the microbial flora of the small intestine.

The enteroendocrine or APUD cells are also found in the epithelium of the villi and intestinal glands. These cells secrete numerous intestinal regulatory hormones that include secretin, cholecystokinin (pancreozymin), and others. The intestinal hormones control gastric and pancreatic secretions, intestinal motility, and contractions of the gallbladder.

A characteristic feature of the first portion of the small intestine, the duodenum, is the presence of mucus-secreting duodenal (Brunner's) glands in the submucosa. The ducts of these glands extend through the muscularis mucosae and open into the bases of the intestinal glands (crypts of Lieberkuhn). When acidic chyme is present, the duodenal glands secrete an alkaline fluid that is rich in bicarbonate ions. This alkaline fluid neutralizes the acidic chyme from the stomach and protects the duodenal surfaces from digestion. The alkaline secretion also provides a more favorable environment for the continued action of the digestive enzymes.

The Large Intestine

The large intestine is situated between the termination of the ileum and the anus. The unabsorbed and undigested food residues in the small intestine are forced by the peristaltic action of the muscles in the small intestine into the large intestine. The residual contents that enter the initial portion of the large intestine are in a semifluid state; however, at the terminal portion of the large intestine, these residues acquire the semisolid consistency of feces.

The principal functions of the large intestine are the absorption of water and minerals from the residual contents and the formation of feces. Consistent with these functions, the epithelium of the large intestine contains both absorptive and mucus-secreting goblet cells. The absorptive functions are carried out by the columnar absorptive cells; these appear similar to those seen in the epithelium of the small intestine. No digestive enzymes are produced by the cells of the large intestine.

The goblet cells appear more numerous in the large intestine than in the small intestine. Their main functions are to produce mucus and to lubricate the lumen for the passage of the hardened feces.

There are no villi or Paneth cells in the large intestine. The deep intestinal glands of the large intestine, however, contain the enteroendocrine or APUD cells.

PLATE 68

SMALL INTESTINE: DUODENUM (LONGITUDINAL SECTION)

PLATE 68

The wall of the duodenum consists of four layers: the **mucosa (13, 14, 15)**, **submucosa (17)**, **muscularis externa (18)**, and **serosa (visceral peritoneum) (19)**. These layers are continuous with those in the stomach and in the small and large intestine.

The small intestine is characterized by the **villi (3, 13)**, a surface epithelium of columnar cells with **striated borders (1)**, **goblet cells (1)**, and short tubular **intestinal glands (crypts of Lieberkühn) (5, 6, 7)** in the **lamina propria (3, 13)**. The presence of the mucous **duodenal (Brunner's) glands (8)** in the submucosa **(17)** is indicative of the upper duodenum. These submucosal glands are absent in the jejunum, ileum, and the entire large intestine.

The villi **(3, 13)** are mucosal surface modifications with **intervillous spaces (2)** between them. The lining epithelium (1) covers the villi, lines the intervillous spaces (2), and continues into the intestinal glands (5, 6, 7). Each villus has a core of lamina propria (3, 13), some smooth muscle fibers (4) that extend from the **muscularis mucosae (15)**, and a central lacteal (not illustrated). (See Plate 70, Fig. 2, for detailed structure of a villus.)

Located in the **lamina propria (14)** are the intestinal glands (crypts of Lieberkühn) (6, 7), which open into the intervillous spaces (5). In certain sections, exten-sions of submucosal duodenal (Brunner's) glands (8, 17) are seen in the lamina propria (8, upper leader, and **16**). The lamina propria (3, 13) also contains fine connective tissue fibers with reticular cells, diffuse lymphatic tissue, or lymphatic nodules deep in the lamina propria.

The **submucosa (17)** is almost completely filled with highly branched tubular duodenal (Brunner's) glands (8, 17). The muscularis mucosae (15) may be disrupted if these glands penetrate into the mucosal lamina propria, and strands of smooth muscle may be observed in the **glandular area (9)**. The duodenal glands open into the bottom of the intestinal glands (6, 7).

The **muscularis externa (18)** consists of an inner circular and outer longitudinal layer of smooth muscle. Parasympathetic ganglion cells of the **myenteric (Auerbach's) plexus (12)** are seen in the connective tissue between the two muscle layers; this nerve plexus is found between these muscle layers throughout the small and large intestine. Similar but smaller ganglion cells (submucosal or Meissner's plexus) are likewise found in the submucosa (17) throughout the small and large intestine.

The **serosa (visceral peritoneum) (19)** forms the outermost layer of the small intestine.

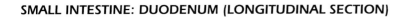

SMALL INTESTINE: DUODENUM (LONGITUDINAL SECTION)

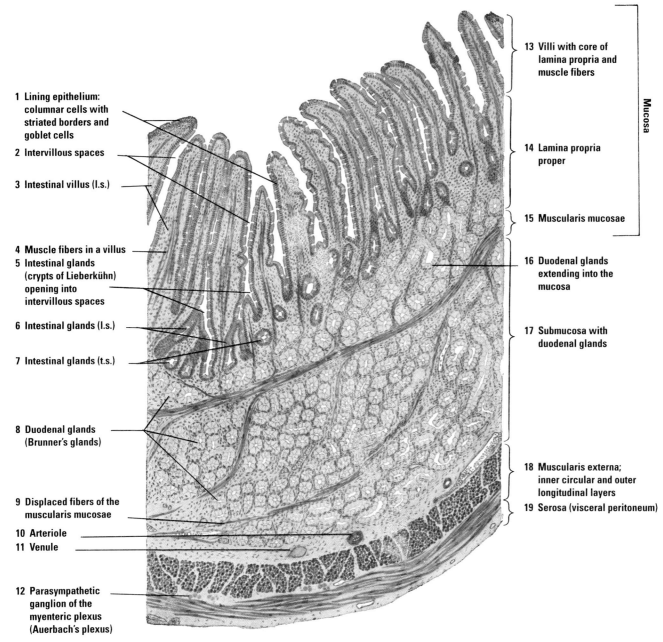

1 Lining epithelium: columnar cells with striated borders and goblet cells

2 Intervillous spaces

3 Intestinal villus (l.s.)

4 Muscle fibers in a villus

5 Intestinal glands (crypts of Lieberkühn) opening into intervillous spaces

6 Intestinal glands (l.s.)

7 Intestinal glands (t.s.)

8 Duodenal glands (Brunner's glands)

9 Displaced fibers of the muscularis mucosae

10 Arteriole

11 Venule

12 Parasympathetic ganglion of the myenteric plexus (Auerbach's plexus)

13 Villi with core of lamina propria and muscle fibers

14 Lamina propria proper

15 Muscularis mucosae

16 Duodenal glands extending into the mucosa

17 Submucosa with duodenal glands

18 Muscularis externa; inner circular and outer longitudinal layers

19 Serosa (visceral peritoneum)

Mucosa

Stain: hematoxylin-eosin. 50×.

179

PLATE 69

■ FIG. 1
SMALL INTESTINE: JEJUNUM-ILEUM (TRANSVERSE SECTION)

The histology of the lower duodenum, jejunum, and ileum remains similar to that of the upper duodenum illustrated in Plate 68. The only exception are the duodenal glands (of Brunner); these are usually limited to submucosa in the upper part of the duodenum. The villi exhibit variable shapes and lengths in the different regions of the small intestine; however, this is not usually apparent in histologic sections. Also, in the lower regions of the ileum, large aggregates of lymphatic nodules (Peyer's patches) are observed at different intervals (See Plate 70, Fig. 1).

This figure illustrates numerous **villi (2)** sectioned in different planes and a prominent, permanent fold of the small intestine, the **plica circulares (10).** Both the mucosa and **submucosa (4, 16)** constitute the plica circulares (10). In the lumen, each villus (2) exhibits a typical structure: a columnar **lining epithelium (1)** with striated border and goblet cells, a core of **lamina propria (3)** with diffuse lymphatic tissue, and strips of smooth muscle fibers from the **muscularis mucosae (6).**

Within the villi are also seen a central lacteal and small blood vessels; these are illustrated on Plate 70, Fig. 2. The **intestinal glands** (crypts of Lieberkühn) **(5, 12)** extend into the lamina propria (3). These glands are closely packed and in the figure are seen in both the longitudinal and cross sections. The intestinal glands (5, 12) open into the **intervillous spaces (11).** A **lymphatic nodule (14)** is seen extending from the lamina propria (3) of the mucosa into the submucosa (16), disrupting the surrounding **muscularis mucosae (15).**

The appearance and distribution of the muscularis mucosae (6, 15), submucosa (4, 16), **muscularis externa (7, 8),** and **serosa (18)** are typical of the small intestine. Parasympathetic ganglion cells of the **myenteric plexus (17)** are seen in the connective tissue between the inner circular smooth muscle layer (7) and the outer longitudinal muscle layer (8) of the muscularis externa. Ganglion cells of the submucosal plexuses are also present in the small intestine but are not illustrated in this figure.

■ FIG. 2
INTESTINAL GLANDS WITH PANETH CELLS AND ENTEROENDOCRINE CELLS

Adjacent to the smooth muscle of the **muscularis mucosae (5, 10)** are illustrated several **intestinal glands (7).** The characteristic **goblet cells (2)** and the cells with striated borders are seen in the glands. At the base of these glands are also found pyramid-shaped cells with large, acidophilic granules, which fill most of the cytoplasm and displace the nucleus toward the base of the cell. These cells are the **Paneth cells (4, 9)** and are found throughout the small intestine.

Interspersed among the intestinal gland cells, **mitotic gland cells (1, 6),** goblet cells (2), and the Paneth cells

(4, 9), are also the **enteroendocrine cells (3, 8).** These cells are characterized by fine granules located in the basal portions of the cytoplasm, and the nucleus is situated above the granules. Most of the enteroendocrine cells take up and decarboxylate precursors of biogenic monoamines and are therefore considered part of a larger group of cells designated as the amine precursor uptake and decarboxylation (APUD) cell series. The APUD cell types are found in the epithelia of the gastrointestinal tract (stomach, small, and large intestines), respiratory tract, pancreas, and thyroid glands.

SMALL INTESTINE

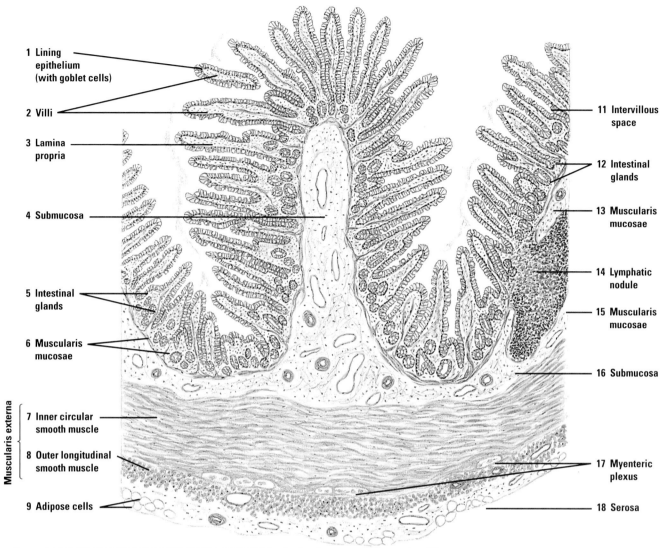

1 Lining epithelium (with goblet cells)

2 Villi

3 Lamina propria

4 Submucosa

5 Intestinal glands

6 Muscularis mucosae

Muscularis externa

7 Inner circular smooth muscle

8 Outer longitudinal smooth muscle

9 Adipose cells

11 Intervillous space

12 Intestinal glands

13 Muscularis mucosae

14 Lymphatic nodule

15 Muscularis mucosae

16 Submucosa

17 Myenteric plexus

18 Serosa

FIG. 1. JEJUNUM-ILEUM (TRANSVERSE SECTION). Stain: hematoxylin-eosin. 50 ×

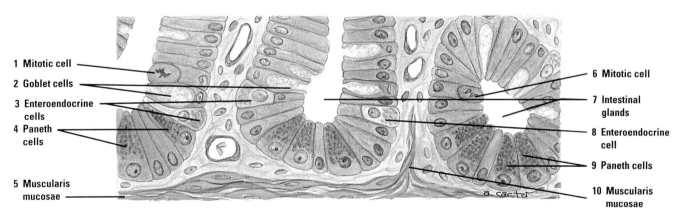

1 Mitotic cell

2 Goblet cells

3 Enteroendocrine cells

4 Paneth cells

5 Muscularis mucosae

6 Mitotic cell

7 Intestinal glands

8 Enteroendocrine cell

9 Paneth cells

10 Muscularis mucosae

FIG. 2. INTESTINAL GLANDS WITH PANETH CELLS AND ENTEROENDOCRINE CELLS. Stain: hematoxylin-eosin, plastic section.

181

PLATE 70

■ **FIG. 1**

SMALL INTESTINE: ILEUM WITH AGGREGATED NODULES (PEYER'S PATCH) (TRANSVERSE SECTION)

This cross section of the ileum illustrates the four coats of the intestinal wall **(9 through 16** inclusive). The **villi (1, 2, 9)** have been sectioned in various planes and thus appear irregular. The **intestinal glands (crypts of Lieberkühn) (3, 10)** are located in the lamina propria; two of these glands are illustrated opening into an intervillous space (upper leader 3, upper leader 10).

A characteristic feature of the ileum are the aggregations of lymphatic nodules called the **Peyer's patches (5).** Each Peyer's patch is an aggregation of ten or more lymphatic nodules, which are located in the wall of the ileum opposite the attachment of the mesentery. The portion of the Peyer's patch illustrated in this figure shows nine lymphatic nodules (4, 5, and others), most of which exhibit **germinal centers (5).** The lymphatic nodules coalesce and the boundaries between them are not usually discernible.

The nodules originate in the diffuse lymphatic tissue of the **lamina propria (11).** Villi are absent in the area of the intestinal lumen where the nodules reach the surface of the **mucosa (4).** Typically, the lymphatic nodules extend into the **submucosa (7, 13),** disrupt the **muscularis mucosae (6),** and spread out in the loose connective tissue of the submucosa (7, 13).

■ **FIG. 2**

SMALL INTESTINE: SECTIONS OF VILLI

The distal parts of villi that have been sectioned in different planes are illustrated at a higher magnification. Two of the villi are sectioned longitudinally (left and right). The central **villus (1)** was bent and sectioned in two parts; the apex has been sectioned transversely (1) and the lower portion **tangentially (7)** and **longitudinally (8).**

The **surface epithelium (2)** contains **goblet cells (9, 10, 13)** and columnar cells with **striated borders (14,** 15). A thin **basement membrane (5)** in different areas of the villi is visible between the surface epithelium (2) and the **lamina propria (12).** In the core of the lamina propria (12) are seen reticular cells of the stroma, lymphocytes, and **smooth muscle fibers (4, 16).** Present in each villus (but not always seen in sections) is a **central lacteal (3, 17),** a dilated lymphatic vessel lined with endothelium. Also seen in the villus are arterioles, one or more venules, and numerous **capillaries (11).**

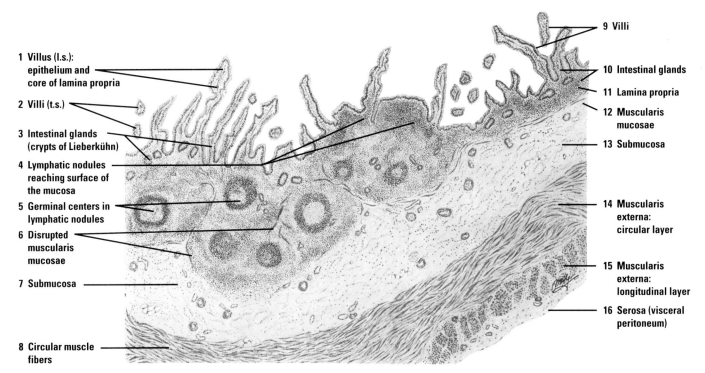

1 Villus (l.s.):
   epithelium and
   core of lamina propria

2 Villi (t.s.)

3 Intestinal glands
   (crypts of Lieberkühn)

4 Lymphatic nodules
   reaching surface of
   the mucosa

5 Germinal centers in
   lymphatic nodules

6 Disrupted
   muscularis
   mucosae

7 Submucosa

8 Circular muscle
   fibers

9 Villi

10 Intestinal glands

11 Lamina propria

12 Muscularis
   mucosae

13 Submucosa

14 Muscularis
   externa:
   circular layer

15 Muscularis
   externa:
   longitudinal layer

16 Serosa (visceral
   peritoneum)

FIG. 1. ILEUM WITH AGGREGATED NODULES (PEYER'S PATCH, TRANSVERSE SECTION). Stain: hematoxylin-eosin. 25×.

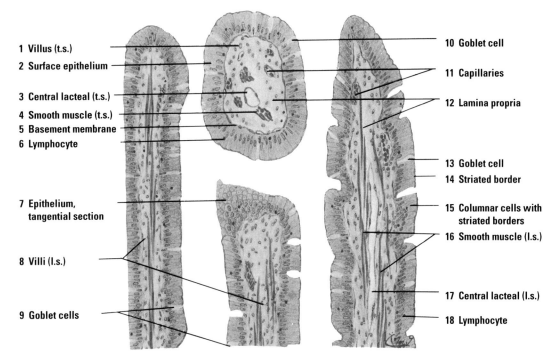

1 Villus (t.s.)

2 Surface epithelium

3 Central lacteal (t.s.)

4 Smooth muscle (t.s.)
5 Basement membrane
6 Lymphocyte

7 Epithelium,
   tangential section

8 Villi (l.s.)

9 Goblet cells

10 Goblet cell

11 Capillaries

12 Lamina propria

13 Goblet cell
14 Striated border

15 Columnar cells with
   striated borders
16 Smooth muscle (l.s.)

17 Central lacteal (l.s.)

18 Lymphocyte

FIG. 2. SMALL INTESTINE: VILLI. Stain: hematoxylin-eosin. 200×.

PLATE 71

LARGE INTESTINE: COLON AND MESENTERY (PANORAMIC VIEW, TRANSVERSE SECTION)

The colon has the same basic wall layers as the small intestine. These are the **mucosa (5, 6), submucosa (4), muscularis externa (1, 15, 16)** with two smooth muscle layers, and **serosa (2)** (in the regions of the transverse and sigmoid colon). Plate 72 illustrates in greater detail the characteristic features of each layer.

There are, however, several distinct modifications in the colon histology that distinguish it from other regions of the digestive tract. The colon does not have villi and the luminal surface of the mucosa is smooth. Plicae circularis are also absent from the colon; however, **temporary folds (7)** of the submucosa and mucosa are seen when the colon is undistended. The outer longitudinal layer of the muscularis externa is condensed into three broad, longitudinal bands of muscle called **taeniae coli (3, 12, 19).** In the rest of the colon wall, an extremely thin muscle layer is found between the taeniae coli (1, upper leader, 15); this muscle layer is often discontinuous. Between these two muscle layers of the muscularis externa are found the ganglion cells of the **myenteric (Auerbach's) plexus (18).**

Both the transverse and sigmoid portions of the colon are attached to the body wall by a **mesentery (9).** As a result, the serosa (2) becomes the outermost layer in these regions of the colon. The mesentery contains loose connective tissue, adipose tissue, blood vessels, and **nerves (10).**

LARGE INTESTINE: COLON (PANORAMIC VIEW, TRANSVERSE SECTION) AND MESENTERY

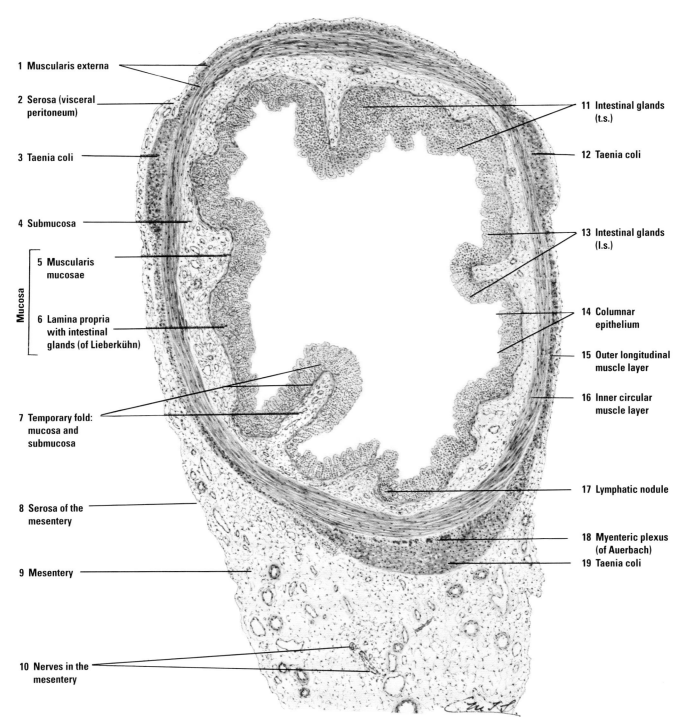

1 Muscularis externa

2 Serosa (visceral peritoneum)

3 Taenia coli

4 Submucosa

Mucosa
5 Muscularis mucosae

6 Lamina propria with intestinal glands (of Lieberkühn)

7 Temporary fold: mucosa and submucosa

8 Serosa of the mesentery

9 Mesentery

10 Nerves in the mesentery

11 Intestinal glands (t.s.)

12 Taenia coli

13 Intestinal glands (l.s.)

14 Columnar epithelium

15 Outer longitudinal muscle layer

16 Inner circular muscle layer

17 Lymphatic nodule

18 Myenteric plexus (of Auerbach)
19 Taenia coli

Stain: hematoxylin-eosin. 20×.

185

PLATE 72

LARGE INTESTINE: COLON WALL (TRANSVERSE SECTION)

A small section of an undistended colon wall is illustrated in greater detail. The four layers of the wall are the **mucosa (2, 3, 4), submucosa (5), muscularis externa (6),** and **serosa (7).** These layers are continuous with those of the small intestine. This section of the colon wall shows the **temporary fold (9)** of the mucosa (2, 3, 4) and submucosa (5).

The villi are absent in the colon. The mucosa, however, is indented by long tubular **intestinal glands** (crypts of Lieberkühn) **(1, 10),** which extend through the **lamina propria (3)** to the **muscularis mucosae (4, 11).**

The **lining epithelium (2)** in the colon is primarily columnar, with thin striated borders and numerous goblet cells. This epithelium continues into the intestinal glands (1, 10), where the goblet cells are abundant. Some of the intestinal glands (1, 10) may be seen sectioned in longitudinal, transverse, or oblique planes.

The lamina propria (2), similar to that in the small intestine, contains abundant diffuse lymphatic tissue. A distinct **lymphatic nodule (13)** is seen deep in the lamina propria (2). Some of the larger lymphatic nodules may extend through the muscularis mucosae (4, 11) into the submucosa (5).

The appearance and distribution of the muscularis mucosae (4, 11), submucosa (5), and serosa (7) are typical for the digestive tract. The muscularis externa (6), however, appears atypical. In this section, the longitudinal layer of the muscularis externa (6) is arranged into strips or bands of smooth muscle called the **taeniae coli (15).** The parasympathetic ganglia of the **myenteric plexus (8, 14)** are seen between the muscle layers in the muscularis externa (6).

The serosa (7) covers the transverse and sigmoid colon; however, the ascending and descending colon are retroperitoneal and the outer layer on their posterior surface is the adventitia.

LARGE INTESTINE: COLON (WALL, TRANSVERSE SECTION)

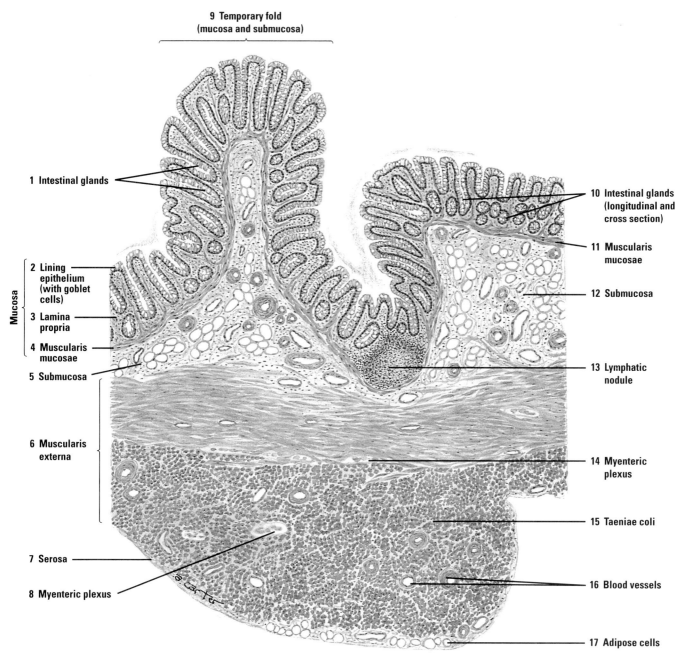

9 Temporary fold
(mucosa and submucosa)

1 Intestinal glands

Mucosa

2 Lining epithelium (with goblet cells)

3 Lamina propria

4 Muscularis mucosae

5 Submucosa

6 Muscularis externa

7 Serosa

8 Myenteric plexus

10 Intestinal glands (longitudinal and cross section)

11 Muscularis mucosae

12 Submucosa

13 Lymphatic nodule

14 Myenteric plexus

15 Taeniae coli

16 Blood vessels

17 Adipose cells

Stain: hematoxylin and eosin.

187

PLATE 73

APPENDIX (PANORAMIC VIEW, TRANSVERSE SECTION)

The figure illustrates a cross section of the vermiform appendix at low magnification. It is structurally similar to the colon except for certain modifications that are characteristic of the appendix.

In comparing the appendix with the colon, one sees that the mucosa exhibits a similar **lining epithelium (1)** with numerous goblet cells, the underlying **lamina propria (3)** containing the **intestinal glands (5)** (crypts of Lieberkühn), and the **muscularis mucosae (2).** The intestinal glands (5) in the appendix are less well developed, shorter, and often spaced farther apart than those in the colon. **Diffuse lymphatic tissue (6)** in the lamina propria (3) is abundant and is often observed in the adjacent **submucosa (8).**

Lymphatic nodules (4, 9) with germinal centers are very numerous and highly characteristic of the appendix. These nodules originate in the lamina propria (3); however, because of their large size, the nodules may extend from the surface epithelium (1) to the submucosa (8).

The submucosa (8) is highly vascular and exhibits numerous **blood vessels (11).** The **muscularis externa (7)** consists of the characteristic **inner circular (7a)** and **outer longitudinal layers (7b)** of smooth muscle; these muscle layers may vary in thickness. The **parasympathetic ganglia (12)** of the **myenteric plexus (12)** are seen between the inner and outer smooth muscle layers. **Serosa (10)** in the appendix is the outermost layer.

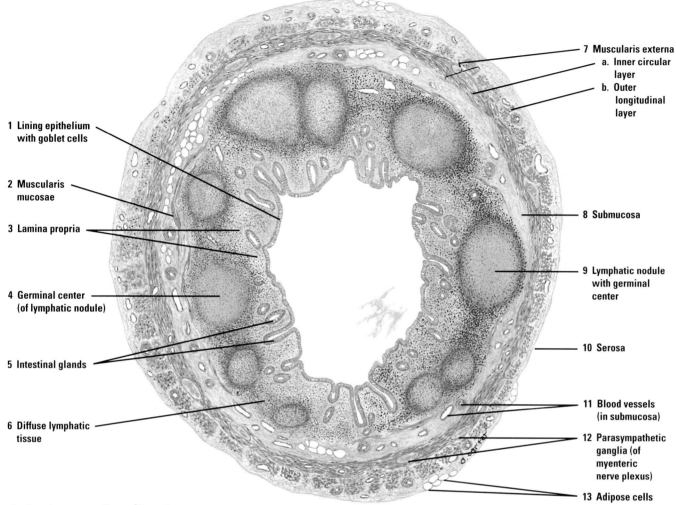

1 Lining epithelium with goblet cells

2 Muscularis mucosae

3 Lamina propria

4 Germinal center (of lymphatic nodule)

5 Intestinal glands

6 Diffuse lymphatic tissue

7 Muscularis externa
a. Inner circular layer
b. Outer longitudinal layer

8 Submucosa

9 Lymphatic nodule with germinal center

10 Serosa

11 Blood vessels (in submucosa)

12 Parasympathetic ganglia (of myenteric nerve plexus)

13 Adipose cells

Stain: hematoxylin and eosin.

PLATE 74

RECTUM: PANORAMIC VIEW, TRANSVERSE SECTION

This figure illustrates a transverse section through the upper rectum. The histology of the rectum is similar to that of the colon; the same **layers** are present in the wall **(3, 9, 12–15)** and the same components are found in each layer. Except for the **longitudinal muscle layer (14),** this figure could be a section of the colon.

The **surface epithelium (8)** is lined by columnar cells with striated borders and goblet cells. The **intestinal glands (10, 11)** in the wide **lamina propria (9)** are similar to those in the colon; however, the glands (10, 11) are longer, closer together, and contain almost all goblet cells.

Temporary **longitudinal folds (4)** may appear in the upper rectum and colon. These folds contain a core of submucosa **(12)** and are covered by **mucosa (4).** Permanent transversal folds of the rectum, if present in a section, would contain smooth muscle fibers from the circular layers of the muscularis externa. Permanent longitudinal folds (rectal columns) are found in the lower rectum, the anal canal.

Taeniae coli of the colon continue into the rectum where the **muscularis externa (13, 14)** again acquires the typical inner circular and outer longitudinal smooth muscle layers.

Adventitia (15) covers part of the rectum and serosa the remainder.

RECTUM (PANORAMIC VIEW, TRANSVERSE SECTION)

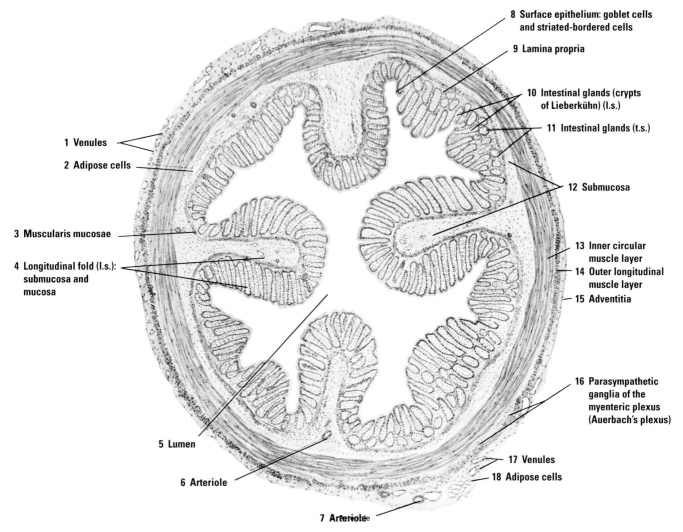

8 Surface epithelium: goblet cells and striated-bordered cells

9 Lamina propria

10 Intestinal glands (crypts of Lieberkühn) (l.s.)

11 Intestinal glands (t.s.)

1 Venules

2 Adipose cells

12 Submucosa

3 Muscularis mucosae

13 Inner circular muscle layer

14 Outer longitudinal muscle layer

4 Longitudinal fold (l.s.): submucosa and mucosa

15 Adventitia

16 Parasympathetic ganglia of the myenteric plexus (Auerbach's plexus)

5 Lumen

17 Venules

6 Arteriole

18 Adipose cells

7 Arteriole

Stain: hematoxylin-eosin. 40×.

191

PLATE 75

ANAL CANAL (LONGITUDINAL SECTION)

The **upper portion of the anal canal (A),** above the **anal valves (11),** represents the lowermost part of the rectum. The **lower part of the anal canal (B),** below the anal valves (11), shows the transition from the simple columnar epithelium to the stratified squamous epithelium of the skin. The change from the rectal mucosa to the anal mucosa occurs at the apex of the anal valves (**10,** 11). This region is the **anorectal junction (10).**

The **rectal mucosa (4–8)** is similar to the mucosa of colon; however, the **intestinal glands (7)** are shorter and farther apart. As a result, the **lamina propria (8)** is more prominent, diffuse lymphatic tissue more abundant, and solitary **lymphatic nodules (6)** more numerous.

The **muscularis mucosae (5, 12)** and the intestinal glands (7) of the digestive tract terminate in the vicinity of the anal valve (11). The lamina propria (8) of the rectum is replaced by the dense irregular connective tissue of the **lamina propria of the anal canal (13, lower leader).** The **submucosa (9)** of the rectum merges with the connective tissue in the lamina propria of the anal canal, a region that is highly vascular; the **internal hemorrhoidal plexus of veins (15)** lies in the mucosa of the anal canal. Blood vessels from this region continue into the submucosa (9) of the rectum. Internal hemorrhoids develop from chronic dilation of these vessels. External hemorrhoids develop from vessels of the external venous plexus of the anus (not illustrated in this figure).

The circular smooth muscle layer of the **muscularis externa (1)** increases in thickness in the upper region of the anal canal (A) and forms the **internal anal sphincter (1, 14).** Lower in the anal canal, this sphincter is replaced by skeletal muscles, the **external anal sphincter (16).** External to this sphincter is the skeletal **levator ani muscle (3).** The longitudinal muscle layer of the **muscularis externa (2)** becomes thin and disappears in the connective tissue of the external anal sphincter.

ANAL CANAL (LONGITUDINAL SECTION)

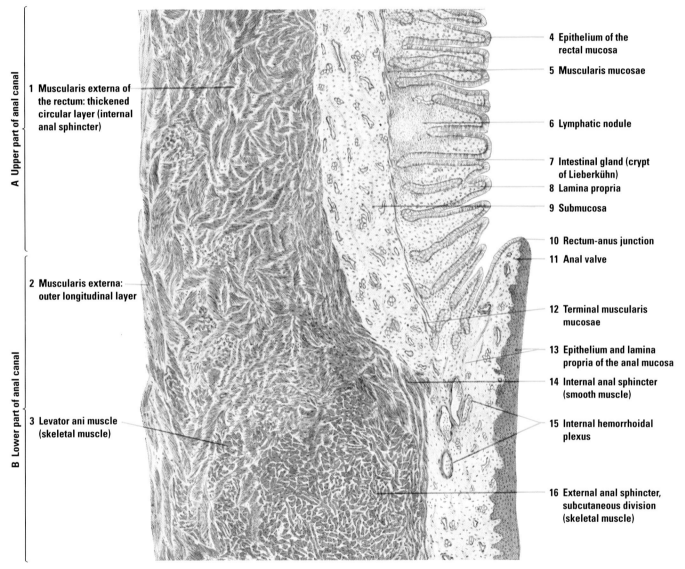

A Upper part of anal canal

B Lower part of anal canal

1 Muscularis externa of the rectum: thickened circular layer (internal anal sphincter)

2 Muscularis externa: outer longitudinal layer

3 Levator ani muscle (skeletal muscle)

4 Epithelium of the rectal mucosa

5 Muscularis mucosae

6 Lymphatic nodule

7 Intestinal gland (crypt of Lieberkühn)

8 Lamina propria

9 Submucosa

10 Rectum-anus junction

11 Anal valve

12 Terminal muscularis mucosae

13 Epithelium and lamina propria of the anal mucosa

14 Internal anal sphincter (smooth muscle)

15 Internal hemorrhoidal plexus

16 External anal sphincter, subcutaneous division (skeletal muscle)

Stain: hematoxylin-eosin. 25×.

THE DIGESTIVE SYSTEM: THE ACCESSORY DIGESTIVE ORGANS

The liver, gallbladder, and pancreas are the accessory digestive organs that are associated with the small intestine. The cells of the liver and pancreas secrete numerous products for digestion; these are then delivered into the duodenum by a duct common to both organs.

The Liver

The liver has a highly strategic location in the body. All venous blood that returns from the digestive organs and spleen by way of the portal vein first percolates through the liver. Because venous blood is poor in oxygen, the liver is also supplied by the hepatic artery. Thus, the liver has a dual blood supply.

The mixing of the venous and arterial blood occurs only in the hepatic sinusoids of the liver as it flows toward the central vein of the liver lobule. The liver sinusoids are dilated blood channels lined by a discontinuous layer of fenestrated endothelial cells, which are separated from the underlying liver cells, the hepatocytes, by a perisinusoidal space (of Disse). As a result of this arrangement, the material carried in the blood percolates through the discontinuous endothelial wall and comes in direct contact with the hepatocytes. This allows for a more efficient exchange of materials between the blood and hepatocytes and vice versa.

The hepatocytes are highly versatile cells that perform numerous vital functions. They are exocrine cells because they synthesize and release a secretory product (bile) into a system of ducts. The hepatocytes are also endocrine cells because many of their products are released directly into the blood stream as the blood percolates through the sinusoids. Thus, the liver cells perform both endocrine and exocrine functions.

The main exocrine function of the hepatocytes is the secretion of bile, which enters tiny bile canaliculi located between adjacent hepatocytes. In the liver, the bile flows toward the bile duct located at the periphery of the liver lobule and exactly in the opposite direction to the flow of blood. The bile salts that are present in the bile emulsify the fats that enter the small intestine from the stomach. This action of the bile promotes easier digestion of the fats by the fat-digesting enzymes, the lipases, and their subsequent absorption by the cells in the small intestine. Bile salts also solubilize cholesterol and facilitate its excretion from the body.

The endocrine functions of the liver are related to the synthesis of numerous plasma proteins, among which are the blood clotting factors prothrombin and fibrinogen, and albumen. Liver also stores fats, various vitamins, and glucose as glycogen. When the cells of the body need glucose, glycogen that is stored in the liver is converted back into glucose and released into the blood stream. Liver cells also detoxify various drugs and harmful chemicals. Also, specialized cells located in the hepatic sinusoids (called Kupffer cells) remove from the blood and phagocytize particulate material and cellular debris. In the fetus, the liver cells are involved in hemopoietic functions. Thus, the liver is essential to life.

The Gallbladder

The gallbladder is a small, hollow organ attached to the inferior surface of the liver. Its main functions are to receive, store, and concentrate bile by absorbing its water. In response to the presence of fats in the small intestine, a hormone, cholecystokinin, is released into the blood stream by the enteroendocrine (APUD) cells located in the intestinal mucosa. Cholecystokinin causes the contraction of the smooth muscles in the wall of the gallbladder and forces the bile into the duodenum by way of the common bile duct.

The Pancreas

The pancreas is the main accessory digestive organ that produces an alkaline fluid with numerous digestive enzymes that break down proteins, fats, and carbohydrates into smaller molecules for absorption in the small intestine. Most of the pancreas consists of exocrine secretory units or acinar cells; these cells secrete the pancreatic enzymes. Pancreatic secretions are regulated by both hormones and vagal stimulation. Two intestinal hormones, secretin and cholecystokinin, which are secreted by the enteroendocrine (APUD) cells of the duodenal mucosa into the blood stream, regulate the pancreatic secretions. In response to acidic chyme in the duodenum, secretin release stimulates the pancreatic cells (probably the duct cells) to secrete large amounts of watery fluid rich in sodium bicarbonate ions. The function of this fluid is to neutralize the acidic chyme for activity of the pancreatic enzymes. In response to presence of fats and proteins in the duodenum, cholecystokinin release stimulates the acinar cells in the pancreas to secrete large amounts of different digestive enzymes. The pancreatic enzymes are released into the duodenum in an inactive form and then activated by a hormone secreted by duodenal mucosa.

Scattered throughout the secretory acini in the pancreas are pale-staining, spherical units of cells called the islets of Langerhans; these islets constitute the endocrine portion of the pancreas. With special stains, three main types of cells can be identified in the islets of Langerhans: alpha, beta, and delta. The islet cells produce two very important hormones, insulin and glucagon. The alpha cells produce glucagon, whose main physiologic function is to increase the levels of glucose in the blood. This function is primarily accomplished by accelerating the conversion of glycogen, amino acids, and fatty acids in the liver into glucose; these actions elevate the sugar levels in the blood. The beta cells of the islets produce insulin. The main physiologic function of insulin is to lower the glucose levels in the blood by accelerating membrane transport of glucose into cells, especially into the muscle fibers (cells). Insulin also accelerates the conversion of glucose into glycogen. The effects of insulin on the levels of blood glucose are just the opposite of those of glucagon.

PLATE 76

■ **FIG. 1**
PIG'S LIVER (PANORAMIC VIEW, TRANSVERSE SECTION)

■ **FIG. 2**
PRIMATE LIVER

PLATE 76

■ **FIG. 1**
PIG'S LIVER (PANORAMIC VIEW, TRANSVERSE SECTION)

The connective tissue from the liver hilus extends between the liver lobes as interlobular septa. In the pig's liver, the individual **hepatic (liver) lobules (7)** are well defined. To illustrate the boundaries of the hepatic lobules, a section of pig's liver was stained with Mallory-Azan stain, which stains the connective tissue septa dark blue.

This figure illustrates, in transverse section, a complete hepatic lobule (on the left) and parts of several adjacent **hepatic lobules (7).** The blue-staining **interlobular septa (5, 9)** contain interlobular branches of the **portal vein, bile duct,** and **hepatic artery (2, 3, 4, 11, 12, 13).** These regions around the hepatic lobule are collectively considered **portal canals** or **areas.** Around the periphery of each lobule can be seen several portal canals within the interlobular septa (5, 9). The interlobular septa (5, 9) also contain small lymphatic vessels

and nerves; however, these structures are small, inconspicuous, and seen only occasionally.

In the center of each hepatic lobule (7) is a **central vein (1, 8).** Radiating from the central vein (1, 8) toward the periphery of the lobule are **plates of hepatic cells (6).** Located between the hepatic plates (6) are the **hepatic sinusoids (10).** On entering the liver, arterial and venous blood mixes in these sinusoids and then flows toward the central veins (1, 8) of the lobule (7). Bile is formed in the liver cells and flows through the minute bile canaliculi in the opposite direction into the interlobular **bile ducts (2, 12)** (See also Plate 77, Fig. 3).

The interlobular vessels and bile ducts (2, 3, 4, 11, 12, 13) exhibit numerous branches in the liver parenchyma. Thus, in a cross section of the liver lobule, it is possible to see more than one section of each of these structures within a portal area.

■ **FIG. 2**
PRIMATE LIVER

In the primate or human liver, the connective tissue septa between individual **hepatic lobules (8)** are not as conspicuous as in the pig's liver. As a result, the liver sinusoids are continuous from one lobule to the next. Despite these differences, portal areas containing the interlobular branches of the **portal veins, hepatic arteries,** and **bile ducts (1, 2, 3, 11, 12, 13)** are visible around the peripheries of different lobules.

This figure illustrates numerous hepatic lobules (8). In the center of each hepatic lobule (8) is the **central vein (6, 9).** The **hepatic sinusoids (5)** are seen between the **hepatic plates (7)** that radiate from the central veins (6, 9) toward the periphery of the hepatic lobule (8). As illustrated in Fig. 1, numerous branches of interlobular vessels and bile ducts are seen within the portal areas of a given hepatic lobule (8).

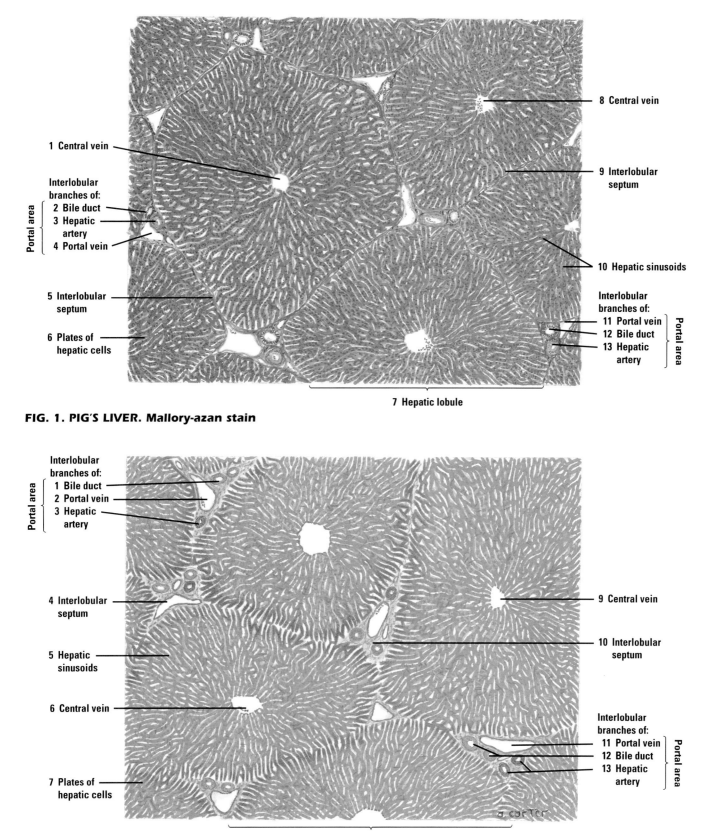

1 Central vein

Interlobular
branches of:
Portal area
2 Bile duct
3 Hepatic artery
4 Portal vein

5 Interlobular septum

6 Plates of hepatic cells

8 Central vein

9 Interlobular septum

10 Hepatic sinusoids

Interlobular
branches of:
11 Portal vein
12 Bile duct
13 Hepatic artery
Portal area

7 Hepatic lobule

FIG. 1. PIG'S LIVER. Mallory-azan stain

Interlobular
branches of:
Portal area
1 Bile duct
2 Portal vein
3 Hepatic artery

4 Interlobular septum

5 Hepatic sinusoids

6 Central vein

7 Plates of hepatic cells

9 Central vein

10 Interlobular septum

Interlobular
branches of:
11 Portal vein
12 Bile duct
13 Hepatic artery
Portal area

FIG. 2. PRIMATE LIVER. Hematoxylin-eosin stain

PLATE 77

■ **FIG. 1**
HEPATIC (LIVER) LOBULE (SECTIONAL VIEW, TRANSVERSE SECTION)

A portion of a hepatic lobule between the **central vein (1)** and the peripheral **interlobular septum (9)** is illustrated in greater detail and higher magnification than on Plate 76.

The central vein (1) is a venule lined with **endothelium (3)**. At the periphery of the lobule is the **interlobular septum (9)** with the portal area, which consists of a **portal vein (8)**, two **branches of the hepatic artery (6, 12)**, four sections of the **bile duct (7, 14)** and a **lymphatic vessel (13)**.

The hepatic lobule consists of **plates of hepatic cells (11)**. These plates branch and anastomose within the lobule. At the periphery of the lobule, the hepatic cells form a solid **limiting plate (10)**, which separates the hepatic plates and sinusoids from the interlobular con-

nective tissue septum (9). The portal venules and hepatic arterioles penetrate the connective tissue to form the **sinusoids (2, 5)**.

The hepatic cells (11) are polygonal, vary in size, contain a large, round vesicular nucleus, and may occasionally be binucleate. The cells have a granular acidophilic cytoplasm which varies with their functional state (see also Fig. 2).

The **sinusoids (2, 5)** are situated between plates of hepatic cells, and follow their branchings and anastomoses. The sinusoids (2, 5) are lined with a discontinuous type of endothelium (3). Also present in the sinusoid wall are fixed macrophages, the Kupffer cells (see Fig. 2). The blood in the sinusoids, containing **erythrocytes (4)** and leukocytes, drains into the central vein (1).

■ **FIG. 2**
LIVER: KUPFFER CELLS (INDIA INK PREPARATION)

To demonstrate the phagocytic system in the **sinusoids (2)** of the liver, a rabbit liver was intravenously injected with India ink. The **Kupffer cells (1, 5)**, because of their phagocytosis of carbon particles, appear prominent in the sinusoids between the **hepatic cells (4)**. The phagocytic Kupffer cells (1, 5) are large with several

processes, and exhibit an irregular or stellate outline. Because of the increased phagocytosis, the nucleus is obscured by the accumulation of ingested carbon particles. **Endothelial cells (3)** are also visible in the sinusoids (2); they are smaller and usually only the nucleus is visible.

■ **FIG. 3**
LIVER: BILE CANALICULI (OSMIC ACID PREPARATION)

A section of liver was fixed in osmic acid and the sections prepared and stained with hematoxylin-eosin. Osmic acid fixation reveals the **bile canaliculi (2, 8)**, which are minute channels between individual cells in the **hepatic plates (1, 6)**. The canaliculi follow an irregular course between the hepatic cells and branch freely

within the hepatic plates (1, 6). In this figure, some canaliculi (8) are illustrated in a transverse plane.

The **sinusoids (4, 5)** are lined by **endothelial cells (7)** with small nuclei and a **Kupffer cell (9)** with a larger nucleus and branched cytoplasm. Also illustrated is a sinusoid (4, upper leader) opening into a central vein.

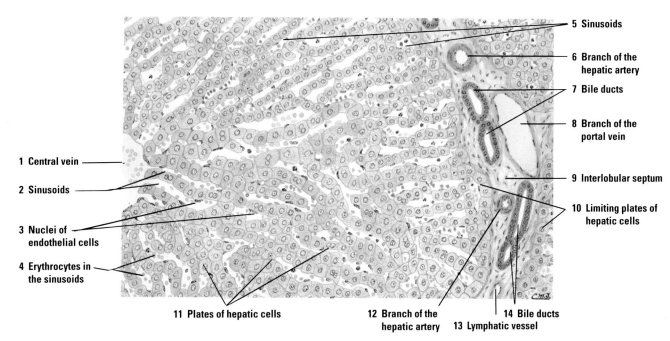

5 Sinusoids

6 Branch of the hepatic artery

7 Bile ducts

8 Branch of the portal vein

9 Interlobular septum

10 Limiting plates of hepatic cells

1 Central vein

2 Sinusoids

3 Nuclei of endothelial cells

4 Erythrocytes in the sinusoids

11 Plates of hepatic cells

12 Branch of the hepatic artery

13 Lymphatic vessel

14 Bile ducts

FIG. 1. LIVER LOBULE (SECTIONAL VIEW, TRANSVERSE SECTION). Stain: hematoxylin-eosin. 285×.

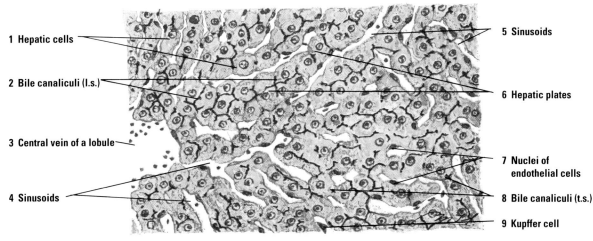

1 Kupffer cells gorged with carbon particles

2 Sinusoids

3 Endothelial cell (nucleus)

4 Hepatic cells

5 Kupffer cells gorged with carbon particles

FIG. 2. LIVER: KUPFFER CELLS (INDIA INK PREPARATION). Stain: hematoxylin-eosin. 350×.

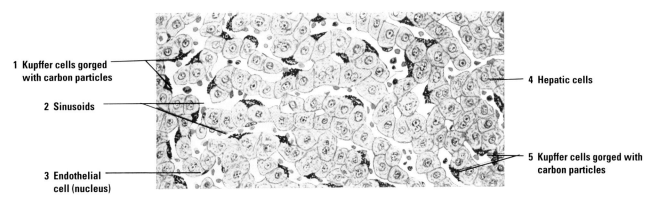

1 Hepatic cells

2 Bile canaliculi (l.s.)

3 Central vein of a lobule

4 Sinusoids

5 Sinusoids

6 Hepatic plates

7 Nuclei of endothelial cells

8 Bile canaliculi (t.s.)

9 Kupffer cell

FIG. 3. LIVER: BILE CANALICULI (OSMIC ACID PREPARATION). Stain: hematoxylin-eosin. 300×.

PLATE 78

■ **FIG. 1**
MITOCHONDRIA AND FAT DROPLETS IN LIVER CELLS (ALTMANN'S STAIN)

This liver section was fixed in potassium bichromate and osmic acid, and then stained with acid fuchsin and picric acid. This preparation stains **mitochondria (2)** red. The **fat droplets (1)** usually stain black after osmic acid fixation, but in this preparation stain blue.

■ **FIG. 2**
GLYCOGEN IN LIVER CELLS (BEST'S CARMINE STAIN)

Staining the liver sections with alcohol and ammonia solution of carmine demonstrates **glycogen (1)** as red granules that exhibit an irregular distribution within the cytoplasm. If the sections are previously stained with Meyer's hemalum, the nuclei appear violet.

■ **FIG. 3**
RETICULAR FIBERS IN A HEPATIC LOBULE (DEL RIO HORTEGA'S STAIN)

The Del Rio Hortega modification of ammonium silver carbonate method for silver impregnation demonstrates the fine fibrillar structure of the liver stroma. The reticular fibers stain black and the liver cells pale violet.

The reticular fibers form most of the supporting connective tissue of the liver. They line the liver **sinusoids** **(1)** between the hepatocytes and the discontinuous endothelial cells, and form a dense network of **fibers (3)** around the **central vein (2).**

The collagenous fibers in the dense irregular connective tissue of the **interlobular septa (4)** stain dark brown; the reticular fibers merge with these fibers.

LIVER

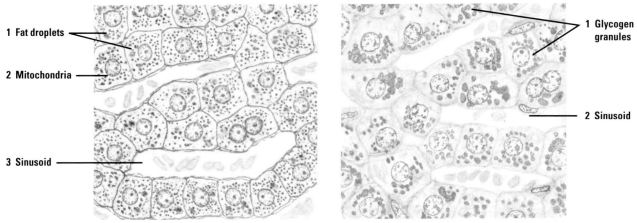

1 Fat droplets

2 Mitochondria

3 Sinusoid

1 Glycogen granules

2 Sinusoid

FIG. 1. MITOCHONDRIA (RED) AND FAT DROPLETS (BLUE) IN LIVER CELLS (ALTMANN'S STAIN). Fixation in Champy's fluid. 800×.

FIG. 2. GLYCOGEN IN LIVER CELLS. Best's carmine stain. 800×.

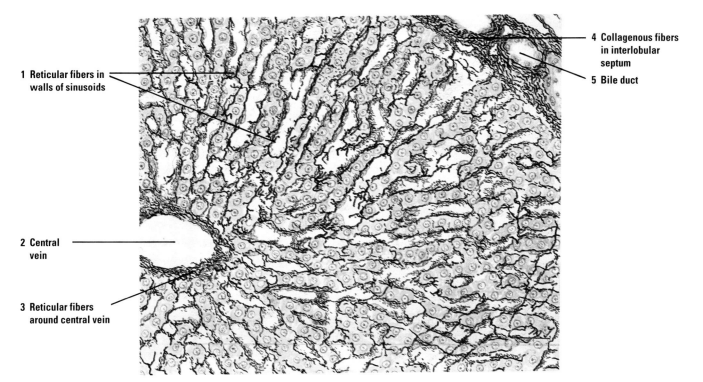

1 Reticular fibers in walls of sinusoids

4 Collagenous fibers in interlobular septum

5 Bile duct

2 Central vein

3 Reticular fibers around central vein

FIG. 3. RETICULAR FIBERS IN A HEPATIC LOBULE. Stain: Del Rio Hortega. 300×.

PLATE 79

GALLBLADDER

The wall of the gallbladder consists of a **mucosa (3, 4, 5)**, a **fibromuscular layer (2)**, a perimuscular **connective tissue layer (1, 10)**, and a **serosa (6)** on all of its surface except the hepatic, where an adventitia attaches it to the liver.

The mucosa exhibits temporary **folds (15)**, which disappear when the gallbladder is distended with bile. These folds resemble the villi in the small intestine; however, they vary in size, shape and irregular arrangement. The **crypts** or **diverticula (16)** between the folds often form deep indentations in the mucosa. In cross section, these **diverticula (18)** in the lamina propria resemble tubular glands; however, there are no glands in the gallbladder proper (except in the neck region).

The **lining epithelium (5, 14, 20)** is a simple tall columnar epithelium with lightly stained cytoplasm and basal nuclei. The **lamina propria (4, 17)** contains loose connective tissue and some diffuse lymphatic tissue.

The **smooth muscle fibers (7)** in the fibromuscular layer (2) are interspersed within the layers of loose connective tissue that are rich in **elastic fibers (8).** In contrast to other organs in which a serosa or adventitia covers the muscular layer, the gallbladder has a wide layer of perimuscular loose connective tissue (1, 10), which contain **blood vessels (11, 13)**, lymphatics, and **nerves (12);** serosa (6) is the outermost layer and covers all of these structures.

GALLBLADDER

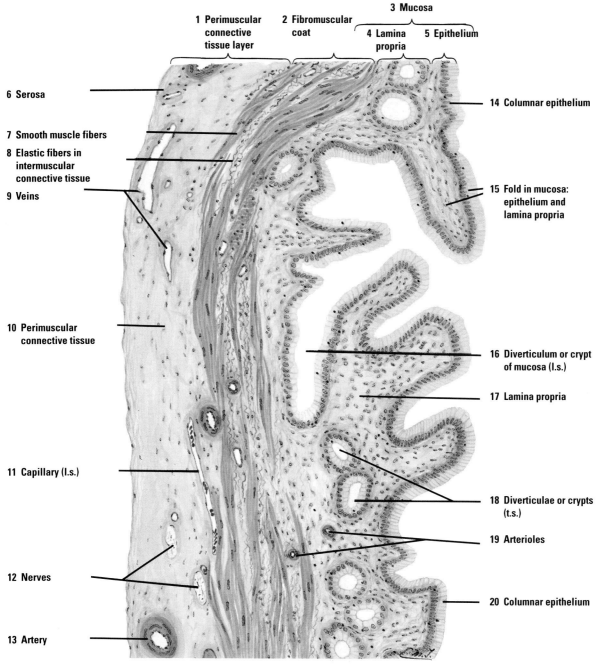

1 Perimuscular connective tissue layer

2 Fibromuscular coat

3 Mucosa

4 Lamina propria

5 Epithelium

6 Serosa

7 Smooth muscle fibers

8 Elastic fibers in intermuscular connective tissue

9 Veins

10 Perimuscular connective tissue

11 Capillary (l.s.)

12 Nerves

13 Artery

14 Columnar epithelium

15 Fold in mucosa: epithelium and lamina propria

16 Diverticulum or crypt of mucosa (l.s.)

17 Lamina propria

18 Diverticulae or crypts (t.s.)

19 Arterioles

20 Columnar epithelium

Stain: hematoxylin-eosin. 120×.

PLATE 80

■ **FIG. 1**
PANCREAS (SECTIONAL VIEW)

The pancreas consists of **serous acini (2, 15)** arranged into numerous small lobules and surrounded by intralobular and interlobular connective tissue with their corresponding **ducts (1, 5, 20; 10, 11)**. Within the masses of serous acini are found isolated **pancreatic islets (of Langerhans) (4, 8, 9)**, which are characteristic features of the organ.

A **pancreatic acinus (2, 15, I)** consists of pyramidal **secretory (zymogenic) cells (I, 21)** and small **centroacinar cells (22)** within its lumen. The secretory products from individual acini are drained by long, narrow **intercalated ducts (intralobular ducts) (1, 5, 20, II)**, which exhibit small lumina and are lined by low cuboidal cells. The ductal epithelium extends into individual acini and is visible as the pale-staining cen-troacinar cells (22). The intercalated ducts then drain into larger **interlobular ducts (11, 19, III)**, which are lined with columnar epithelium and found in the **connective tissue septa (10)**.

The **pancreatic islets (of Langerhans) (4, 8, 9)** are round masses of endocrine cells of varying size that are demarcated from the surrounding acinar tissue by thin layer of reticular fibers; the islets are normally larger than the individual acini. Under higher magnification (IV), the islets appear as compact clusters of **epithelial cells (23)** permeated by a rich network of **capillaries (24)**.

Located in the connective tissue septa of the pancreas are **blood vessels (6, 7, 12, 13, 18)**, **nerves (14, 17)**, occasional small ganglia, and **Pacinian corpuscles (16)**.

■ **FIG. 2**
PANCREATIC ACINI (SPECIAL PREPARATION)

With special staining of pancreatic acini with Gomori's chrome hematoxylin-phloxine, the **zymogen granules (1)** stain red and the **basophilic (chromophilic) substance (2)** stains blue. The upper triangle of the figure is similar to Figure 1 (90X). The lower tri-angle has a higher magnification (450X) and illustrates the zymogen granules (1) filling the apical portion of the cells (storage phase). In the basal portion of the cells, this stain illustrates the basophilic cytoplasm and its striations (2). The nucleus lies in this zone.

■ **FIG. 3**
PANCREATIC ISLETS (SPECIAL PREPARATION)

In a pancreatic islet (of Langerhans), the Gomori's chrome hematoxylin-phloxine stain distinguishes the **alpha (A) cells (1)** and the **beta (B) cells (2)**. Granules in alpha (A) cells (1) stain red, while the granules of beta (B) cells (2) stain blue. Cell membranes are usually more distinguishable in alpha cells (1). Also, the alpha (A) cells (1) are situated more peripherally in the islet and the beta (B) cells (2), in general, lie deeper. In addi-tion, the beta (B) cells (2) are the predominant cell type of the pancreatic islets and constitute about 60% of their mass. The delta (D) cells (not illustrated) are also seen in the islets. These cells are least abundant, have variable cell shape, and may occur anywhere in the pancreatic islet.

Numerous **capillaries (3)** are clearly visible, demonstrating the rich vascularity of the pancreatic islets.

PANCREAS

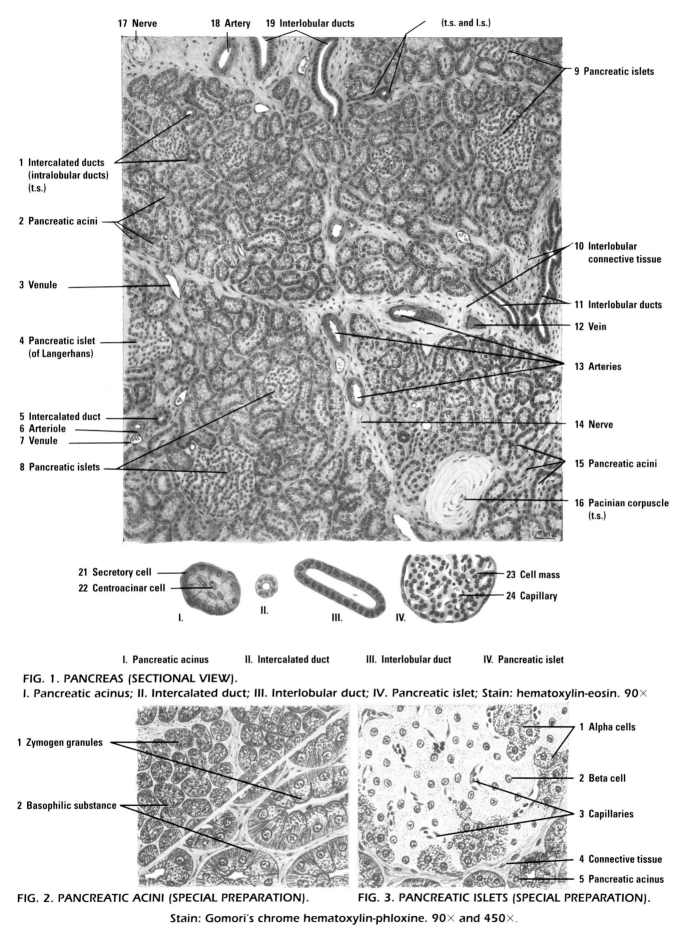

17 Nerve   18 Artery   19 Interlobular ducts   (t.s. and l.s.)

9 Pancreatic islets

1 Intercalated ducts
(intralobular ducts)
(t.s.)

2 Pancreatic acini

3 Venule

4 Pancreatic islet
(of Langerhans)

5 Intercalated duct
6 Arteriole
7 Venule

8 Pancreatic islets

10 Interlobular
connective tissue

11 Interlobular ducts

12 Vein

13 Arteries

14 Nerve

15 Pancreatic acini

16 Pacinian corpuscle
(t.s.)

21 Secretory cell
22 Centroacinar cell

23 Cell mass
24 Capillary

I.   II.   III.   IV.

I. Pancreatic acinus   II. Intercalated duct   III. Interlobular duct   IV. Pancreatic islet

FIG. 1. PANCREAS (SECTIONAL VIEW).
I. Pancreatic acinus; II. Intercalated duct; III. Interlobular duct; IV. Pancreatic islet; Stain: hematoxylin-eosin. 90×

1 Zymogen granules

2 Basophilic substance

1 Alpha cells

2 Beta cell

3 Capillaries

4 Connective tissue
5 Pancreatic acinus

FIG. 2. PANCREATIC ACINI (SPECIAL PREPARATION).   FIG. 3. PANCREATIC ISLETS (SPECIAL PREPARATION).

Stain: Gomori's chrome hematoxylin-phloxine. 90× and 450×.

THE RESPIRATORY SYSTEM

The respiratory system consists of two lungs and numerous tubes that lead to and from each lung. The respiratory system is normally divided into an air-conducting portion and a respiratory portion. The epithelium in the extrapulmonary passages and in the larger tubes is pseudostratified ciliated epithelium with numerous goblet cells. As the conducting tubes enter the lungs and become progressively smaller, the height of the epithelium and the amount of goblet cells gradually diminish. In those regions of the lungs where gaseous exchange takes place, the epithelium is simple squamous and the goblet cells are absent.

The Conducting Portion

The conducting portion of the respiratory system consists of extrapulmonary nasal cavities, pharynx, larynx, trachea, bronchi, and a series of intrapulmonary bronchi and bronchioles with decreasing diameters, culminating in the terminal bronchioles. Hyaline cartilage plays an important supporting role in the conducting system by providing support for the structures and keeping their passageways patent (open). In the trachea, incomplete cartilage rings encircle its lumen. As the trachea divides into bronchi and the bronchi enter the lungs, the cartilage rings are replaced by cartilage plates. As the bronchi become smaller, the cartilage plates become reduced in size and number. Cartilage plates disappear from the conducting passageways when the size of the bronchioles is reduced to about 1 mm in diameter. The final air passageways of the conducting system are the terminal bronchioles, whose diameters range from 0.5 mm to 1.00 mm.

The main functions of the conducting portion of the respiratory system are to condition and deliver air from the external environment to the respiratory portion in the lungs. Here an exchange of oxygen and carbon dioxide takes place between the blood and inspired air. Mucus plays an important role in conditioning the air. It is constantly produced by the goblet cells in the respiratory epithelium and mucous glands in the lamina propria; the mucous layer covers the luminal surfaces in most of the conducting tubes. As a result, air that enters the conducting portion from the external environment is warmed, humidified, and cleansed of particulate matter, infectious microorganisms, or other airborne matter. Goblet cells,

however, lack in the epithelium that lines the bronchioles.

The Olfactory Portion

The roof of the nasal cavity contains an area of epithelium that is specialized for reception and transmission of smell. This region is the olfactory epithelium. Some cells in the olfactory epithelium are the sensory bipolar neurons; these cells end at the surface of the olfactory epithelium as small olfactory vesicles. Radiating from each olfactory vesicle are long, nonmotile cilia that lie flat on the epithelial surface in the overlying mucus and function as odor receptors. For an individual to smell or to detect odor, the odoriferous substances must first be dissolved. For this reason, the olfactory epithelium is always kept moist by a thin, watery secretion produced by the Bowman's glands located below the epithelium in the lamina propria. The secretion from these glands continuously washes over the surface of the olfactory epithelium and in this manner, allows the receptor cells to respond to new odors.

The Respiratory Portion

The respiratory portion is the distal continuation of the conducting portion. It consists of the respiratory bronchioles, alveolar ducts, alveolar sacs, and alveoli. The terminal bronchioles give rise to respiratory bronchioles. These bronchioles represent the transitional structures between the conducting and respiratory portions of the respiratory system because the respiratory bronchioles contain thin-walled outpocketings, the alveoli. Respiration or gaseous exchange can only occur in the alveoli because the barrier between the inspired air in the alveoli and blood in the capillaries is extremely thin. Thus, the functional units of the lung are the alveoli.

The alveoli consist of two types of cells. The most abundant cells are the Type I pneumocytes or squamous alveolar cells. These cells are thin and line all of the alveolar surfaces. The remaining cells interspersed among the squamous alveolar cells singly or in small groups are the type II pneumocytes or great alveolar cells. These cells are secretory in nature and secrete a phospholipid-rich product called pulmonary surfactant. As surfactant is released from the cells, it spreads over the alveolar cell surfaces and lowers the surface tension in the alveoli. Decreased surface tension in the alveoli stabilizes their diameters and prevents their collapse during the respiratory processes. During fetal development, surfactant is secreted by type II pneumocytes during the last weeks of gestation.

Alveolar macrophages or dust cells, which are derived from the blood monocytes, are also associated with the alveoli. They are found in the alveolar septa and on the surface of the alveoli. The primary function of the alveolar macrophages is protection; they clean the alveoli of the lungs of invading microorganisms and inhaled particulate matter.

PLATE 81

■ **FIG. 1**
OLFACTORY MUCOSA AND SUPERIOR CONCHA, RHESUS MONKEY, (GENERAL VIEW)

■ **FIG. 2**
OLFACTORY MUCOSA: DETAIL OF A TRANSITIONAL AREA

PLATE 81

■ **FIG. 1**
OLFACTORY MUCOSA AND SUPERIOR CONCHA, RHESUS MONKEY (GENERAL VIEW)

The **olfactory mucosa (2, 5)** is illustrated on the surface of the **superior concha (1)**, one of the bony shelves in the nasal cavity.

The respiratory epithelium in the nasal cavity is pseudostratified ciliated columnar with goblet cells. The **olfactory epithelium (2, 5;** Fig. 2) is specialized for reception of smell and therefore differs from the respiratory epithelium; it is pseudostratified tall columnar epithelium without goblet cells. The olfactory epithelium is found in the roof of each nasal cavity, on each side of the septum, and in the upper nasal conchae.

The underlying **lamina propria (2)** contains the branched tubuloacinar **olfactory glands** of **Bowman (3, 6)**. These glands produce a serous secretion, in contrast to mixed mucous and serous secretion produced by the glands in the rest of the nasal cavity. Numerous small nerves found in the connective tissue of the lamina propria are the olfactory nerves or **fila olfactoria (4, 7)**. These nerves represent the aggregated axons of the olfactory cells. The lamina propria (2) merges with the periosteum of the bone.

■ **FIG. 2**
OLFACTORY MUCOSA: DETAIL OF A TRANSITIONAL AREA

This illustration depicts a transitional area between the **olfactory (1)** and **respiratory epithelia (9)**. In this region, the histologic differences between these two important epithelia become obvious. The olfactory epithelium (1) is tall, pseudostratified columnar epithelium, composed of three different cell types: the supporting, basal, and neuroepithelial olfactory cells. The individual cell outlines are difficult to distinguish in a routine histologic preparation; however, the location and shape of nuclei allow some identification of different cell types that comprise the olfactory epithelium (1).

The **supportive or sustentacular cells (3)** are elongated, with their oval nuclei situated more apically or superficially in the epithelium than the nuclei of the **olfactory cells (4)**. The broad apical surfaces of the olfactory cells (4) contain slender microvilli that protrude into the overlying layer of surface **mucus (2)**; basally, the cells are slender.

The olfactory cells (4) have oval or round nuclei that occupy a region in the epithelium that is somewhat between the nuclei of the supportive cells (3) and **basal cells (5)**. The apices of the olfactory cells (4) are slender and pass to the epithelial surface. Extending from the slender cell bases are axons that pass into the underlying connective tissue or **lamina propria (6)**, where they aggregate into small bundles of unmyelinated olfactory nerves, the **fila olfactoria (14)**. These nerves ultimately leave the nasal cavity and pass into the olfactory bulbs at the base of the brain. The **basal cells (5)** are short, small cells located at the base of the epithelium and between the bases of supportive (3) and olfactory cells (4).

The transition from the olfactory (1) to the respiratory (9) epithelium is abrupt. In this illustration, the respiratory epithelium (9) is pseudostratified columnar epithelium with distinct surface **cilia (10)** and an abundance of **goblet cells (11)**; the goblet cells are not present in the olfactory epithelium (1). Also, in the transition area, the height of the respiratory epithelium appears similar to that of the olfactory; however, in other regions of the respiratory tract, the epithelial height is much reduced in comparison to olfactory epithelium.

Beneath the olfactory epithelium (1) is the lamina propria (6), containing a rich supply of capillaries, lymphatic vessels, **arterioles (8)**, and **venules (13)**. In addition to olfactory nerves (14), the lamina propria also contains branched, tubuloacinar **olfactory glands (of Bowman) (7)**. These serous glands deliver their secretions through narrow **ducts (12)**, which penetrate the olfactory epithelium (1) and open onto the surface. The secretions from these glands moisten the olfactory mucosa and provide the necessary solvent, in which the odoriferous substances dissolve and stimulate the olfactory receptor cells (3).

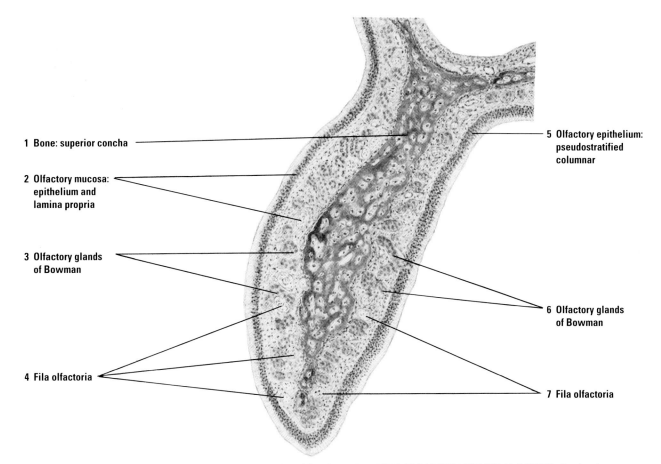

1 Bone: superior concha

2 Olfactory mucosa: epithelium and lamina propria

3 Olfactory glands of Bowman

4 Fila olfactoria

5 Olfactory epithelium: pseudostratified columnar

6 Olfactory glands of Bowman

7 Fila olfactoria

FIG. 1. OLFACTORY MUCOSA AND SUPERIOR CONCHA, RHESUS MONKEY (GENERAL VIEW). Stain: hematoxylin-eosin. 60×.

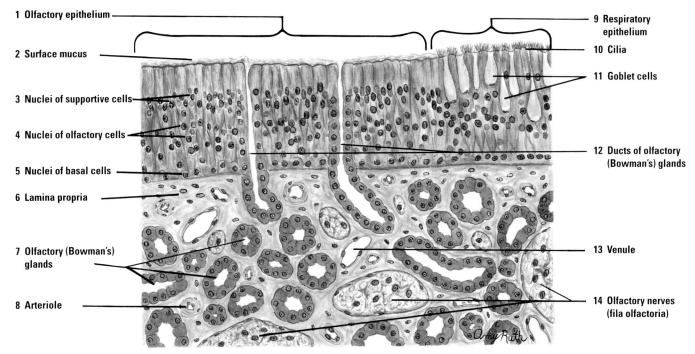

1 Olfactory epithelium

2 Surface mucus

3 Nuclei of supportive cells

4 Nuclei of olfactory cells

5 Nuclei of basal cells

6 Lamina propria

7 Olfactory (Bowman's) glands

8 Arteriole

9 Respiratory epithelium

10 Cilia

11 Goblet cells

12 Ducts of olfactory (Bowman's) glands

13 Venule

14 Olfactory nerves (fila olfactoria)

FIG. 2. OLFACTORY MUCOSA: DETAIL OF A TRANSITION AREA. Stain: hematoxylin-eosin. 500×

213

PLATE 82

EPIGLOTTIS (LONGITUDINAL SECTION)

The epiglottis is the superior portion of the larynx; it projects upward from its anterior wall as a flat flap.

A central **epiglottic (elastic) cartilage (7)** forms the framework of the epiglottis. Its **anterior** or **lingual surface (6)** is covered with a noncornified **stratified squamous epithelium (9).** The underlying **lamina propria (4)** merges with the **perichondrium (8)** of the epiglottic cartilage (7).

The anterior or lingual mucosa (6) covers the apex of the epiglottis and more than half of the posterior or laryngeal surface (2). The **stratified squamous epithelium (3),** however, is lower; the connective tissue papillae disappear, and a transition is made to a respiratory epithelium, which is **pseudostratified ciliated columnar epithelium (5)** with goblet cells.

Tubuloacinar mucous, serous, or mixed glands are present in the lamina propria (4). Occasional **taste buds (1)** are seen in the epithelium. Solitary lymphatic nodules may be present in the lingual or laryngeal mucosa.

EPIGLOTTIS (LONGITUDINAL SECTION)

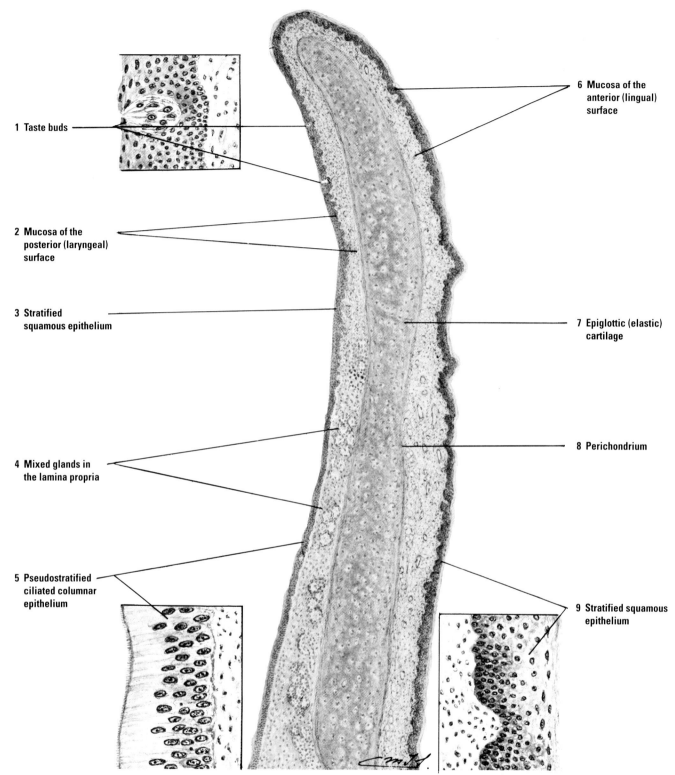

1 Taste buds

2 Mucosa of the posterior (laryngeal) surface

3 Stratified squamous epithelium

4 Mixed glands in the lamina propria

5 Pseudostratified ciliated columnar epithelium

6 Mucosa of the anterior (lingual) surface

7 Epiglottic (elastic) cartilage

8 Perichondrium

9 Stratified squamous epithelium

Stain: hematoxylin-eosin. 25× and **300×**.

PLATE 83

LARYNX (FRONTAL SECTION)

A vertical section through the larynx shows the two prominent **vocal folds (13, 18–20)**, the supporting **cartilages (8, 11)**, and **muscles (10, 20)**.

The **superior or false vocal fold (13)** of the larynx is formed by the mucosa and is continuous with the **posterior surface of the epiglottis (12)**. The lining epithelium is **pseudostratified ciliated columnar (14)** with goblet cells. Below the epithelium in the **lamina propria (3)** are found **mixed glands (15)**, which are predominantly mucous. **Excretory ducts (16)**, which open onto the epithelial surface, are seen among the acini of the glands **(15)**. **Lymphatic nodules (7)** are located in the lamina propria **(3)** on the ventricular side of the vocal fold.

The **ventricle (17)** is a deep indentation and recess separating the **false vocal fold (13)** from the **true vocal fold (18–20)**. The mucosa in the **lateral wall (3, 4, 5, 6)** of the ventricle **(17)** is similar to that of the false vocal fold **(13)**. Lymphatic nodules are more numerous in this area and are sometimes called the **"laryngeal tonsils" (7)**. The lamina propria **(3)** blends with the **perichondrium (9)** of the **thyroid cartilage (8)**; there is no distinct submucosa. The lower wall of the ventricle makes the transition to a true vocal fold **(18–20)**.

The mucosa of the true vocal fold **(18–20)** consists of noncornified, **stratified squamous epithelium (18)** and a thin, dense lamina propria devoid of glands, lymphatic tissue, or blood vessels. At the apex of the true vocal fold is the **vocal ligament (19)**, consisting of dense elastic fibers that spread out into the adjacent lamina propria and the skeletal **vocalis muscle (20)**. The skeletal **thyroarytenoid muscle (10)** and the **thyroid cartilage (8)** comprise the remaining wall.

The epithelium in the lower larynx changes to **pseudostratified ciliated columnar (21)**, and the underlying lamina propria contains **mixed glands (22)**. The **cricoid cartilage (11)** is the lowermost cartilage of the larynx.

LARYNX (FRONTAL SECTION)

1 Adipose tissue

2 Arteriole and venule

3 Lamina propria of ventricular wall

4 Serous acini

5 Mucous acini

6 Excretory duct

7 Lymphatic nodules (laryngeal tonsils)

8 Thyroid cartilage (hyaline)

9 Perichondrium

10 Thyroarytenoid muscle (skeletal muscle)

11 Cricoid cartilage (hyaline)

12 Posterior surface of the epiglottis

13 False (superior) vocal fold

14 Pseudostratified ciliated columnar epithelium

15 Mixed glands

16 Excretory duct

17 Ventricle

18 Stratified squamous epithelium

19 Vocal ligament

20 Vocalis muscle (skeletal muscle)

True (inferior) vocal fold

21 Pseudostratified ciliated columnar epithelium

22 Mixed glands in the lamina propria of the lower larynx

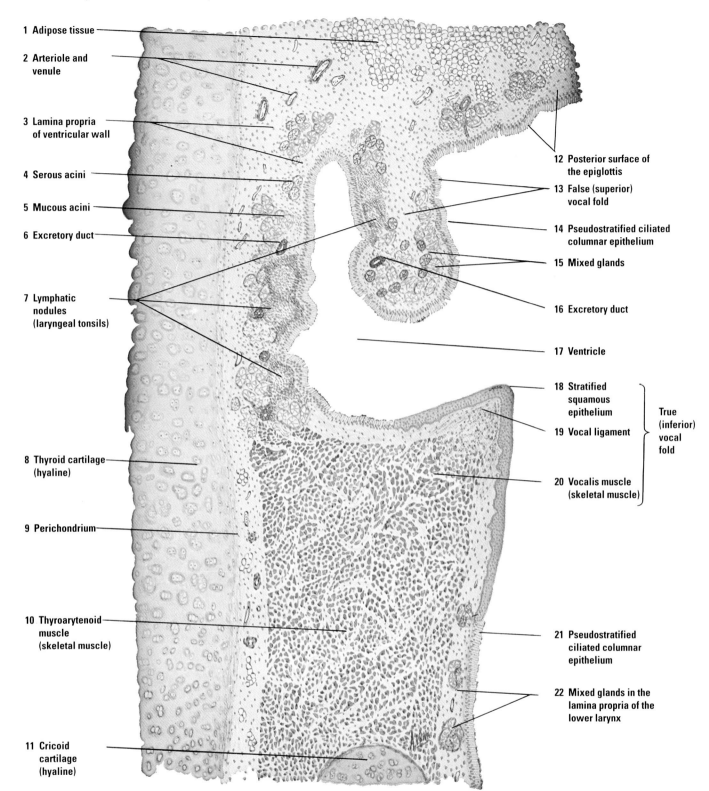

Stain: hematoxylin-eosin. 35×.

217

PLATE 84

■ FIG. 1
TRACHEA (PANORAMIC VIEW, TRANSVERSE SECTION)

The wall of the trachea consists of a mucosa, submucosa, hyaline cartilage, and adventitia. The cartilage in the trachea is a series of C-shaped rings between whose ends lies the smooth **trachealis muscle (9).**

A section of the trachea is illustrated in Figure 1. The mucosa consists of **pseudostratified ciliated columnar epithelium (13)** with goblet cells. The **lamina propria (11, 14)** contains fine connective tissue fibers, diffuse **lymphatic tissue (14),** and occasional solitary lymphatic nodules. Deep in the lamina propria (11), the elastic fibers form a longitudinal **elastic membrane (15).** In the loose connective tissue of the **submucosa (16)** are mixed **tubuloacinar glands (4, 5)** whose **ducts (10, 17)** pass through the lamina propria (11) to the tracheal lumen.

The **hyaline cartilage (3)** is surrounded by dense connective tissue, the **perichondrium (2),** which merges with the submucosa (16) on one side and the **adventitia (1)** on the other side. Numerous **blood vessels and nerves (6)** course in the adventitia (1) and provide smaller branches to the outer layers.

The **mucosa (12)** exhibits folds along the posterior wall of the trachea where the cartilage is absent. The trachealis muscle (9) lies deep to the elastic membrane of the mucosa and is embedded in the fibroelastic tissue that occupies the area between the ends of the cartilage rings. Most of the trachealis muscle fibers (9) insert into the perichondrium of the cartilage (2, upper leader). Mixed glands are present in the submucosa; these can intermingle with the muscle fibers and extend into the adventitia **(8).**

■ FIG. 2
TRACHEA (SECTIONAL VIEW)

A small section of trachea is illustrated at a higher magnification and stained with hematoxylin-eosin to show details of the wall. The pseudostratified surface epithelium contains **ciliated (5)** and **goblet cells (10),** the irregular location of the nuclei, and the thickened **basement membrane (6).** A longitudinal **elastic membrane (7)** is visible in the deeper region of the lamina propria; in this illustration, the fibers are cut in transverse plane. Also seen in the lamina propria are a group of **mucous acini (9)** of the tracheal glands and their **duct (8).** In the adjacent **cartilage (2),** the larger lacunae and **chondrocytes (3)** in the interior become progressively flatter toward the **perichondrium (1)** while the matrix gradually blends with the connective tissue.

■ FIG. 3
TRACHEA (SECTIONAL VIEW): ELASTIC FIBER STAIN

This section of the trachea has been stained with Gallego's method to demonstrate the **elastic fibers (8)** in the elastic membrane, which stain red with carbolfuchsin. Collagen fibers stain blue with aniline blue and provide a contrast where they intermix with the elastic fibers. Collagenous fibers are also demonstrated in the **perichondrium (1, lower leader), submucosa (3),** and **superficial lamina propria (9).**

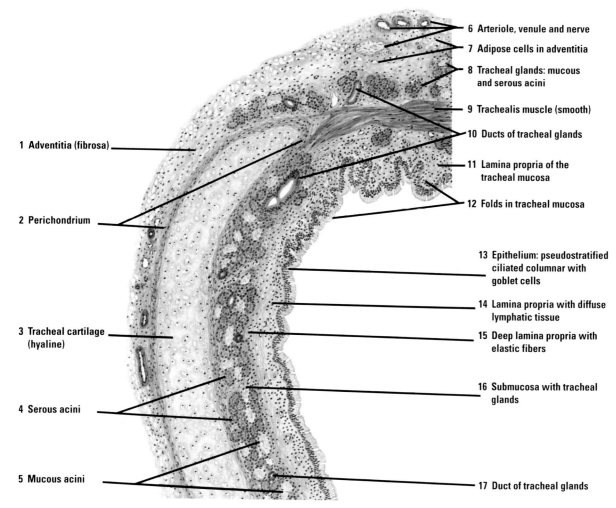

1 Adventitia (fibrosa)

2 Perichondrium

3 Tracheal cartilage (hyaline)

4 Serous acini

5 Mucous acini

6 Arteriole, venule and nerve

7 Adipose cells in adventitia

8 Tracheal glands: mucous and serous acini

9 Trachealis muscle (smooth)

10 Ducts of tracheal glands

11 Lamina propria of the tracheal mucosa

12 Folds in tracheal mucosa

13 Epithelium: pseudostratified ciliated columnar with goblet cells

14 Lamina propria with diffuse lymphatic tissue

15 Deep lamina propria with elastic fibers

16 Submucosa with tracheal glands

17 Duct of tracheal glands

FIG. 1. TRACHEA (PANORAMIC VIEW, TRANSVERSE SECTION). Stain: hematoxylin-eosin. 50×.

1 Perichondrium

2 Cartilage: matrix

3 Flattened chondrocytes

4 Cartilage: territorial matrix

5 Epithelium: pseudostratified ciliated columnar

6 Basement membrane

7 Elastic fibers, t.s. (elastic membrane)

8 Duct of a tracheal gland (t.s.)

9 Mucous acinus with a serous demilune

10 Goblet cell

FIG. 2. TRACHEA (SECTIONAL VIEW). Stain: hematoxylin-eosin. 220×.

1 Cartilage and perichondrium

2 Mixed acinus; mucous acinus; serous acinus

3 Submucosa

4 Duct of tracheal glands

5 Goblet cell

6 Ciliated cell

7 Basement membrane

8 Elastic fibers (elastic membrane) in the deeper lamina propria

9 Superficial lamina propria

FIG. 3. TRACHEA (SECTIONAL VIEW). Stain: Gallego's method for elastic fibers. 220×.

PLATE 85

LUNG (PANORAMIC VIEW)

The respiratory system consists of the lungs and the air passages, which are divided into the conducting portion and the respiratory portion. The conducting portion consists of the nasal cavity, nasopharynx, larynx, trachea, bronchi, bronchioles, and terminal bronchioles. The respiratory portion consists of the respiratory bronchioles, alveolar ducts, alveolar sacs, and alveoli. Plate 86 illustrates the histology of these divisions in greater detail and higher magnification and the characteristic features of the lung are illustrated in this panoramic view. All cartilage in the lung is hyaline.

The histology of the extrapulmonary bronchi is similar to that of the trachea. In the intrapulmonary bronchi, the C-shaped cartilage rings are replaced by cartilage plates that encircle the bronchi. The smooth muscle spreads out from the trachealis muscle to surround the lumina of the bronchi.

The **intrapulmonary bronchus (33** and Plate 81, Fig. 1) is normally identified by several cartilage plates located in close proximity to each other. The **epithelium (32)** is pseudostratified columnar ciliated epithelium with goblet cells. The rest of the wall consists of a thin lamina propria, a narrow layer of **smooth muscle (31)**, a submucosa with scattered bronchial glands, **hyaline cartilage plate (30),** and adventitia.

As the intrapulmonary bronchi branch and become smaller bronchi, there is a decrease in the epithelial height and the amount of cartilage. Farther down the airway tube, only occasional small pieces of cartilage are seen. In bronchi that are about 1 mm in diameter, cartilage is no longer visible.

In **bronchioles (16),** the epithelium is low, pseudostratified columnar ciliated epithelium with occasional goblet cells. The mucosa is normally folded and the smooth muscle surrounding the lumen is prominent. Glands and cartilage plates are no longer present, and adventitia surrounds these structures.

The **terminal bronchioles (6, 12)** exhibit a wavy mucosal lining and ciliated epithelium that is now columnar; goblet cells are lacking in the terminal bronchioles. Still present, however, are a thin lamina propria, a layer of smooth muscle, and an adventitia.

The **respiratory bronchioles (5, 8, 17, 23, 26, 27)** have a direct connection with the alveolar ducts and alveoli. In these bronchioles, the epithelium is low columnar or cuboidal (5, 8) and may be ciliated in the proximal portion of the tubules. A minimal amount of connective tissue supports the band of intermixed smooth muscle, the elastic fibers of the lamina propria, and the accompanying blood vessels. Individual **alveoli (25)** appear in the wall of the respiratory bronchioles (26) as small outpockets. Alveoli increase in number distally in the tubules. The epithelium and smooth muscle in the distal respiratory bronchioles appear as small, intermittent areas between the openings of the numerous alveoli (5, upper leader; 17, 23, 24, 25).

The terminal portion of each respiratory bronchiole branches into several **alveolar ducts (2, 15, 22);** in histologic sections only one such alveolar duct may be seen (5 and 2, lower leader; 23, upper leader and 22, middle leader). The walls of the alveolar ducts (2, 15, 22) are formed by a series of alveoli situated adjacent to each other. A cluster of alveoli that open into an alveolar duct is called an **alveolar sac (14, 20).** The **alveoli (4, 21, 25)** form the parenchyma of the lung, giving it the appearance of fine lace (See Fig. 4, Plate 86 for details). In this illustration, a plane of section shows a continuous passageway from the terminal bronchiole (6) to the respiratory bronchiole (5, 26, 27) into the alveolar duct (lowest leader of 2; middle leader of 22).

The **pulmonary artery (28)** branches repeatedly to accompany the divisions of the bronchial tree. Large pulmonary vein branches also accompany the bronchi and bronchioles; numerous small branches of the vein are seen in the lung **trabeculae (3).** Pulmonary arterioles (7, 10) supply the walls of various bronchi, bronchioles, (6, 12) and other areas of the lung. Small **bronchial veins (29)** may be seen in the walls of the larger **bronchi (33).**

The **visceral pleura (1)** adheres closely to lungs. It is composed of a thin layer of pleural **connective tissue (19)** and **pleural mesothelium (18).**

LUNG (PANORAMIC VIEW)

1 Visceral pleura

2 Alveolar ducts (l.s.)

3 Trabecula with pulmonary vein

4 Alveolus (t.s.)

5 Respiratory bronchiole (distal and proximal portions)

6 Terminal bronchiole

7 Pulmonary arteriole
8 Respiratory bronchiole (t.s.)
9 Alveolar duct (t.s.)

10 Pulmonary arteriole
11 Lymphatic nodule
12 Terminal bronchiole

13 Smooth muscle

14 Alveolar sac

15 Alveolar duct (l.s.)

16 Bronchiole

17 Respiratory bronchiole (distal portion, l.s.)

18 Pleural mesothelium
19 Pleural connective tissue

20 Alveolar sac

21 Alveoli

22 Alveolar ducts (l.s.)

23 Respiratory bronchioles (distal)

24 Simple columnar epithelium
25 Alveoli in distal respiratory bronchiole
26 Respiratory bronchiole (proximal)
27 Respiratory bronchiole (t.s.)

28 Pulmonary artery

29 Bronchial vein

30 Cartilage (hyaline)

31 Smooth muscle
32 Pseudostratified columnar ciliated epithelium
33 Intrapulmonary bronchus

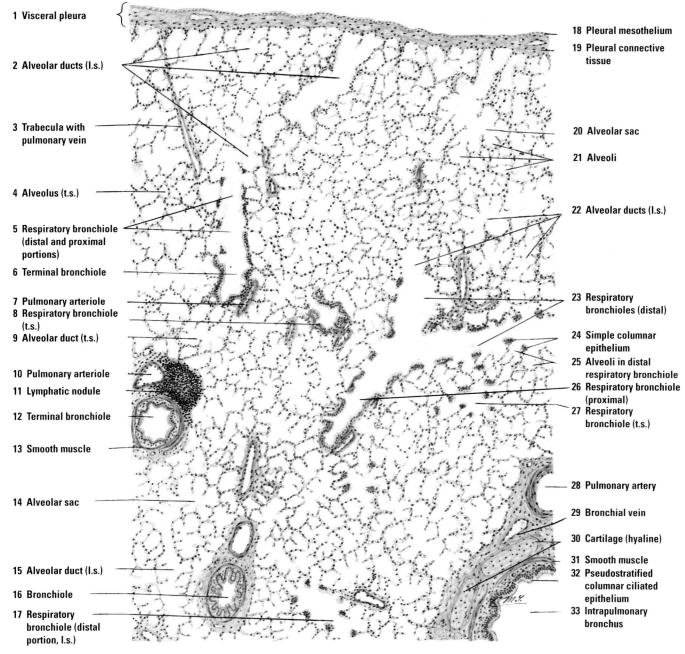

Stain: hematoxylin-eosin. 30×.

PLATE 86

■ FIG. 1
INTRAPULMONARY BRONCHUS

The primary or extrapulmonary bronchi divide and give rise to a series of smaller intrapulmonary bronchi. Such bronchi are lined by pseudostratified columnar ciliated **epithelium (12)**, a thin **lamina propria (13)** of fine connective tissue with many elastic fibers (not illustrated), and a few lymphocytes. **Ducts (2)** from the submucosal **bronchial glands (5, 8, 10)** pass through lamina propria (13) to open into the bronchial lumen. A thin layer of **smooth muscle (6)** surrounds the lamina propria (13). The submucosa contains glands of either **serous (5, 8), mucous,** or **mucoserous acini (10).** In the mixed glands, serous demilunes may be seen.

The **cartilage plates (4)** are distributed close together around the periphery of the bronchus; the plates become smaller and farther apart as the bronchi continue to divide and their size continues to decrease. Between the **cartilage plates (4),** the submucosal connective tissue blends with the well-developed **adventitia (3).**

The accompanying branch of the **pulmonary artery (15)** is located either adjacent to the bronchi or in the outer adventitia (14). A smaller branch of another **pulmonary artery (7)** probably accompanies a small bronchus or bronchiole which is located in another plane of section.

Bronchial vessels are seen in the connective tissue of a bronchus: an **arteriole (16),** a **venule (11),** and **capillaries (9).**

■ FIG. 2
TERMINAL BRONCHIOLE

The terminal bronchioles have small diameters, about 1 mm or less. **Mucosal folds (4)** are prominent and the epithelium is low pseudostratified columnar ciliated with few goblet cells. In the terminal bronchioles, the **epithelium (5)** is columnar ciliated and the goblet cells are absent. A well-developed **smooth muscle (3)** layer surrounds the thin lamina propria which is, in turn, surrounded by the **adventitia (2).** Cartilage plates, glands, and goblet cells are absent.

Adjacent to the bronchiole is a small branch of the **pulmonary artery (6);** the bronchiole is surrounded by the **alveoli (7)** of the lung.

■ FIG. 3
RESPIRATORY BRONCHIOLE

The wall of the respiratory bronchiole is lined with cuboidal **epithelium (4).** Cilia may be present in the epithelium of the proximal but disappear in the distal portion of the respiratory bronchiole. **Smooth muscle (3)** is located adjacent to the epithelium. A small branch of the **pulmonary artery (5)** accompanies the respiratory bronchiole.

An **alveolar duct (2)** arises from the respiratory bronchiole and numerous **alveoli (1)** open into the **alveolar duct (2).**

■ FIG. 4
ALVEOLAR WALLS: INTERALVEOLAR SEPTA

The oval **alveoli (5)** are lined by simple squamous epithelium, which is not very obvious at this magnification. Adjacent alveoli share a common **interalveolar septum (4).** Located in the thin septum (4) are **capillary plexuses (1, 3)** supported by fine connective tissue fibers, fibroblasts, and other cells. As a result of the thin interalveolar septum (4) and its contents, the capillaries are in close proximity to the squamous cells of the adjacent alveoli, separated from the epithelium only by the sparse connective tissue. In routine preparation of lung tissue, it is difficult to distinguish between the nuclei of squamous cells in the alveoli (5), endothelial cells in the **blood vessels (capillaries) (1, 3),** and the **fibroblasts (6)** in the interalveolar septum (4).

At the free ends of the interalveolar septa (4) and around the open ends of the alveoli are narrow bands of **smooth muscle (2),** which is a continuation from the muscle layer of the respiratory bronchiole.

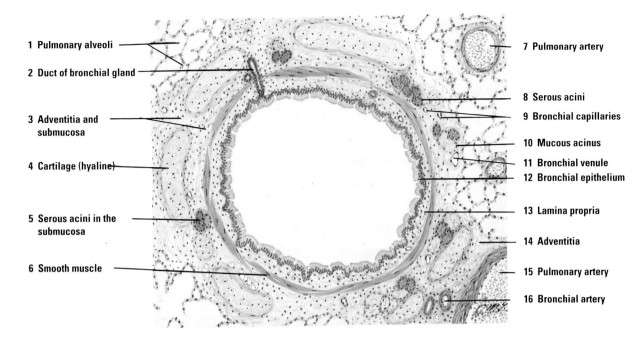

1 Pulmonary alveoli

2 Duct of bronchial gland

3 Adventitia and submucosa

4 Cartilage (hyaline)

5 Serous acini in the submucosa

6 Smooth muscle

7 Pulmonary artery

8 Serous acini

9 Bronchial capillaries

10 Mucous acinus

11 Bronchial venule

12 Bronchial epithelium

13 Lamina propria

14 Adventitia

15 Pulmonary artery

16 Bronchial artery

FIG. 1. INTRAPULMONARY BRONCHUS. Stain: hematoxylin-eosin. 50X

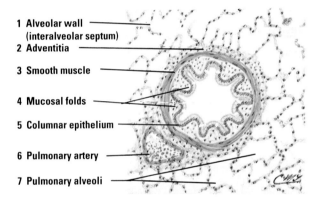

1 Alveolar wall (interalveolar septum)

2 Adventitia

3 Smooth muscle

4 Mucosal folds

5 Columnar epithelium

6 Pulmonary artery

7 Pulmonary alveoli

FIG. 2. TERMINAL BRONCHIOLE. Stain: hematoxylin-eosin. 50X

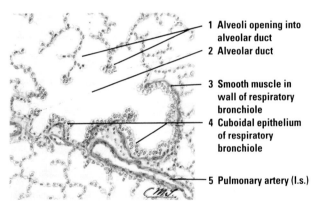

1 Alveoli opening into alveolar duct

2 Alveolar duct

3 Smooth muscle in wall of respiratory bronchiole

4 Cuboidal epithelium of respiratory bronchiole

5 Pulmonary artery (l.s.)

FIG. 3. RESPIRATORY BRONCHIOLE. Stain: hematoxylin-eosin. 80X

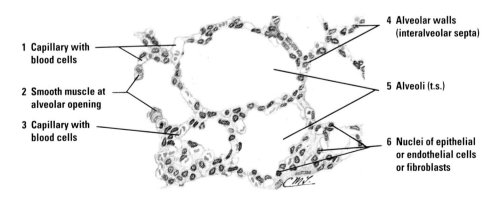

1 Capillary with blood cells

2 Smooth muscle at alveolar opening

3 Capillary with blood cells

4 Alveolar walls (interalveolar septa)

5 Alveoli (t.s.)

6 Nuclei of epithelial or endothelial cells or fibroblasts

FIG. 4. ALVEOLAR WALLS (INTERALVEOLAR SEPTA). Stain: hematoxylin-eosin. 700X

223

The urinary system consists of kidneys, ureters, urinary bladder, and urethra. The kidneys perform numerous vital functions in maintaining homeostasis of the body. They regulate blood pressure, blood composition, and fluid volume of the body; produce urine; and maintain acid-base balance. In addition, the cells of the kidneys produce two important hormones, renin and erythropoietin. Renin functions in regulating the blood pressure to maintain proper kidney functions and erythropoietin influences red blood cell formation in the red bone marrow.

The Nephron

The functional unit of the kidney is the uriniferous tubule, which consists of a nephron and a collecting duct into which the contents of the nephron empty. The nephron has two major components, the renal corpuscle and renal tubule. The renal corpuscle consists of a tuft of capillaries, the glomerulus, surrounded by a double layer of epithelial cells, the glomerular (Bowman's) capsule.

The main function of the renal corpuscle is to filter blood through the capillaries of the glomerulus into the capsular (urinary) space, which is located between the two epithelial layers. Filtration of blood is facilitated by the glomerular endothelium. This endothelium is porous (fenestrated) and highly permeable to many substances in the blood, except to the formed elements and plasma proteins. Thus, the glomerular filtrate that enters the capsular space is similar to that of plasma, except for the absence of proteins.

There are two types of nephrons. Those located in the cortex of the kidney are called the cortical nephrons and those situated near the corticomedullary junction are the juxtamedullary nephrons; all nephrons participate in urine formation. The juxtamedullary nephrons are important because they produce a hypertonic environment in the interstitium of the medulla, a condition that is necessary for the production of concentrated (hypertonic) urine.

The glomerular filtrate flows from the glomerular capsule into the renal tubule, which extends from the glomerular capsule to the collecting tubule. The renal tubule is highly convoluted and has several distinct histologic and functional regions. It consists of the proximal convoluted tubule, loop of Henle, and distal convoluted tubule. In the juxtamedullary nephrons, the loop of Henle is long; it descends from the cortex deep into the medulla and then loops back to ascend into the cortex. The Henle's loop consists of a thick, descending portion of the proximal tubule, a long thin segment, and a thick, ascending portion of the distal tubule.

The proximal convoluted tubule arises at the urinary pole of the renal corpuscle. Its main function is to absorb, by means of the microvilli in the brush border of its cells, all the glucose, amino acids, and about 85% of water and sodium chloride from the glomerular filtrate. In addition, the proximal convoluted tubule excretes certain metabolites, dyes, and drugs into the glomerulate filtrate.

The loop of Henle is necessary for the production of hypertonic urine. This is accomplished by concentrating sodium chloride in the interstitial tissue of the kidney medulla by means of a complex countercurrent multiplier system. As a result of this ionic concentration, a high osmotic pressure or hypertonic extracellular fluid is produced. The hypertonicity of the extracellular fluid in the medulla removes the water from the glomerular filtrate as it flows through the collecting tubules, resulting in the production of concentrated urine.

The distal convoluted tubule is shorter and less convoluted than the proximal tubule. It functions in the active resorption of sodium ions from the filtrate. The resorptive activity is coupled with the excretion of the hydrogen or potassium ions into the filtrate or tubular urine. The functions of the distal convoluted tubule are vital for maintaining a proper acid-base balance in the body.

The glomerular filtrate flows from the distal convoluted tubule to the collecting tubule, which is normally not permeable to water. During the presence of an antidiuretic hormone (ADH) in the system, however, the epithelium of the collecting tubule becomes highly permeable to water. Consequently, as the glomerular filtrate in the collecting tubule flows through the medulla, water is drawn out from the filtrate because of the high osmotic pressure created by the hypertonic extracellular fluid. The retained water is then returned to the general circulation by way of the blood vessels and the glomerular filtrate in the collecting tubules becomes a more concentrated urine. In the absence of the circulating ADH, water does not leave the collecting tubule because the epithelium becomes impermeable to water. As a result, the expelled urine is dilute and contains more water. The ADH is secreted by the neurohypophysis of the pituitary gland in response to a limited intake of water.

The Juxtaglomerular Apparatus

Situated adjacent to the renal corpuscle and the distal convoluted tubule is the juxtaglomerular apparatus, consisting of juxtaglomerular cells and macula densa. The juxtaglomerular cells are modified smooth muscle cells in the wall of the afferent arteriole just before it enters the glomerular capsule. The macula densa consists of modified epithelial cells of the distal convoluted tubule, which are situated adjacent to the afferent arteriole with the juxtaglomerular cells.

The juxtaglomerular apparatus performs an important role in maintaining normal systemic blood pressure. The juxtaglomerular cells are believed to respond to changes in the systemic blood pressure, and the macula densa cells probably respond to the changes in the sodium concentration of the glomerular filtrate in the distal convoluted tubule.

A decrease in systemic blood pressure causes the juxtaglomerular cells to release the hormone renin into the blood stream. Renin converts the plasma protein angiotensinogen to angiotensin I, which in turn is converted to angiotensin II by a blood enzyme present in the endothelial cells of the lung. Angiotensin II is a powerful vasoconstrictor that initially produces arterial constriction, thereby increasing the systemic blood pressure. In addition, angiotensin II stimulates the release of the hormone aldosterone from the adrenal cortex. Aldosterone acts mostly on the cells of the distal convoluted tubules in the kidney to increase their reabsorption of sodium and chloride ions. The increased retention of sodium ions increases the fluid volume in the circulatory system and raises the systemic blood pressure.

PLATE 87

KIDNEY: CORTEX AND PYRAMID (PANORAMIC VIEW)

PLATE 87

KIDNEY: CORTEX AND PYRAMID (PANORAMIC VIEW)

The kidney is subdivided into an outer region, the **cortex (20)** and an inner region, the **medulla (21)**. Externally, the cortex is covered with a connective tissue **capsule (19)** and the perirenal connective and **adipose tissues (18)**.

In the cortex are found **convoluted tubules (3), glomeruli (2, 8), straight tubules (4),** and **medullary rays (5)**. The cortex also contains renal corpuscles (glomerular or Bowman's capsules and glomeruli), adjacent proximal and distal **convoluted tubules (3)** of the nephrons, and the interlobular **arteries (6)** and **veins (7)**. The **medullary rays (5)** contain straight portions of nephrons and collecting tubules. Medullary rays do not extend to the kidney capsule because of a narrow zone of **convoluted tubules (1)**.

The medulla is composed of a number of renal pyramids. Each pyramid is situated with its **base (11)** adjacent to the cortex (20) and its apex directed inward. The apices of renal pyramids form the **papilla (16),** which projects into a **minor calyx (14)**. The medulla also contains the loops of Henle (straight or descending proximal tubules, thin segments, and straight or ascending distal tubules) and collecting tubules. The collecting tubules join each other in the medulla to form large papillary ducts (Plate 89).

The papilla (16) is usually covered with a simple **columnar epithelium (12)**. As this epithelium reflects on to the outer wall of the calyx, it becomes **transitional epithelium (13)**. A thin layer of connective tissue and smooth muscle (not illustrated) is found under this epithelium, which then merges with the connective tissue of the **renal sinus (17)**.

In the renal sinus (17), between the pyramids, are branches of the renal artery and vein, the **interlobar vessels (15)**. These vessels enter the kidney and then arch over the base of the pyramid at the corticomedullary junction as the **arcuate vessels (9)**. The arcuate vessels give rise to smaller, **interlobular arteries and veins (6, 7, 10)**. The arcuate arteries (9) pass radially into the kidney cortex (20) and give off numerous afferent glomerular arteries to the glomeruli.

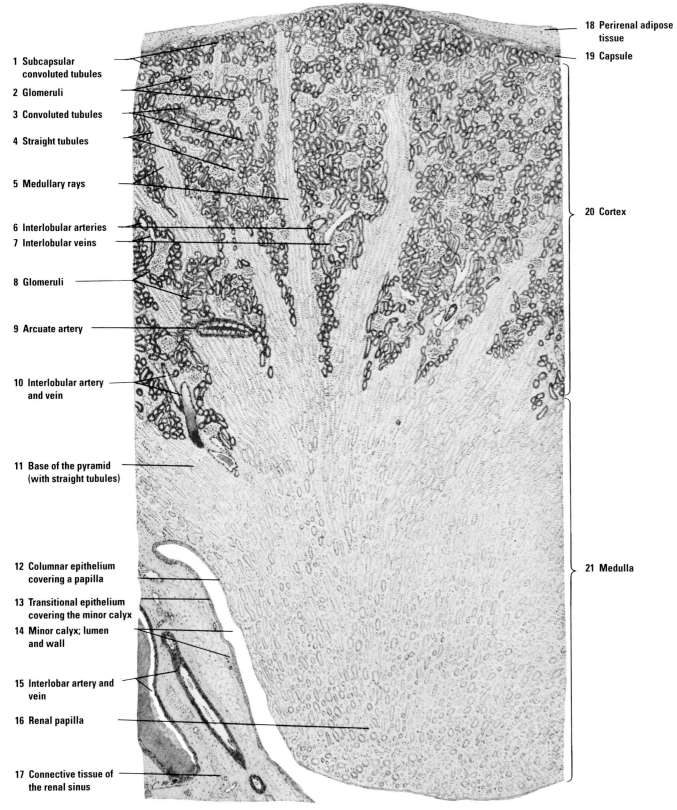

1 Subcapsular convoluted tubules

2 Glomeruli

3 Convoluted tubules

4 Straight tubules

5 Medullary rays

6 Interlobular arteries

7 Interlobular veins

8 Glomeruli

9 Arcuate artery

10 Interlobular artery and vein

11 Base of the pyramid (with straight tubules)

12 Columnar epithelium covering a papilla

13 Transitional epithelium covering the minor calyx

14 Minor calyx; lumen and wall

15 Interlobar artery and vein

16 Renal papilla

17 Connective tissue of the renal sinus

18 Perirenal adipose tissue

19 Capsule

20 Cortex

21 Medulla

Stain: hematoxylin-eosin. 25×.

PLATE 88

■ **FIG. 1**
KIDNEY: DEEP CORTICAL AREA AND OUTER MEDULLA

A higher magnification of the kidney cortex reveals greater details of the renal corpuscle. Each corpuscle consists of a **glomerulus (3)** and a glomerular or Bowman's **capsule (2, 17).** The glomerulus (3) is a tuft of capillaries formed from the afferent glomerular arterioles and supported by fine connective tissue.

The **visceral layer (17)** of the glomerular capsule consists of modified epithelial cells called the podocytes. These cells closely follow the contours of the glomerulus and invest the capillary tufts. At the vascular pole, the visceral epithelium reflects to become the **parietal layer (17)** of the glomerular capsule. The space between the visceral and parietal layers of the capsule is the capsular space, which becomes continuous with the lumen of the proximal convoluted tubule at the urinary pole (See Fig. 2). At the urinary pole, the squamous epithelium of the parietal layer changes to cuboidal epithelium of the **proximal convoluted tubule (9).**

Numerous tubules, sectioned in various planes, lie adjacent to the renal corpuscles. The tubules are primarily of two types, the **proximal convoluted (4, 10, 15, 21)** and **distal convoluted (1, 14, 21)**; these tubules are the initial and terminal segments of the nephron, respectively. The proximal convoluted tubules are numerous in the cortex, exhibit a small, uneven lumen, and contain a single layer of large cuboidal cells with intensely eosinophilic, granular cytoplasm. The well-developed **brush borders (15)** are present but are not always well preserved in sections.

Distal convoluted tubules (14) are fewer in number and exhibit a larger lumen with smaller, cuboidal cells. The cytoplasm stains less intensely and the brush borders are not present (14, compare with 15).

Renal corpuscles and their associated tubules constitute the kidney cortex. The cortex surrounds the medullary rays, which are composed of straight portions of the nephrons and collecting tubules. The medullary rays include three types of tubules. The straight (descending) segments of the **proximal tubules (6),** the straight (ascending) segments of the **distal tubules (11, 20),** and the **collecting tubules (5, 19).** The straight segments of the proximal tubules are similar to the proximal convoluted tubules and the straight segments of the distal tubules are similar to distal convoluted tubules, respectively. Collecting tubules are distinct because of lightly stained cuboidal cells and visible cell membranes.

The medulla contains only straight portions of tubules and thin segments of Henle's loops. In the outer medullary region are illustrated thin segments of **Henle's loops (13, 23)** lined with squamous epithelium, straight segments of distal tubules (20), and the collecting tubules (12, 22).

■ **FIG. 2**
KIDNEY CORTEX: THE JUXTAGLOMERULAR APPARATUS

A small area of the kidney cortex at a higher magnification illustrates the renal corpuscle, adjacent tubules, and juxtaglomerular apparatus.

The renal corpuscle exhibits the **glomerular capillaries (2), parietal (10a)** and **visceral (10b)** epithelium of glomerular (Bowman's) **capsule (10),** and the **capsular space (13).** Conspicuous brush borders and acidophilic cells distinguish the **proximal convoluted tubules (6, 14)** from the **distal convoluted tubules (1, 15)** whose smaller, less intensely stained cells lack brush borders. The cells of the **collecting tubules (8)** are cuboidal with distinct cell outlines and clear, pale cytoplasm. Distinct **basement membranes (9)** surround these tubules.

Each renal corpuscle exhibits a vascular pole on one side where the **afferent glomerular arterioles (12)** enter and efferent glomerular arterioles exit. On the opposite side of the corpuscle is the **urinary pole (11),** where the capsular space (13) becomes continuous with the lumen of the proximal convoluted tubule (6, 14). The plane of section through the renal corpuscle, as illustrated in this figure, is seen only occasionally in the kidney cortex; however, illustration of both vascular and urinary poles represents an important structural association of the renal corpuscle with the region of blood filtration, glomerular filtrate accumulation, and initial stages of filtrate modification in urine formation.

At the vascular pole, the smooth muscle cells in the tunica media of the afferent glomerular arteriole (12) are replaced by highly modified epithelioid cells with cytoplasmic granules. These are the **juxtaglomerular cells (4).** In the adjacent segment of the distal convoluted tubules, the cells that border the juxtaglomerular area are narrower and more columnar than elsewhere in the tubules. This area of darker, more compact cell arrangement is called the **macula densa (5).** The juxtaglomerular cells in the afferent glomerular arteriole (12) and the **macula densa (5)** cells in the distal convoluted tubule together constitute the juxtaglomerular apparatus.

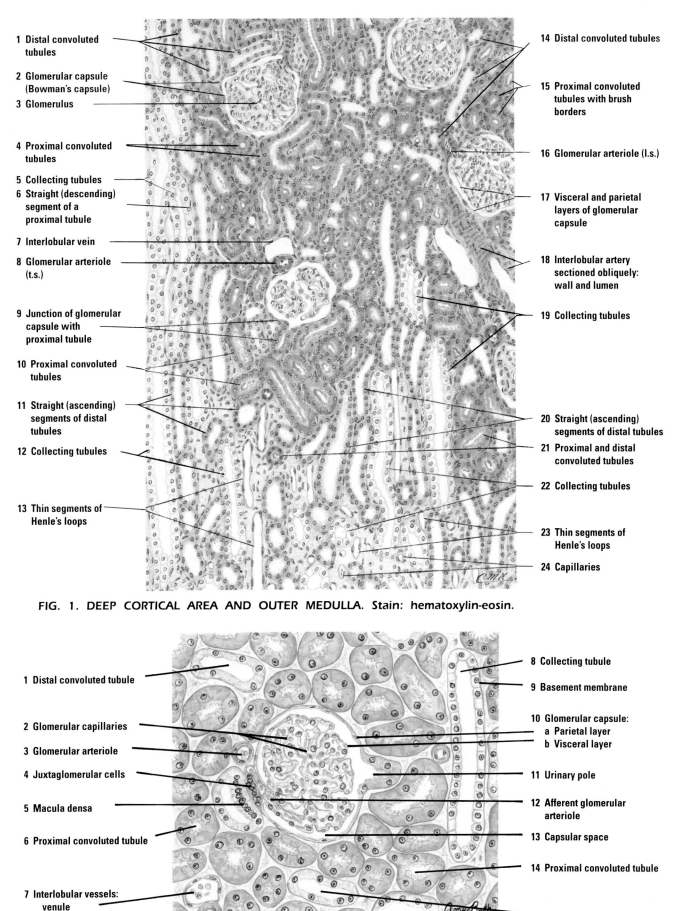

1 Distal convoluted tubules
2 Glomerular capsule (Bowman's capsule)
3 Glomerulus
4 Proximal convoluted tubules
5 Collecting tubules
6 Straight (descending) segment of a proximal tubule
7 Interlobular vein
8 Glomerular arteriole (t.s.)
9 Junction of glomerular capsule with proximal tubule
10 Proximal convoluted tubules
11 Straight (ascending) segments of distal tubules
12 Collecting tubules
13 Thin segments of Henle's loops

14 Distal convoluted tubules
15 Proximal convoluted tubules with brush borders
16 Glomerular arteriole (l.s.)
17 Visceral and parietal layers of glomerular capsule
18 Interlobular artery sectioned obliquely: wall and lumen
19 Collecting tubules
20 Straight (ascending) segments of distal tubules
21 Proximal and distal convoluted tubules
22 Collecting tubules
23 Thin segments of Henle's loops
24 Capillaries

FIG. 1. DEEP CORTICAL AREA AND OUTER MEDULLA. Stain: hematoxylin-eosin.

1 Distal convoluted tubule
2 Glomerular capillaries
3 Glomerular arteriole
4 Juxtaglomerular cells
5 Macula densa
6 Proximal convoluted tubule
7 Interlobular vessels: venule arteriole

8 Collecting tubule
9 Basement membrane
10 Glomerular capsule:
   a Parietal layer
   b Visceral layer
11 Urinary pole
12 Afferent glomerular arteriole
13 Capsular space
14 Proximal convoluted tubule
15 Distal convoluted tubule

FIG. 2. KIDNEY CORTEX: THE JUXTAGLOMERULAR APPARATUS. Stain: periodic acid-Schiff and hematoxylin.

231

PLATE 89

■ **FIG. 1**
KIDNEY MEDULLA: PAPILLA (TRANSVERSE SECTION)

The papilla of the kidney contains the terminal portions of the collecting tubules, the **papillary ducts (2, 5, 6).** These ducts have large diameters and wide lumina and are lined by tall, pale-staining columnar cells. Also seen in this region are cross sections of the thin segments of the **loops of Henle (3, 8)** and the ascending straight portions of the **distal tubules (7). Connective tissue (10)** is more abundant in this region than elsewhere in the kidney, and the collecting tubules are not as close together. Numerous small **blood vessels (4, 9)** are also present. The thin segments of Henle's loop (3, 8) in cross section resemble the capillaries or venules (4, 9).

■ **FIG. 2**
PAPILLA ADJACENT TO A CALYX (LONGITUDINAL SECTION)

Several collecting tubules merge in the medulla to form large, straight tubules called **papillary ducts (5),** which open at the tip of the papilla. Their numerous openings on the surface of the papilla produce a sievelike appearance; this is the area cribrosa. In this illustration, the papilla is covered by a **stratified cuboidal epithelium (8).** At the area cribrosa, however, the covering epithelium is usually a simple columnar epithelium which is continuous with the lining of the papillary ducts. Also illustrated are thin segments of **Henle's loops (3, 4, 6)** and ascending straight portion of the **distal tubule (1).** Abundant **connective tissue (7)** and many **capillaries (2)** are also seen.

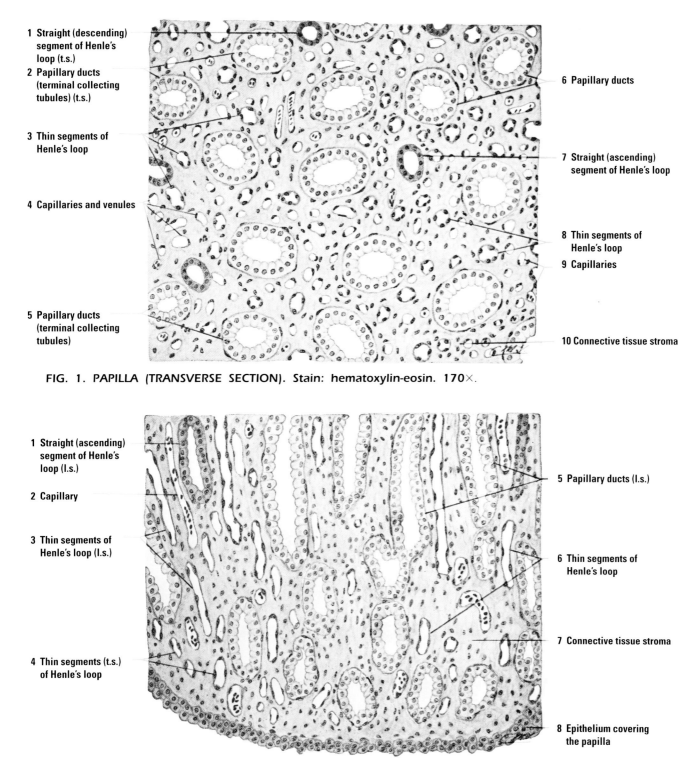

1 Straight (descending) segment of Henle's loop (t.s.)

2 Papillary ducts (terminal collecting tubules) (t.s.)

3 Thin segments of Henle's loop

4 Capillaries and venules

5 Papillary ducts (terminal collecting tubules)

6 Papillary ducts

7 Straight (ascending) segment of Henle's loop

8 Thin segments of Henle's loop

9 Capillaries

10 Connective tissue stroma

FIG. 1. PAPILLA (TRANSVERSE SECTION). Stain: hematoxylin-eosin. 170×.

1 Straight (ascending) segment of Henle's loop (l.s.)

2 Capillary

3 Thin segments of Henle's loop (l.s.)

4 Thin segments (t.s.) of Henle's loop

5 Papillary ducts (l.s.)

6 Thin segments of Henle's loop

7 Connective tissue stroma

8 Epithelium covering the papilla

FIG. 2. PAPILLA ADJACENT TO A CALYX, LONGITUDINAL SECTION. Stain: hematoxylin-eosin. 120×.

233

PLATE 90

■ **FIG. 1**
URETER: TRANSVERSE SECTION

An undistended ureter exhibits a convoluted lumen, formed by the longitudinal mucosal folds. The wall of the ureter consists of mucosa, muscularis, and adventitia.

The mucosa consists of **transitional epithelium (9, 10)** and a wide **lamina propria (5).** The transitional epithelium has several cell layers, with the outermost layer characterized by large cuboidal cells (9). The intermediate cells are polyhedral in shape, whereas the basal cells are low columnar or cuboidal (10). The basal surface of the epithelium is smooth and there are no indentations by the connective tissue papillae.

The lamina propria (5) contains fibroelastic connective tissue, which is denser with more fibroblasts under the epithelium and looser near the muscularis. Diffuse lymphatic tissue and occasional small lymphatic nodules may be observed in the lamina propria.

In the upper ureter, the muscularis consists of an inner **longitudinal (3)** smooth muscle layer and an outer **circular (2)** smooth muscle layer; these layers are not always distinct. An additional outer, longitudinal layer of smooth muscle is found in the lower third of the ureter.

The **adventitia (6)** blends with the surrounding fibroelastic **connective tissue** and **adipose tissue (1, 12),** which contains numerous **arteries (8), venules (11),** and small **nerves (7).**

■ **FIG. 2**
URETER WALL: TRANSVERSE SECTION

A higher magnification of the ureter wall illustrates greater structural details and layers. The **transitional epithelium (8, 9, 10)** exhibits the same cell layers as described in Fig. 1. The outermost cells often stain deeper than the remaining cells. The surface membrane, illustrated as a narrow acidophilic band (9), serves as an osmotic barrier between urine and tissue fluids.

In the **lamina propria (12),** fibroblasts are more numerous in the connective tissue under the epithelium than in the deeper region.

The **muscularis layer (7, 11)** appears often as loosely arranged smooth muscle bundles surrounded by abundant connective tissue, as illustrated in the inner **longitudinal layer (11).**

The **adventitia (5)** merges with the **connective tissue (6)** of the posterior abdominal wall in which the ureter is embedded.

URETER

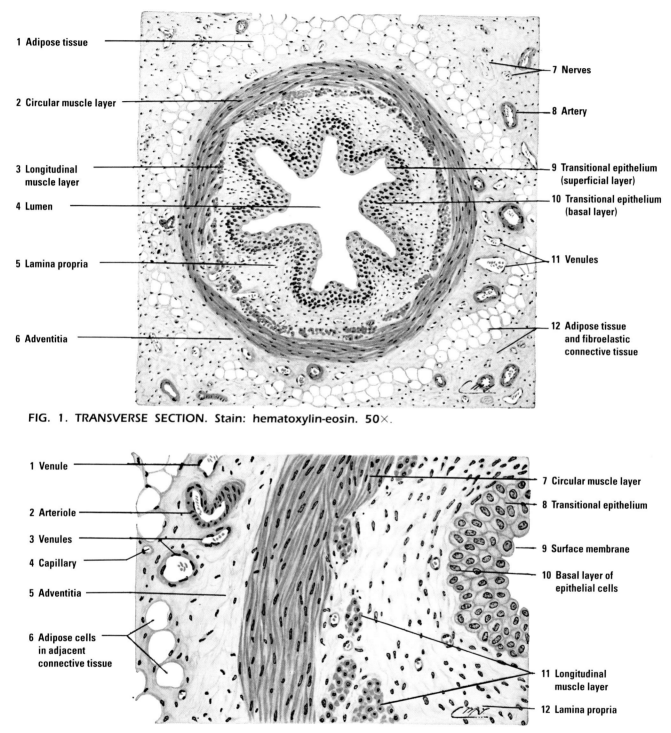

1 Adipose tissue

2 Circular muscle layer

3 Longitudinal muscle layer

4 Lumen

5 Lamina propria

6 Adventitia

7 Nerves

8 Artery

9 Transitional epithelium (superficial layer)

10 Transitional epithelium (basal layer)

11 Venules

12 Adipose tissue and fibroelastic connective tissue

FIG. 1. TRANSVERSE SECTION. Stain: hematoxylin-eosin. 50×.

1 Venule

2 Arteriole

3 Venules

4 Capillary

5 Adventitia

6 Adipose cells in adjacent connective tissue

7 Circular muscle layer

8 Transitional epithelium

9 Surface membrane

10 Basal layer of epithelial cells

11 Longitudinal muscle layer

12 Lamina propria

FIG. 2. URETER WALL, TRANSVERSE SECTION. Stain: hematoxylin-eosin. 150×.

PLATE 91

■ **FIG. 1**
URINARY BLADDER, SUPERIOR SURFACE: WALL (TRANSVERSE SECTION)

The **smooth muscle (1)** layers in the bladder wall are similar to those in the ureter except for their thickness. The bladder wall consists of a **mucosa (6, 7, 8)**, a **muscularis (1, 9)** and a **serosa (4, 5)** on the superior surface of the bladder. The inferior surface of the bladder is covered by adventitia, which merges with the connective tissue of adjacent structures.

The mucosa in an empty bladder exhibits numerous **folds (6)**; however, these folds disappear during bladder distension. The **transitional epithelium (7)** contains more cell layers and the **lamina propria (8)** is wider than in the ureter. The loose connective tissue in the deeper zone contains more elastic fibers.

The muscularis (1, 9) is thick, and in the neck of the bladder, the three layers are arranged in anastomosing bundles (1) between which is found **loose connective tissue (2)**. In this section, muscle bundles are seen in various planes of section (1) and the three distinct muscle layers are difficult to distinguish. The interstitial connective tissue merges with the connective tissue of the serosa (4); **mesothelium (5)** is the outermost layer.

■ **FIG. 2**
URINARY BLADDER: MUCOSA (TRANSVERSE SECTION)

The mucosa of the bladder is illustrated at a higher magnification.

In an empty bladder, the superficial cells of the **transitional epithelium (5)** are low **cuboidal or columnar (6)**. When the bladder is full and the transitional epithelium is stretched, the cells exhibit a **squamous (9)** appearance. The acidophilic surface **membrane (7)** of the superficial cells may be prominent. The deeper layers of cells in the epithelium are round (5) and basal cells more columnar (See also Plate 4).

In the **lamina propria (2)** are two zones, as in the ureter, but more pronounced. The subepithelial region is denser with fine fibers and numerous fibroblasts (2, upper leader). The deeper zone (2, lower leader) contains typical loose or moderately dense irregular connective tissue, which extends between the muscle fibers as interstitial connective tissue.

URINARY BLADDER (SUPERIOR SURFACE)

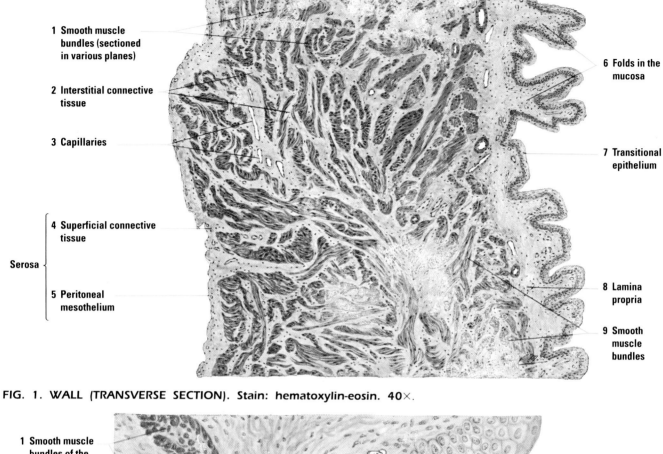

1 Smooth muscle bundles (sectioned in various planes)

2 Interstitial connective tissue

3 Capillaries

4 Superficial connective tissue

5 Peritoneal mesothelium

Serosa

6 Folds in the mucosa

7 Transitional epithelium

8 Lamina propria

9 Smooth muscle bundles

FIG. 1. WALL (TRANSVERSE SECTION). Stain: hematoxylin-eosin. 40×.

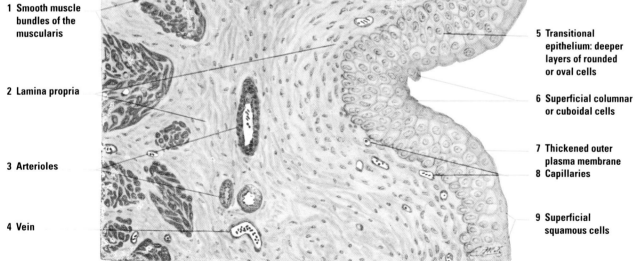

1 Smooth muscle bundles of the muscularis

2 Lamina propria

3 Arterioles

4 Vein

5 Transitional epithelium: deeper layers of rounded or oval cells

6 Superficial columnar or cuboidal cells

7 Thickened outer plasma membrane

8 Capillaries

9 Superficial squamous cells

FIG. 2. MUCOSA (TRANSVERSE SECTION). Stain: hematoxylin-eosin. 160×.

237

The endocrine system consists of cells, tissues, and/or organs that synthesize and secrete different chemicals or hormones into the blood or lymph capillaries. The chemicals are then transported by the vascular system to distant target organs, where they exert an influence on their structure and function.

The endocrine organs include the hypophysis (pituitary), thyroid, adrenal (suprarenal), and parathyroid glands. Their structure and function are described below. The individual endocrine cells or tissues that are part of mixed organs are discussed with these organs.

The Hypophysis (Pituitary Gland)

The structure and function of the hypophysis reflect its embryological origin from two distinct regions of the body. The epithelium of the pharyngeal roof (oral cavity) forms an outward outpocketing, detaches, and gives rise to the glandular portion of the hypophysis, the adenohypophysis. At the same time, the downgrowth of the developing brain forms the neural portion, the neurohypophysis. The formed hypophysis remains attached to the brain by a neural stalk. As a result of this dual origin, the structure and function of these two portions of the hypophysis are different from each other.

Although the hypophysis produces a variety of hormones, their synthesis and/or release from the hypophysis are directly controlled by the hypothalamus of the brain. The hypothalamic hormones that control the function of the adenohypophysis are the specific releasing factors (hormones) or the inhibitory factors (hormones). These factors are carried to the adenohypophysis by way of the blood vessels of the hypothalamohypophyseal portal system. On reaching the adenohypophysis, these factors then influence the secretion of specific hormones from different cells.

Adenohypophysis

The adenohypophysis contains two main categories of cells, the chromophobes and chromophils. The chromophils are further subdivided into acidophils and basophils, based on the affinity of their granules for specific stains. There are two types of acidophils, the somatotrophs and mammotrophs. The hormones that are produced by the acidophils and their specific effects on different organs of the body are described in the following paragraphs. The chromophobes are believed to be degranulated chromophilic cell types.

Chromophils—Acidophils

Growth hormone (somatotropin or GH). This hormone is produced by the somatotrophs. Its main function is to stimulate general body growth, especially the proliferation of the cartilage cells in the epiphyseal plates of the long bones.

Prolactin. This hormone, produced by mammotrophs, stimulates mammary gland development and maintenance of milk production during lactation.

There are three types of basophils, the thyrotrophs, gonadotrophs, and corticotrophs. The hormones produced by basophils and their specific effects on different organs of the body are described as follows.

Chromophils—Basophils

1. Thyroid-stimulating hormone (thyrotropin or TSH) is produced by the thyrotrophs. This hormone stimulates the synthesis and secretion of the thyroid hormones thyroxin and triiodothyronine from the thyroid gland.

2. Follicle-stimulating hormone (FSH) is produced by the gonadotrophs. FSH promotes the growth and maturation of the ovarian follicles in the ovaries and stimulates spermatogenesis in the seminiferous tubules of the testes.

3. Luteinizing hormone (LH) is also produced by the gonadotrophs. LH functions in association with FSH to promote the final maturation of the ovarian follicles and to induce ovulation. LH is also responsible for the formation of corpus luteum in the ovary following ovulation and the secretion of progesterone from the formed corpus luteum. In males, LH maintains and stimulates the interstitial cells (of Leydig) in the testes to produce the male hormone testosterone.

4. Adrenocorticotropic hormone (ACTH), produced by corticotrophs, influences the function of cells in the adrenal cortex of the adrenal gland. ACTH stimulates the synthesis and release of glucocorticoids from the zona fasciculata and zona reticularis of the adrenal cortex.

The adenohypophysis also contains pars intermedia. In lower vertebrates (amphibians and fishes), this area is well developed and produces melanocyte-stimulating hormone (MSH). In these animals, MSH increases pigmentation of the skin by causing dispersion of the melanin granules. In most mammals and humans, this region of the hypophysis is rudimentary.

The release of the listed hormones into the blood stream is influenced by the releasing factors or hormones produced by the hypothalamus. In addition, the hypothalamus elaborates inhibitory factors or hormones. The inhibitory factors are the growth hormone inhibitory factor and the prolactin inhibitory factor.

Neurohypophysis

The neurohypophysis is primarily composed of unmyelinated axons that originate from the neurosecretory cells in the hypothalamus and the supporting neuroglial cells, the pituicytes. Two hormones, oxytocin and vasopressin or antidiuretic hormone (ADH), are released by the neurohypophysis. These two hormones are first synthesized by the cells in the hypotha-lamus and then transported along the unmyelinated axons for storage in the axon terminals of the neurohy-pophysis as Herring bodies.

On release into the blood stream from the axon ter-minals, oxytocin stimulates the contraction of smooth muscles in the uterus, especially during the final stages of pregnancy and parturition. In addition, oxytocin causes the contraction of myoepithelial cells around the secretory alveoli and ducts in the lactating mammary glands. Stimulation of the myoepithelial cells causes the ejection of milk into the excretory ducts of the mammary gland and is part of the milk-ejection reflex. The initiation of this reflex is triggered by the suckling action of the infant on the nipple.

Release of the vasopressin or ADH into the blood stream stimulates contraction of the smooth muscle layers in small arteries and arterioles. This action nar-rows the lumina of these blood vessels and increases the blood pressure. The main action of ADH, however, is to increase the permeability to water of the distal convoluted tubules and collecting tubules in the kid-ney. This effect allows more water to be resorbed by the kidney tubules and retained in the body while at the same time increasing the concentration of the urine.

The Thyroid Gland

The thyroid gland is characterized by spherical struc-tures filled with secretory product. These structures are called follicles and are the structural and functional units of the thyroid gland. The follicular cells that sur-round the follicles secrete and store their secretory product extracellularly in the lumen of the follicles as a gelatinous substance called colloid. The colloid is com-posed of thyroglobulin, a glycoprotein that contains several iodinated amino acids; colloid is also the stor-age form of the thyroid hormone.

The activity of the follicular cells in the thyroid gland is controlled by the thyroid-stimulating hormone (TSH) of the adenohypophysis. This highly complex activity includes the synthesis of the thyroglobulin, iodination of the thyroglobulin, temporary storage of the thy-roglobulin in the follicular lumen, and release of the thyroid hormones. In response to the secretory stimu-lus, the follicular cells in the thyroid gland engulf and hydrolyze the iodinated thyroglobulin, and then release the thyroid hormones into the blood stream.

The thyroid hormones are thyroxine or T4 and tri-iodothyronine or T3. Release of these hormones into general circulation accelerates the metabolic rate of the body, increases cell metabolism, growth, differentia-tion, and development throughout the body. In addi-tion, the thyroid hormones increase the rate of protein, carbohydrate, and fat metabolism.

The thyroid gland also contains parafollicular cells. These cells lie adjacent to the follicles but do not extend to or contact the follicular lumen and its colloid. The parafollicular cells produce the hormone thyrocalci-tonin or calcitonin. The main function of this hormone

is to lower blood calcium levels in the body. This effect is accomplished by decreasing bone resorption. Secretion and release of thyrocalcitonin by the parafol-licular cells depends primarily on elevated blood calci-um levels and not the hormones from the pituitary gland.

The Parathyroid Gland

In mammals, there are usually four parathyroid glands. These small glands are situated on the posterior surface of the thyroid gland, but are separated from the thyroid gland by a thin connective tissue capsule.

The chief cells of the parathyroid glands produce the parathyroid hormone or parathormone, whose main function is to maintain a proper calcium level in the body. This function is accomplished by raising the cal-cium levels in the blood, an action that is opposite or antagonistic to that produced by thyrocalcitonin (calci-tonin) of the thyroid gland. The parathyroid hormone stimulates the activity and proliferation of the osteo-clasts in the bones. As a result of the increased osteolyt-ic activities of the bone osteoclasts, more calcium is released into the blood, thereby maintaining the nor-mal calcium levels.

In addition to raising blood calcium levels, the parathyroid hormone influences the renal tubules to decrease their clearance of calcium and increase the elimination of phosphate, sodium, and potassium in the urine.

The secretion and release of parathyroid hormone depends primarily on the concentration of calcium lev-els in the blood and not on the hormones from the pitu-itary gland. Because the hormone of the parathyroid glands maintains the optimal levels of calcium in the blood, these glands are essential to life.

The Adrenal (Suprarenal) Gland

The adrenal (suprarenal) glands are paired and are situated near the superior pole of the kidneys. Each gland is surrounded by a connective tissue capsule and consists of an outer cortex and an inner medulla. Although these two regions of the adrenal gland are in one organ and are linked by a common blood supply, they have different embryologic origin, structure, and function.

The Cortex

The adrenal cortex exhibits three concentric zones: zona glomerulosa, zona fasciculata, and zona reticu-laris. The cells of these zones in the adrenal cortex pro-duce three classes of steroid hormones. These are the mineralocorticoids, glucocorticoids, and steroid sex hormones.

The cells of the zona glomerulosa produce mineralo-corticoid hormones, of which aldosterone is the most potent. The major function of aldosterone is to increase sodium resorption from the glomerular filtrate by the distal tubules of the kidney and to increase potassium excretion in urine. The secretion of aldosterone is initiated by way of the renin-angiotensin system in response to a decrease in blood pressure and plasma levels of sodium, as detected by the juxtaglomerular apparatus in the kidney. Release of aldosterone causes increased retention of sodium and water in the body. This action increases fluid volume in the circulation and raises the blood pressure.

The cells of zona fasciculata and probably of zona reticularis secrete glucocorticoids, of which cortisol and cortisone are the most important. The secretion of glucocorticoids is an important response of the body to stress; glucocorticoids have a major effect on protein, fat, and carbohydrate metabolism, especially in increasing blood sugar levels. Glucocorticoids suppress the inflammatory responses in the body; they suppress the immune system by arresting mitotic activities in the lymphoid tissues and decreasing the production of antibodies.

Although the cells of the zona reticularis are believed to produce sex steroids, the amount of the hormones produced has little effect on normal physiologic processes.

Glucocorticoid secretion and the secretory functions of zona fasciculata and zona reticularis are regulated by the pituitary gland adrenocorticotropic hormone (ACTH).

The Medulla

The cells of adrenal medulla produce catecholamines (primarily epinephrine and norepinephrine). Their release from the adrenal medulla is under direct control of the autonomic nervous system. The effects of these catecholamines are similar to those produced by the stimulation of the sympathetic division of the autonomic nervous system.

PLATE 92

■ FIG. 1
HYPOPHYSIS OR PITUITARY GLAND (PANORAMIC VIEW, SAGITTAL SECTION)

The hypophysis consists of two major subdivisions, the adenohypophysis and neurohypophysis. The adenohypophysis is further subdivided into **pars distalis (anterior lobe) (5), pars tuberalis (9),** and **pars intermedia (10).** The neurohypophysis is divided into **pars nervosa** or **infundibular process (11), infundibular stalk (8),** and tuber cinerum of the median eminence (not illustrated). The pars tuberalis (9) of the adenohypophysis surrounds the infundibular stalk (8) and is, therefore, visible above and below the stalk in a sagittal section; it extends higher on the anterior than the posterior surface of the hypophysis. The infundibular stalk (8) connects the hypophysis with the central nervous system (base of the brain).

The pars distalis (5) is the largest of the four divisions of the hypophysis and contains two main types of cells, the **chromophobe cells (1)** and chromophil cells. The **chromophils** are subdivided into **acidophils (alpha) (3)** and **basophils (beta) cells (4).** (These are illustrated at a higher magnification in Fig. 2 below). It is currently believed that the chromophobes represent acidophil or basophil cells in an inactive state following degranulation.

The pars nervosa (11) is the second largest of the four divisions. Pars intermedia (10) and pars nervosa (11) form the posterior lobe of the hypophysis, which consists primarily of unmyelinated nerve fibers and supporting cells, the pituicytes. The **connective tissue septa (12)** that arise from the surrounding capsule penetrate into the gland.

The pars intermedia (10) is situated between the pars distalis and pars nervosa. This region contains colloid-filled cysts lined by different cells, with basophils predominant.

The neurohypophysis develops as ventral evagination or extension from the floor of brain. The adenohypophysis develops from the oral ectoderm diverticulum, the pouch of Rathke, and includes pars distalis (5), pars intermedia (10) and pars tuberalis (9).

■ FIG. 2
HYPOPHYSIS OR PITUITARY GLAND (SECTIONAL VIEW)

Under higher magnification, numerous **sinusoidal capillaries (6)** and different cell types are visible in the pars distalis. The **chromophobe cells (4)** exhibit a light-staining, homogeneous cytoplasm. They are normally smaller than the chromophils and are found in groups. The cytoplasm of chromophils stains red in **acidophils (3)** and blue in **basophils (5).**

The pars intermedia contains colloid-filled cysts or **vesicles (7)** lined by low columnar cells; some cells in these vesicles contain basophilic granules while others do not exhibit any granules in their cytoplasm. Follicles lined with **basophils (8)** are often seen in pars intermedia, with some cells exhibiting secretory granules in their cytoplasm (8, lower leader).

Also illustrated is a portion of **pars nervosa (9).** This region is characterized by unmyelinated axons and cytoplasmic processes of the **pituicytes (9, 10),** both of which stain lightly. Oval nuclei of the pituicytes are seen (10), but not the scanty cytoplasm.

HYPOPHYSIS (PITUITARY GLAND)

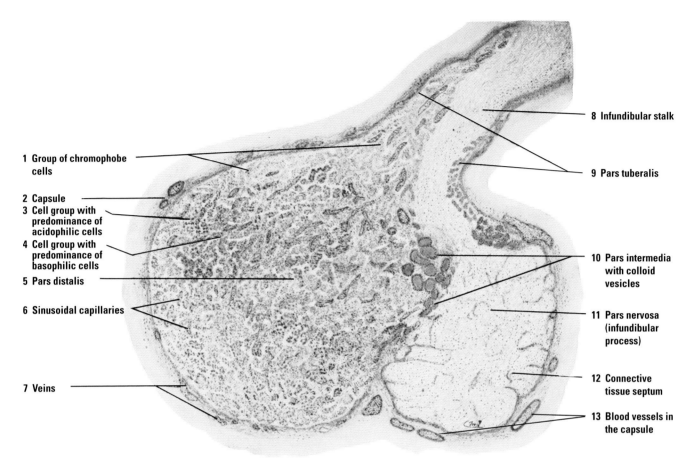

1 Group of chromophobe
   cells

2 Capsule

3 Cell group with
   predominance of
   acidophilic cells

4 Cell group with
   predominance of
   basophilic cells

5 Pars distalis

6 Sinusoidal capillaries

7 Veins

8 Infundibular stalk

9 Pars tuberalis

10 Pars intermedia
   with colloid
   vesicles

11 Pars nervosa
   (infundibular
   process)

12 Connective
   tissue septum

13 Blood vessels in
   the capsule

FIG. 1. PANORAMIC VIEW (SAGITTAL SECTION). Stain: hematoxylin-eosin. 22×.

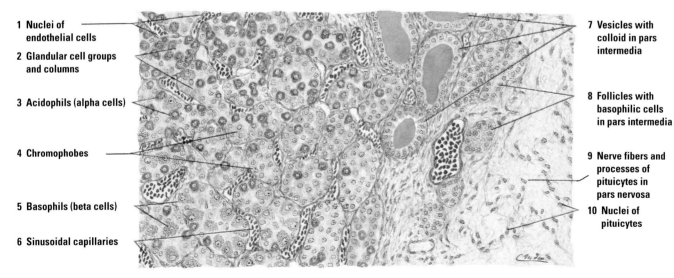

1 Nuclei of
   endothelial cells

2 Glandular cell groups
   and columns

3 Acidophils (alpha cells)

4 Chromophobes

5 Basophils (beta cells)

6 Sinusoidal capillaries

7 Vesicles with
   colloid in pars
   intermedia

8 Follicles with
   basophilic cells
   in pars intermedia

9 Nerve fibers and
   processes of
   pituicytes in
   pars nervosa

10 Nuclei of
   pituicytes

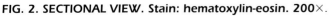

FIG. 2. SECTIONAL VIEW. Stain: hematoxylin-eosin. 200×.

243

PLATE 93

■ **FIG. 1**
HYPOPHYSIS: PARS DISTALIS (AZAN STAIN)

Different cell types in pars distalis can be readily identified following special fixation and/or staining. In the illustration, the hypophysis was fixed with a corrosive sublimate mixture, and the section stained with azocarmine and differentiated with aniline oil. Phosphotungstic acid was then used to destain the connective tissue, followed by aniline blue and orange G as cytoplasmic stains. The cytoplasmic granules stain red, orange or blue, depending on their respective affinities; the nuclei of all cells stain orange.

Chromophobes (3) usually stain light after any stain. Their nuclei stain pale, the cytoplasm stains pale orange, and the cell outlines are poorly defined. The aggregation of chromophobes in groups or clumps is apparent in this illustration.

Two types of **acidophils (1, 6)** can be distinguished (although not as clearly as after other specific stains) by their staining reaction; cells with coarse granules stain red with azocarmine (1) and those with smaller granules stain with orange G (6).

The **basophils (2, 5)** are readily recognized by blue-stained granules, whereas the different types of basophils are not distinguishable. The degree of granularity and the stain density vary in different cells.

■ **FIG. 2**
HYPOPHYSIS: CELL GROUPS (AZAN STAIN)

Different cell types of the hypophysis are illustrated at higher magnification after azan staining. Nuclei of all cells are stained orange-red.

In the **chromophobes (a),** the light orange stain of the cytoplasm indicates that they are nongranular and their cell boundaries indistinct. In the **acidophils (b),** the cytoplasmic granules stain intense red and the cell outlines are distinct. A sinusoid capillary is in close proximity to the acidophils.

The **basophils (c)** exhibit variable round, polyhedral, or angular shapes. The blue granules vary in size and are not as compact as in the acidophils.

The **pituicytes (d)** of pars nervosa exhibit variable shape and size of the cells and **nuclei (1).** The small, orange-stained cytoplasm has diffuse **cytoplasmic processes (2).**

HYPOPHYSIS

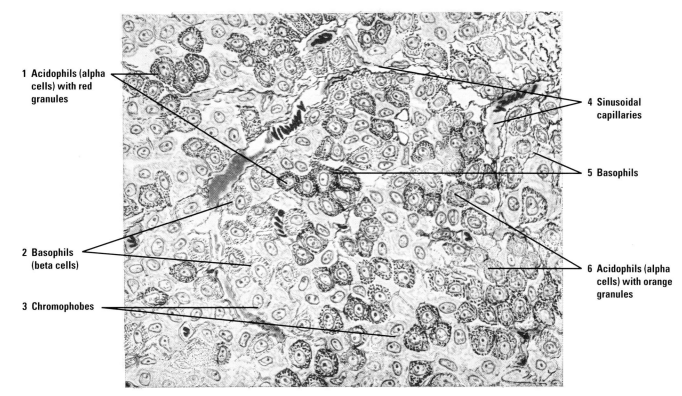

1 Acidophils (alpha cells) with red granules

2 Basophils (beta cells)

3 Chromophobes

4 Sinusoidal capillaries

5 Basophils

6 Acidophils (alpha cells) with orange granules

FIG. 1. PARS DISTALIS (AZAN STAIN).
Sectional view. Nuclei: orange; cytoplasmic granules of alpha cells: red or orange; cytoplasmic granules of beta cells: deep blue; collagenous and reticular fibers: blue; erythrocytes: bright red; hemolyzed blood: deep yellow. About 500×.

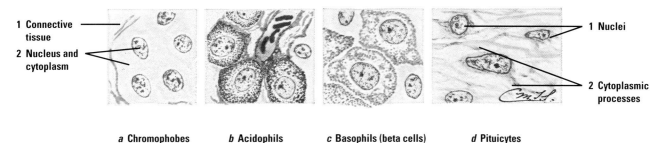

1 Connective tissue

2 Nucleus and cytoplasm

1 Nuclei

2 Cytoplasmic processes

a Chromophobes   *b* Acidophils (alpha cells)   *c* Basophils (beta cells)   *d* Pituicytes

FIG. 2. CELL GROUPS (AZAN STAIN) 800×.

245

PLATE 94

■ **FIG. 1**
THYROID GLAND (GENERAL VIEW)

The thyroid gland is characterized by various-sized, spherical **follicles (1, 2, 5)** containing acidophilic **colloid (2)** material in their lumina. The follicular epithelium is simple columnar or cuboidal epithelium and consists primarily of the follicular or principal cells with large round nuclei. In routine histologic preparations, the colloid material often retracts from the follicular wall (1). The follicles that are **sectioned tangentially (4)** do not have a lumen.

Connective tissue septa (6) from the thyroid gland capsule penetrate and divide the gland into groups of follicles or lobules. The connective tissue contains well developed **capillary plexuses (3)** that are closely associated with the follicular epithelium. Relatively little **interfollicular connective tissue (7)** is found between individual **follicles (2).**

■ **FIG. 2**
THYROID GLAND: FOLLICLES (SECTIONAL VIEW)

At a higher magnification, the epithelium of different follicles exhibits variable height. In some **follicles (1, 2, 5),** the cells are flattened whereas in others, they are cuboidal or low columnar; the nuclei are vesicular. The appearance of the epithelium, the amount of colloid material, and the size of the follicles vary with functional states of the thyroid gland.

Most follicles are filled with acidophilic **colloid material (5).** In some follicles, the **colloid (4)** is retracted; in others, the colloid contains **vacuoles (7).** Tangential sections through the walls of **follicles (8)** are seen as clumps of cells without a lumen surrounded by the interfollicular connective tissue. **Capillaries (3)** are prominent in the thyroid gland and are closely associated with individual follicles.

■ **FIG. 3**
THYROID GLAND: PARAFOLLICULAR CELLS

In addition to the **follicular cells (1, 6),** the thyroid gland also contains parafollicular cells. These cells have a comparatively sparse distribution in the gland.

The **parafollicular cells (3, 4)** occur singly or in groups in the gland. They are situated within the follicles, between the follicular cells and the basement membrane. The parafollicular cells (3, 4) are larger than the follicular cells and oval or of variable shape containing light, finely granular cytoplasm; they do not border directly on the follicular lumina.

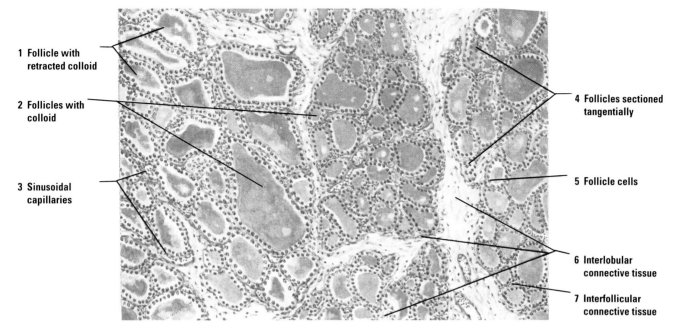

1 Follicle with
retracted colloid

2 Follicles with
colloid

3 Sinusoidal
capillaries

4 Follicles sectioned
tangentially

5 Follicle cells

6 Interlobular
connective tissue

7 Interfollicular
connective tissue

FIG. 1. GENERAL VIEW. Stain: hematoxylin-eosin. 90×.

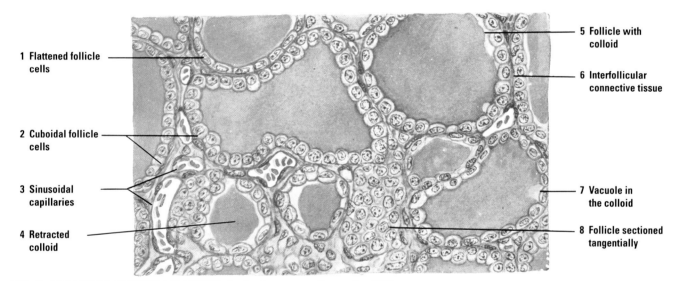

1 Flattened follicle
cells

2 Cuboidal follicle
cells

3 Sinusoidal
capillaries

4 Retracted
colloid

5 Follicle with
colloid

6 Interfollicular
connective tissue

7 Vacuole in
the colloid

8 Follicle sectioned
tangentially

FIG. 2. FOLLICLES (SECTIONAL VIEW). Stain: hematoxylin-eosin. 550×.

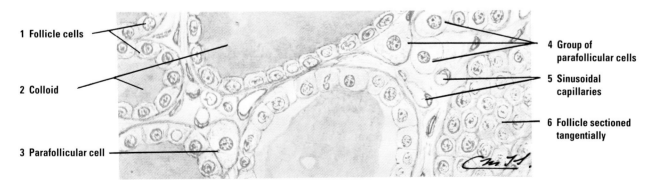

1 Follicle cells

2 Colloid

3 Parafollicular cell

4 Group of
parafollicular cells

5 Sinusoidal
capillaries

6 Follicle sectioned
tangentially

FIG. 3. PARAFOLLICULAR CELLS. Stain: hematoxylin-eosin. 600×.

247

PLATE 95

■ **FIG. 1**
THYROID AND PARATHYROID GLANDS

The location of the **parathyroid gland (9)** in close proximity to the **thyroid gland (7)** allows the examination of their structural relationships and differences in the same histologic section.

The various-sized **follicles (1)** with colloid material characterize the thyroid gland. A thin **connective tissue capsule (2, 8)** with rich capillary plexus separates the thyroid gland (7) from the parathyroid gland (9). This capsule also binds them together. The connective tissue trabeculae (6) from the capsule extend into the parathyroid gland (9) and bring in the larger **blood vessel (6)**, which then branch into extensive capillary network among the parathyroid cells. Nerve fibers accompany the blood vessels and the connective tissue trabeculae may contain **adipose cells (5).**

The cells in the parathyroid gland are not arranged into follicles as seen in the thyroid gland. Instead, the cells are single and arranged close together. Most of the cells in the parathyroid gland are the **principal or chief cells (3).** The larger **oxyphil cells (4),** seen in small groups, appear less frequent than the chief cells (3).

■ **FIG. 2**
PARATHYROID GLAND

The characteristic features of the parathyroid gland are illustrated at a higher magnification.

The **principal (chief) cells (1, 7)** are the most numerous and are arranged in groups; **capillaries (5)** course among the cell groups. The principal cells (1, 7) are round and exhibit a pale, slightly acidophilic cytoplasm with vesicular nuclei. **Oxyphil cells (3, 6)** are seen as single cells or in small clusters. These cells are larger than the principal cells, exhibit granular, acidophilic cytoplasm and smaller, darker staining nuclei. In adults, transitional forms are seen between oxyphils (3, 6) and principal cells (1, 7). In humans, oxyphil cells (3, 6) are not normally present in children under 4 years.

Although not a characteristic feature, **colloid vesicles (2)** are occasionally recorded in the parathyroid gland. **Connective tissue trabeculae (4, 8)** are present in the gland but these do not form distinct lobules as in the thyroid gland.

THYROID AND PARATHYROID GLANDS

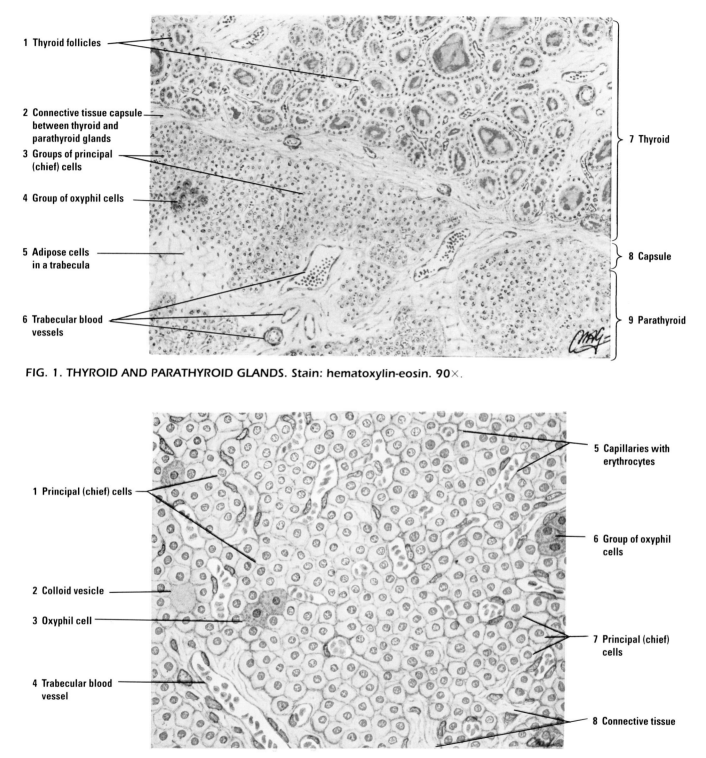

1 Thyroid follicles

2 Connective tissue capsule between thyroid and parathyroid glands

3 Groups of principal (chief) cells

4 Group of oxyphil cells

5 Adipose cells in a trabecula

6 Trabecular blood vessels

7 Thyroid

8 Capsule

9 Parathyroid

FIG. 1. THYROID AND PARATHYROID GLANDS. Stain: hematoxylin-eosin. 90×.

1 Principal (chief) cells

2 Colloid vesicle

3 Oxyphil cell

4 Trabecular blood vessel

5 Capillaries with erythrocytes

6 Group of oxyphil cells

7 Principal (chief) cells

8 Connective tissue

FIG. 2. PARATHYROID GLAND. Stain: hematoxylin-eosin. 550×.

PLATE 96

ADRENAL (SUPRARENAL) GLAND

The adrenal (suprarenal) gland consists of an outer **cortex (2)** and an **inner medulla (3).** The gland is surrounded by a thick connective tissue **capsule (1)** in which are found branches of the main adrenal arteries, veins, **nerves (5)** (largely unmyelinated), and lymphatics. **Connective tissue trabeculae (4)** from the capsule pass into the cortex of the gland and the larger trabeculae carry **arteries (4)** to the **medulla (3). Sinusoidal capillaries (7, 9)** are found throughout the cortex (2) and medulla (3).

The adrenal cortex (2) is subdivided into three concentric zones which are not sharply demarcated from each other. Directly under the connective tissue capsule (1) is the first or the outermost cell layer of the adrenal gland cortex; this is the **zona glomerulosa (2a).** The **cells (6)** in this zone are arranged into ovoid groups. The cytoplasm of these cells (6) contains sparse lipid droplets. In the hematoxylin-eosin preparations, the lipid droplets appear as vacuoles while their nuclei stain dark.

The middle cell layer is the **zona fasciculata (2b),** whose **cells (8)** are arranged into columns or plates with radial arrangement. Increased amount of lipid droplets in the cytoplasm give the cells of zona fasciculata (8) a vacuolated appearance following a normal histologic preparation. The nuclei of these cells are vesicular. **Sinusoidal capillaries (9)** between the cell columns follow a similar radial course.

The third cell layer borders the adrenal medulla and is the **zona reticularis (2c, 15).** The **cells (10)** of this layer form anastomosing cords and are frequently filled with dark-staining, lipofuscin **pigment (11).** The capillaries in this layer exhibit an irregular arrangement.

The **medulla (3)** is not sharply demarcated from the cortex. The cells that constitute the majority of the medulla (3, **14**) are arranged in groups. With normal histologic preparation of the adrenal gland, the cytoplasm in these cells appears clear (14). After tissue fixation in potassium bichromate, however, fine brown granules become visible in the cells of the medulla. This cellular alteration is termed the chromaffin reaction and indicates the presence of the catecholamines epinephrine and norepinephrine in the granules. The medulla also contains **sympathetic ganglion cells (13),** seen singly or in small groups. They exhibit the characteristic vesicular nucleus, prominent nucleolus, and a small amount of peripheral chromatin. Sinusoidal capillaries are also present in the medulla and drain its contents into the **medullary veins (12).**

4 Connective tissue septum with blood vessel (artery)

5 Unmyelinated nerves

1 Capsule

2 Cortex

2a Zona glomerulosa

2b Zona fasciculata

2c Zona reticularis

3 Medulla

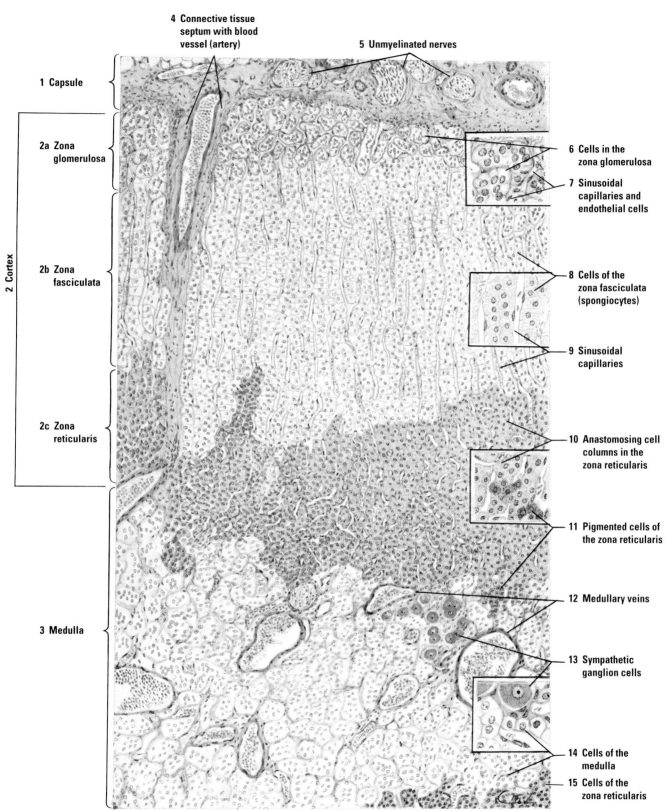

6 Cells in the zona glomerulosa

7 Sinusoidal capillaries and endothelial cells

8 Cells of the zona fasciculata (spongiocytes)

9 Sinusoidal capillaries

10 Anastomosing cell columns in the zona reticularis

11 Pigmented cells of the zona reticularis

12 Medullary veins

13 Sympathetic ganglion cells

14 Cells of the medulla

15 Cells of the zona reticularis

Stain: hematoxylin-eosin. 200×.

THE MALE REPRODUCTIVE SYSTEM

The male reproductive system consists of the gonads or testes, the excretory ducts, the accessory reproductive glands, and the penis. The testes perform two important reproductive functions: they produce the spermatozoa and the male hormone, testosterone.

The Testes

Each testis is subdivided by connective tissue septa into numerous lobules, each containing numerous highly coiled seminiferous tubules. Each seminiferous tubule is lined by the stratified germinal epithelium, which consists of two major cell types: the spermatogenic cells and the supporting or Sertoli cells. The spermatogenic cells divide, differentiate, and produce the spermatozoa by a complex process called spermatogenesis, which involves the following phases: (1) mitotic divisions of spermatogonia to produce successive generations of cells that eventually form spermatocytes; (2) two meiotic divisions, in which the number of chromosomes in the spermatocytes is reduced by half, resulting in the production of spermatids; and (3) spermiogenesis, during which the spermatids undergo differentiation into spermatozoa.

The Sertoli cells perform numerous important functions related to the process of spermatogenesis, among which are: (1) support, protection, and nutrition of the developing sperm cells; (2) phagocytosis of the excess cytoplasm of the spermatozoa (the residual bodies) during spermiogenesis; (3) release of spermatozoa (spermiation) into the seminiferous tubules; and (4) secretion of various hormones, such as the androgen-binding protein and inhibin.

The follicle-stimulating hormone (FSH), released from the adenohypophysis of the pituitary gland, controls the secretion of androgen-binding protein by the Sertoli cells. The androgen-binding protein increases the concentration of testosterone in the seminiferous tubules for proper spermatogenesis. Sertoli cells also secrete inhibin, a hormone believed to suppress or inhibit the production of FSH by the pituitary gland.

Surrounding the seminiferous tubules are fibroblasts, muscle-like cells, nerves, blood vessels and lymphatic vessels. In addition, between seminiferous tubules are clusters of epitheloid cells, the interstitial cells (of Leydig). These cells produce testosterone, a male hormone that is necessary for the development and maintenance of the accessory glands of the male reproductive system and the secondary male sex characteristics.

The normal spermatogenesis in the testes depends on several factors. Proper levels are needed of both the luteinizing hormone (LH) and the follicle-stimulating hormone (FSH); these hormones are produced by the gonadotrophs of the adenohypophysis of the pituitary gland. LH stimulates the production of testosterone by the interstitial cells and FSH stimulates the Sertoli cells to produce the androgen-binding protein. Testosterone binds with androgen-binding protein and enters the lumina of the seminiferous tubules. High levels of testosterone are needed in the seminiferous tubules to sustain the normal process of spermatogenesis.

In addition to the circulating levels of these hormones, proper temperature in the testes is crucial for normal spermatogenesis. Testicular temperature is normally about 2 to 3°C cooler than the core body temperature. Some of this cooling is accomplished by the location of the testes outside of the body in the scrotum. In addition, a venous (pampiniform) plexus surrounds the testicular arteries and provides an important mechanism for a countercurrent heat exchange. By this method, blood in the arteries that flows into the testes is cooled and blood in the veins that returns to the body is warmed.

The Excretory Ducts

The seminiferous tubules in the lobules of the testes terminate as straight tubules, the tubuli recti. Spermatozoa that were released into the tubules pass from here into the rete testis, which then drains into the head of the epididymis by way of the ductuli efferentes (efferent ducts).

The ductuli efferentes are lined with tall ciliated and resorptive nonciliated cells. The cilia in these ducts assist in transporting the sperm to the epididymis and the nonciliated cells absorb some of the fluid that was produced in the seminiferous tubules. As the sperm slowly pass through the highly coiled ducts of the epididymis, the epididymis becomes an important site for sperm storage and sperm maturation. In conjunction with ductuli efferentes, the cells of the epididymis also absorb testicular fluid. During sexual stimulation and ejaculation, strong smooth muscle contractions around the ducts of the epididymis expel the sperm into the ductus deferens, which then conducts the sperm to the urethra.

The Accessory Reproductive Glands

The accessory reproductive glands of the male reproductive tract consist of paired seminal vesicles, paired bulbourethral glands, and a single prostate gland.

The seminal vesicles produce a yellowish, viscous fluid that contains a high concentrations of fructose. The fructose is used by the sperm as a source of energy for their motility following ejaculation.

The prostate gland produces a thin, watery, slightly acidic fluid that is rich in citric acid and acid phosphatase. The enzyme fibrinolysin in the fluid liquefies the congealed semen after ejaculation.

The bulbourethral glands produce a clear, viscid, mucus-like secretion that, during erotic stimulation, functions as a lubricant for the urethra.

PLATE 97

■ **FIG. 1**
TESTIS

■ **FIG. 2**
SEMINIFEROUS TUBULES, STRAIGHT TUBULES,
RETE TESTIS AND DUCTULI EFFERENTES
(EFFERENT DUCTS)

PLATE 97

■ FIG. 1
TESTIS

The testis is enclosed in a thick, connective tissue capsule, the **tunica albuginea (1)**. Internal to this capsule is a vascular layer of loose connective tissue, the **tunica vasculosa (2)**. This layer merges with the stroma of the testis, the **interstitial connective tissue (7)**, which is also rich in **blood vessels (10)**. The fibers of the interstitial connective tissue (7) bind and support the **seminiferous tubules (3, 4, 9)**.

The seminiferous tubules (3, 4, 9) are long, highly convoluted tubules in the testis that are normally observed cut in various planes of section. These tubules are lined with a specialized stratified epithelium called the germinal epithelium, which consists of the spermatogenic and supportive or Sertoli cells. These cells rest on a thin **basement membrane (5)**. (See Plate 98 for details).

Located in the interstitial connective tissue (7) that surrounds the seminiferous tubules are groups of endocrine cells, the **interstitial cells (of Leydig) (8)**. These cells secrete the male sex hormone, testosterone.

■ FIG. 2
SEMINIFEROUS TUBULES, STRAIGHT TUBULES, RETE TESTIS AND DUCTULI EFFERENTES (EFFERENT DUCTS)

In this illustration, the plane of section passes through the connective tissue of the **mediastinum (3)** of the testis, a small portion of the **testis (1)** proper, and the excretory ducts, the **ductuli efferentes (5)**.

The **seminiferous tubules (1)** are represented on the left side of the illustration; they are lined with spermatogenic cells and the supporting Sertoli cells. The interstitial connective tissue of the testis is continuous with the connective tissue of the mediastinum (3). In the mediastinum, the seminiferous tubules of each testicular lobule converge to form **straight tubules (2)**. These tubules are short, narrow ducts lined with cuboidal or low columnar epithelium.

The straight tubules continue into the **rete testis (4, 6)** located in the connective tissue of the mediastinum (3). The rete testis (4, 6) are irregular, anastomosing tubules with wide lumina lined by a single layer of low cuboidal or low columnar epithelium; these tubules become wider near the **ductuli efferentes (efferent ductules) (5)** into which they empty. The ductuli efferentes (5) are straight; however, as they continue into the head of the epididymis, they become highly convoluted. (See Plate 99, Fig. 1).

TESTIS

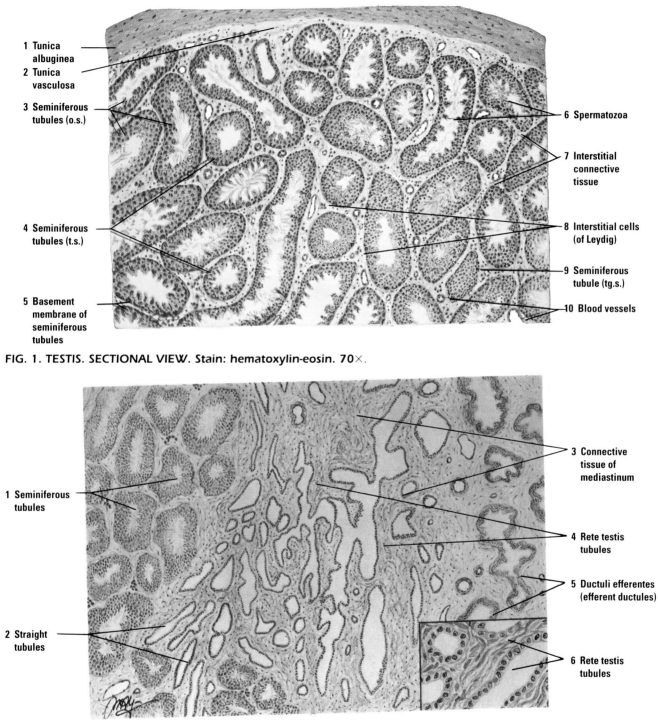

1 Tunica albuginea
2 Tunica vasculosa
3 Seminiferous tubules (o.s.)
4 Seminiferous tubules (t.s.)
5 Basement membrane of seminiferous tubules
6 Spermatozoa
7 Interstitial connective tissue
8 Interstitial cells (of Leydig)
9 Seminiferous tubule (tg.s.)
10 Blood vessels

FIG. 1. TESTIS. SECTIONAL VIEW. Stain: hematoxylin-eosin. 70×.

1 Seminiferous tubules
2 Straight tubules
3 Connective tissue of mediastinum
4 Rete testis tubules
5 Ductuli efferentes (efferent ductules)
6 Rete testis tubules

FIG. 2. SEMINIFEROUS TUBULES, STRAIGHT TUBULES, RETE TESTIS, AND DUCTULI EFFERENTES (EFFERENT DUCTS). Stain: hematoxylin-eosin. 60× and **400×.**

PLATE 98

■ **FIG. 1**
PRIMATE TESTIS: SEMINIFEROUS TUBULES (TRANSVERSE SECTION)

Different stages of spermatogenesis are illustrated in various **seminiferous tubules (3)**. Each tubule (3) is surrounded by an outer layer of connective tissue with **fibroblasts (1)** and an inner **basement membrane (2)**. Between the tubules is the interstitial tissue, consisting of **fibroblasts (18)**, **blood vessels (10)**, nerves, and lymphatics. Also prominent between the seminiferous tubules (3) are the **interstitial cells (of Leydig) (11, 15)**.

The stratified germinal epithelium of the seminiferous tubules consists of the **supporting or Sertoli cells (6, 7, 14)** and the **spermatogenic cells (5, 9, 12)**. The Sertoli cells (6, 7, 14) are slender, elongated cells with irregular outlines extending from the basement membrane to the lumen of the seminiferous tubule (3). The nucleus of the Sertoli cells (6, 7, 14) is generally ovoid or elongated and contains fine, sparse chromatin. A distinct nucleolus in the Sertoli cells (6, 7, 14) distinguishes them from the spermatogenic cells (5, 9, 12), which are arranged in rows between and around the Sertoli cells. In different sections, the spermatogenic cells often appear superimposed on Sertoli cells (6, 7, 14), obscuring their cytoplasm.

The immature spermatogenic cells, the **spermatogonia (12)**, are situated adjacent to the basement membrane (2) of the seminiferous tubules (3). The spermatogonia (12) divide mitotically to produce several generations of cells. Three types of spermatogonia are usually recognized. The **pale type A spermatogonia (12a)** have a light-staining cytoplasm and a round or ovoid nucleus with pale, finely granular chromatin. The **dark type A spermatogonia (12b)** appear similar, but the chromatin stains darker. In type B spermatogonia (not illustrated), the chromatin granules in the spherical nucleus are variable and the nucleolus is centrally located.

Type A spermatogonia (12a) serve as stem cells of the germinal epithelium and give rise to other type A and type B spermatogonia. The final mitosis of type B spermatogonia produces **primary spermatocytes (5, 16)**. The nuclei of these cells have variable appearances because of different states of activity of the chromatin. These cells promptly enter the first meiotic division and the representative meiotic figures are prevalent in the seminiferous tubules (3).

Primary spermatocytes (5, 16) are the most obvious and largest germ cells in the seminiferous tubules (3) and occupy the middle region of the germinal epithelium. Their cytoplasm contains large nuclei with coarse clumps or thin threads of chromatin. The first meiotic division of the primary spermatocytes (Fig. 2, I, 5) produces smaller secondary spermatocytes with less dense nuclear chromatin (Fig. 2, I, 3). The secondary spermatocytes (Fig. 2, I, 3) undergo second meiotic division shortly after their formation and are therefore not frequently seen in sections of the seminiferous tubules (3).

Completion of the second meiotic division produces **spermatids (9, 13, 17)**, which are smaller cells than the primary or secondary spermatocytes (Fig. 2, I, 2, 3, 5). These cells lie in groups in the adluminal portion of the seminiferous tubule in close association with the Sertoli cells (6, 13, 14). In this environment, the spermatids (9, 13, 17) differentiate into **spermatozoa (4, 8)** by a process called spermiogenesis. The small, dark-staining heads of the maturing spermatozoa (4, 8) lie embedded in the cytoplasm of the Sertoli cells (6, 7, 14), and their tails extend into the lumen of the seminiferous tubule (3).

■ **FIG. 2**
PRIMATE TESTIS: STAGES OF SPERMATOGENESIS

Three different stages of spermatogenesis are illustrated in greater detail. In the **left illustration (I)**, the **primary spermatocytes (5)** are undergoing meiotic division to form the **secondary spermatocytes (3)**, which in turn undergo rapid division to form the **spermatids (2)**. In this stage, the **maturing spermatozoa (1)** are embedded deep in the **Sertoli cell (4)** cytoplasm. Adjacent to the basement membrane are the **type A spermatogonia (6)**.

In the **middle illustration (II)**, the **maturing spermatozoa (7)** are located peripherally near the lumen of the seminiferous tubule prior to being released. Also visible are clumps of round **spermatids (8)** and **primary spermatocytes (9)** in close association with the **Sertoli cells (10)**. Near the base of the tubule are found **spermatogonia (11)**.

In the **left illustration (III)**, the mature sperm have been released (spermiation) into the seminiferous tubule and the germinal epithelium contains only **spermatids (8)**, **primary spermatocytes (9)**, **spermatogonia (11)**, and the supporting **Sertoli cells (10)**.

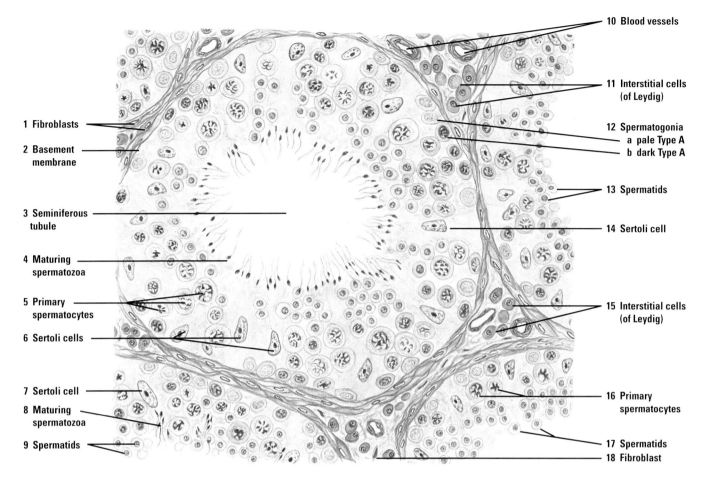

1 Fibroblasts

2 Basement
membrane

3 Seminiferous
tubule

4 Maturing
spermatozoa

5 Primary
spermatocytes

6 Sertoli cells

7 Sertoli cell

8 Maturing
spermatozoa

9 Spermatids

10 Blood vessels

11 Interstitial cells
(of Leydig)

12 Spermatogonia
a pale Type A
b dark Type A

13 Spermatids

14 Sertoli cell

15 Interstitial cells
(of Leydig)

16 Primary
spermatocytes

17 Spermatids

18 Fibroblast

FIG 1. SPERMATOGENESIS IN SEMINIFEROUS TUBULES. PRIMATE TESTIS. PLASTIC SECTION, HEMATOXYLIN AND EOSIN STAIN.

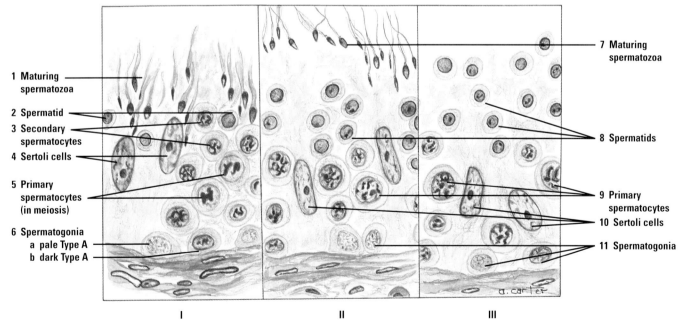

1 Maturing
spermatozoa

2 Spermatid

3 Secondary
spermatocytes

4 Sertoli cells

5 Primary
spermatocytes
(in meiosis)

6 Spermatogonia
a pale Type A
b dark Type A

7 Maturing
spermatozoa

8 Spermatids

9 Primary
spermatocytes

10 Sertoli cells

11 Spermatogonia

I   II   III

FIG 2. STAGES OF SPERMATOGENESIS. PRIMATE TESTIS PLASTIC SECTION, HEMATOXYLIN AND EOSIN STAIN.

259

PLATE 99

■ **FIG. 1**
DUCTULI EFFERENTES AND TRANSITION TO DUCTUS EPIDIDYMIS

The **ductuli efferentes (1, 4, 5)** or efferent ducts emerge from the mediastinum on the posterior-superior surface of the testis and connect the rete testis with the ductus epididymis. The ductuli efferentes are located in the **connective tissue (2)** and form a portion of the head of the **epididymis (7).** Because of the tortuous, spiral course of the tubules, they are seen as isolated tubules cut in various planes of section (1, 5).

The lumina of the ducts exhibit a characteristic irregular contour. The lining epithelium is simple, consisting of alternating groups of tall **ciliated** and shorter **nonciliated cells (4),** which are believed to be absorp-

tive. Occasional basal cells may be present, giving the epithelium a pseudostratified appearance. The basal surface of the tubules has a smooth contour. Located under the basement membrane is a thin layer of connective tissue containing a thin layer of circularly arranged **smooth muscle fibers (3).**

The distal ends of the tubules near the epididymis are lined with columnar cells only **(6),** and the lumina exhibit an even contour. As the ductuli efferentes terminate in the ductus epididymis, there is an abrupt transition of the epithelium to the tall pseudostratified columnar type of the **epididymis (7).**

■ **FIG. 2**
DUCTUS EPIDIDYMIS

The ductus epididymis is a long, highly convoluted tubule surrounded by the **connective tissue (1).** A transverse section through the epididymis shows the **convoluted tubules (2, 5, 6)** in highly varied forms. The individual tubules are surrounded by **smooth muscle fibers (7)** and **connective tissue (1).** Both the internal and external surfaces of the tubules have smooth contours.

The tubular epithelium of ductus epididymis is **pseudostratified (4, 9),** consisting of tall **columnar principal cells (9)** with long, nonmotile **stereocilia (8)** and

small **basal cells (10).** The function of the columnar principal cells (9) with stereocilia (8) is primarily absorption of the tubular fluid; the function of the basal cells is not known. The stereocilia (8) are long, branched microvilli.

The **basement membrane (3)** that surrounds each tubule is distinct. The lamina propria with the circularly arranged smooth muscle fibers (7) is thin and more pronounced than in the ductuli efferentes. Mature spermatozoa are seen in the lumina of some of the tubules.

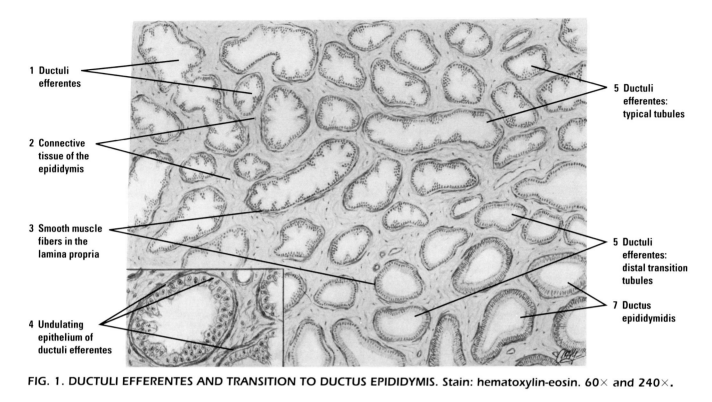

1 Ductuli efferentes

2 Connective tissue of the epididymis

3 Smooth muscle fibers in the lamina propria

4 Undulating epithelium of ductuli efferentes

5 Ductuli efferentes: typical tubules

5 Ductuli efferentes: distal transition tubules

7 Ductus epididymidis

FIG. 1. DUCTULI EFFERENTES AND TRANSITION TO DUCTUS EPIDIDYMIS. Stain: hematoxylin-eosin. 60× and 240×.

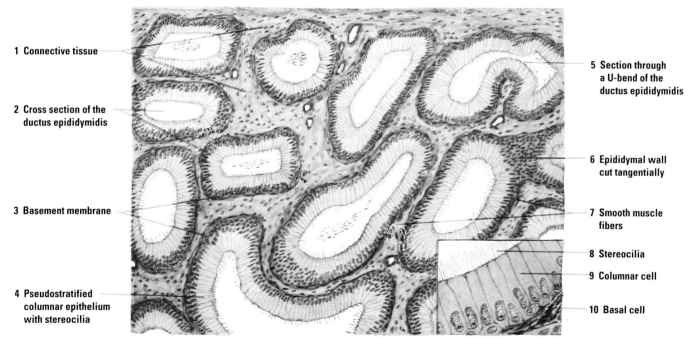

1 Connective tissue

2 Cross section of the ductus epididymidis

3 Basement membrane

4 Pseudostratified columnar epithelium with stereocilia

5 Section through a U-bend of the ductus epididymidis

6 Epididymal wall cut tangentially

7 Smooth muscle fibers

8 Stereocilia

9 Columnar cell

10 Basal cell

FIG. 2. DUCTUS EPIDIDYMIS. Stain: hematoxylin-eosin. 90×.

PLATE 100

■ **FIG. 1**
DUCTUS DEFERENS (TRANSVERSE SECTION)

The ductus deferens exhibits a narrow, irregular lumen, a thin mucosa, a thick muscularis, and adventitia. The irregular outline of the lumen is caused by longitudinal folds of the **lamina propria (5, 6)**, which in transverse section appear as crests or papillae (6). The thin lamina propria (5, 6) consists of compact collagenous fibers and fine elastic network.

The **epithelium** is **pseudostratified columnar (7)** but is somewhat lower than the epithelium lining the ductus epididymis. The epithelium rests on a thin basement membrane and stereocilia is usually seen on the cell apices.

The muscularis consists of a thin **inner longitudinal layer (3)**, a thick **middle circular layer (2)**, and a thin **outer longitudinal smooth muscle layer (1)**. The muscularis is surrounded by **adventitia (4)**, which contains abundant blood vessels and nerves. The adventitia (4) merges with the connective tissue surrounding the spermatic cord.

■ **FIG. 2**
AMPULLA OF THE DUCTUS DEFERENS

The terminal portion of ductus deferens enlarges into an ampulla. The ampulla differs from the ductus deferens mainly in the structure of its mucosa.

The lumen of the ampulla is larger and the mucosa exhibits numerous thin, irregular, branching **folds (6)** with diverticula or **glandular crypts (5, 9)** located between them. The epithelium lining the lumen and the crypts is simple **columnar** or **cuboidal (7)** and is secretory in nature.

The muscularis is similar to the ductus deferens. It consists of a thin **outer longitudinal layer (3)**, a thick **middle layer (2)**, and a thin **inner longitudinal smooth muscle layer (1)** adjacent to the **lamina propria (8)**.

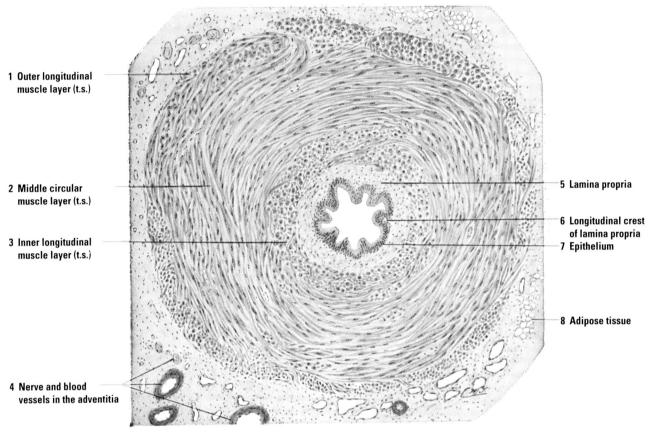

1 Outer longitudinal muscle layer (t.s.)

2 Middle circular muscle layer (t.s.)

3 Inner longitudinal muscle layer (t.s.)

4 Nerve and blood vessels in the adventitia

5 Lamina propria

6 Longitudinal crest of lamina propria

7 Epithelium

8 Adipose tissue

FIG. 1. DUCTUS DEFERENS (TRANSVERSE SECTION). Stain: hematoxylin-eosin. 40×.

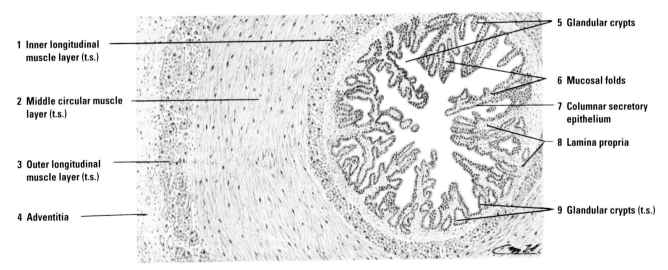

1 Inner longitudinal muscle layer (t.s.)

2 Middle circular muscle layer (t.s.)

3 Outer longitudinal muscle layer (t.s.)

4 Adventitia

5 Glandular crypts

6 Mucosal folds

7 Columnar secretory epithelium

8 Lamina propria

9 Glandular crypts (t.s.)

FIG. 2. AMPULLA OF THE DUCTUS DEFERENS (TRANSVERSE SECTION). Stain: hematoxylin-eosin. 60×.

PLATE 101

■ **FIG. 1**
PROSTATE GLAND WITH PROSTATIC URETHRA

In the prostate gland, the secretory **acini (4, 5)** are part of the many small, irregularly branched tubuloacinar glands; the acini (4, 5) vary in size. The larger-sized acini exhibit wide, irregular lumina (4) and variable epithelium (see Fig. 2). The glands are embedded in a characteristic, **fibromuscular stroma (3)** in which strands of **smooth muscle (6),** collagen, and elastic fibers are oriented in various directions.

The **prostatic urethra (1)** is as a crescent-shaped structure with small **diverticula (8)** in its lumen; the diverticula are especially prominent in the **urethral recesses (9).** The epithelium in the prostatic urethra (1) is usually transitional and a fibromuscular stroma surrounds the urethra (3); however, a thin lamina propria may be present.

A ridge of dense fibromuscular stroma without glands, the **colliculus seminalis (2),** protrudes into the urethral lumen (1), giving it a crescent shape. The **prostatic utricle (7, 10)** is situated in the mass of the colliculus seminalis (2) and is often dilated at its distal end before entering the urethra. Its thin mucous membrane is typically folded, and the epithelium is usually of the simple secretory or pseudostratified columnar type.

■ **FIG. 2**
PROSTATE GLAND (SECTIONAL VIEW, SECTION FROM MAIN PROSTATIC GLANDS IN FIG. 1)

A small section of the prostate gland from Figure 1 is illustrated with more detail and at a higher magnification.

The size of **glandular acini (1)** is variable. Their lumina are wide and typically irregular because of the protrusion of the epithelium-covered connective **tissue folds (5).** A characteristic feature in the acini of the prostate gland are the spherical **prostatic concretions (8)** that are formed by concentric layers of condensed prostatic secretions. The number of prostatic concretions increases with the age of the individual, and they may become calcified.

Although the **glandular epithelium (4)** is usually simple columnar or pseudostratified and the cells are light-staining in the distal regions, there is considerable variation. In some regions, the epithelium may be squamous or cuboidal.

The **ducts (7)** of the glands may resemble the acini and it is often difficult to distinguish the difference between the two structures. In the terminal portions of the ducts (7), the epithelium is usually columnar and stains darker before entering the urethra.

The **fibromuscular stroma (6)** is a characteristic feature of the prostate gland. **Smooth muscle fibers (3)** and the **connective tissue fibers (9)** can, at times, be distinguished; however, they blend together in the **stroma (6)** and are distributed throughout the gland.

PROSTATE GLAND

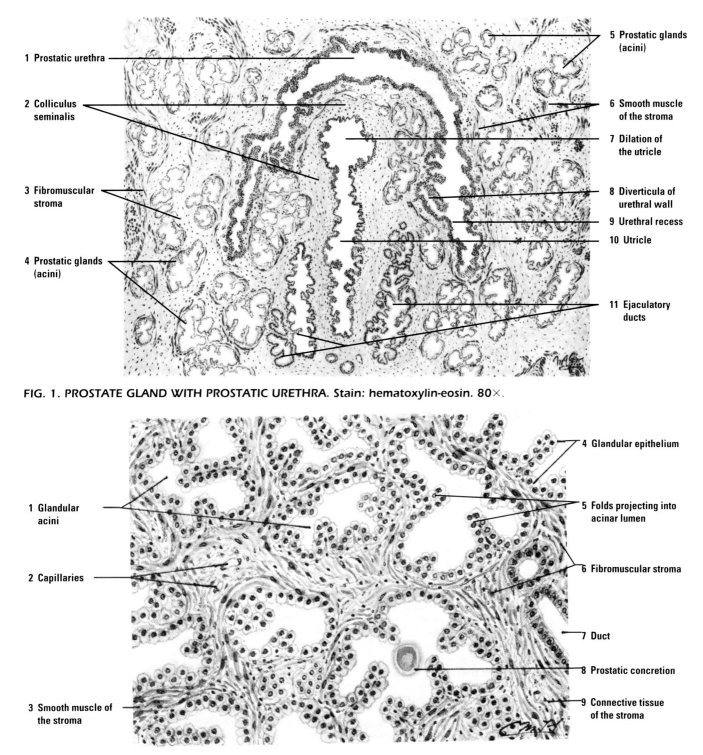

1 Prostatic urethra

2 Colliculus seminalis

3 Fibromuscular stroma

4 Prostatic glands (acini)

5 Prostatic glands (acini)

6 Smooth muscle of the stroma

7 Dilation of the utricle

8 Diverticula of urethral wall

9 Urethral recess

10 Utricle

11 Ejaculatory ducts

FIG. 1. PROSTATE GLAND WITH PROSTATIC URETHRA. Stain: hematoxylin-eosin. 80×.

1 Glandular acini

2 Capillaries

3 Smooth muscle of the stroma

4 Glandular epithelium

5 Folds projecting into acinar lumen

6 Fibromuscular stroma

7 Duct

8 Prostatic concretion

9 Connective tissue of the stroma

FIG. 2. PROSTATE GLAND: SECTIONAL VIEW (SECTION FROM MAIN PROSTATIC GLANDS IN FIG. 1). Stain: hematoxylin-eosin. 180×.

PLATE 102

PLATE 102

■ FIG. 1
SEMINAL VESICLE

The paired seminal vesicles are elongated bodies or sacs with highly convoluted and irregular lumina. A cross section through the gland illustrates the complexity of the **primary folds (5).** These folds branch into numerous **secondary folds (6)** which frequently anastomose, forming **crypts (1)** and cavities. The **lamina propria (7)** projects and forms the core of the larger primary folds (5) and thin stroma of smaller secondary folds (6). These folds extend far into the lumen of the seminal vesicle.

The **glandular epithelium (4)** of the seminal vesicles varies in appearance but is usually of the low pseudostratified type with basal cells and low columnar or cuboidal secretory cells.

The **muscularis (2)** consists of inner circular and outer longitudinal smooth muscle layers. This arrangement of the muscles is often difficult to observe because of the complex folding of the mucosa. The **adventitia (3)** surrounds the muscularis and blends with the connective tissue.

■ FIG. 2
BULBOURETHRAL GLAND

This is a compound tubuloacinar gland. One lobule and portions of other lobules of the gland are illustrated in the figure. The bulbourethral gland is surrounded by **skeletal muscle (2)** and **connective tissue (1).** The skeletal muscle and some smooth muscle fibers are also present in the **interlobular septa (3).**

The secretory units vary in structure and size. Most of the units have **acinar (4)** shape and others exhibit **tubular (5)** or variable other shapes. The secretory product is primarily mucus (4). The secretory cells are cuboidal, low columnar or squamous, and light-staining. Interspersed among the secretory cells are darker-staining acidophilic cells.

Smaller excretory ducts may be lined with secretory cells, whereas the larger **excretory ducts (6)** exhibit pseudostratified or stratified columnar epithelium.

SEMINAL VESICLE AND BULBOURETHRAL GLAND

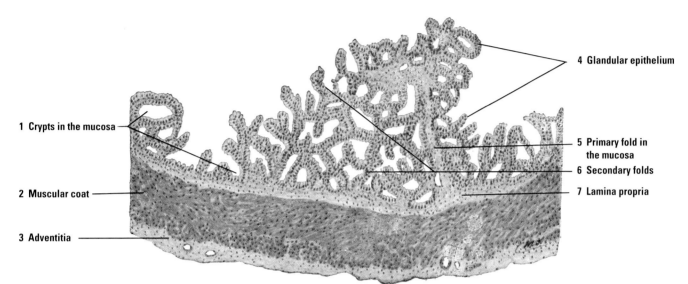

1 Crypts in the mucosa

2 Muscular coat

3 Adventitia

4 Glandular epithelium

5 Primary fold in the mucosa

6 Secondary folds

7 Lamina propria

FIG. 1. SEMINAL VESICLE. Stain: hematoxylin-eosin. 60×.

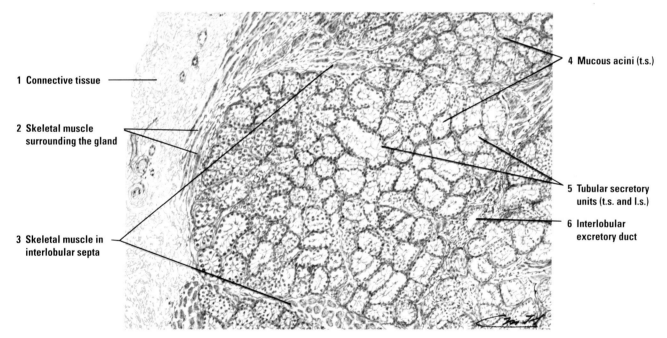

1 Connective tissue

2 Skeletal muscle surrounding the gland

3 Skeletal muscle in interlobular septa

4 Mucous acini (t.s.)

5 Tubular secretory units (t.s. and l.s.)

6 Interlobular excretory duct

FIG. 2. BULBOURETHRAL GLAND. SECTIONAL VIEW. Stain: Masson's stain. 350×.

PLATE 103

■ **FIG. 1**
HUMAN PENIS (TRANSVERSE SECTION)

A cross section of the penis (human) illustrates the three cavernous bodies: the two adjacent **corpora cavernosa (9)** and a single **corpus spongiosum (16)**, through which passes the **urethra (15)**. Surrounding the corpora cavernosa (9) of the penis is a thick, fibrous connective tissue capsule, the **tunica albuginea (5)**; it also extends between the two bodies as the **median septum (10)**. This septum is better developed at the posterior end of the penis than at the anterior end. The **tunica albuginea (6)** surrounding the **corpus spongiosum** (corpus cavernosa urethrae) **(16)** is thinner than that around the corpora cavernosa and contains smooth muscle and elastic fibers.

All three cavernous bodies are surrounded by loose connective tissue, the deep **penile (Buck's) fascia (4)** which, in turn, is surrounded by the connective tissue of the **dermis (2)** that is located immediately under the **epidermis (1)**. Strands of smooth muscle, the **dartos tunic (3)**, and an abundance of peripheral blood vessels are located in the dermis (2). **Sebaceous glands (7)** are present in the dermis on the ventral side of the penis.

The core of each corpus cavernosum (9) is occupied by numerous **trabeculae (14)**, which consist of collagenous, elastic, and smooth muscle fibers. The trabeculae (14) surround the cavernous cavities or **sinuses (veins) (12)** of the corpora cavernosa (9). Nerves and blood vessels are present in the trabeculae (14). The cavernous cavities or sinuses (12) of the corpora cavernosa (9) are lined with endothelium and receive blood from the **dorsal (8)** and **deep arteries (11)** of the penis. Smaller branches from the deep arteries (11) open into the cavernous cavities (12) of the corpora cavernosa (9). The corpus spongiosum (16) receives its blood supply largely from the bulbourethral artery, a branch of the internal pudendal artery. Blood that leaves the cavernous cavities exits mainly through the **superficial veins (13)** in the dermis (2) and the deep dorsal vein.

The urethra (15) is designated as the spongiosa or cavernous urethra. At the base of the penis, the urethra is lined with pseudostratified or stratified columnar epithelium; however, at the external orifice, the epithelium becomes stratified squamous. The urethra also exhibits numerous small but deep invaginations in its mucous membrane. These are the urethral lacunae (of Morgagni) with mucous cells. Branched tubular urethral glands (of Littre) open into these recesses. The lacunae and the urethral glands are not visible at this magnification (see Fig. 2).

■ **FIG. 2**
CAVERNOUS URETHRA (TRANSVERSE SECTION)

A section of the **cavernous urethra (4)** is illustrated with pseudostratified or **stratified columnar epithelium (5)** lining. A thin **lamina propria (3)** merges with the surrounding connective tissue of the corpus spongiosum.

Numerous various-sized mucosal outpockets or the **urethral lacunae (of Morgagni) (9)** give the **urethral lumen (4)** an irregular form. Some of these urethral lacunae (9) contain mucous cells. The deeper urethral lacunae (9) are connected with the branched **urethral glands (of Littre) (7)** located in the lamina propria of the corpus spongiosum (7, lowest leader). The urethral glands (7) are lined with the same type of epithelium that lines the lumen of the cavernous urethra (4) (stratified columnar in this illustration).

The **corpus spongiosum (1)** surrounds the urethra (4); its internal structure is similar to that of the corpora cavernosa described in Figure 1. In the illustration are seen the characteristic **trabeculae (1, 11)** of connective tissue and smooth muscle between the **cavernous veins (2, 8, 10)**.

PENIS AND CAVERNOUS URETHRA

1 Epidermis

2 Dermis

3 Dartos tunic

4 Deep penile fascia

5 Tunica albuginea of
   corpus cavernosum

6 Tunica albuginea of
   corpus spongiosum

7 Sebaceous gland
   in dermis

8 Dorsal artery

9 Corpus cavernosum

10 Median septum

11 Deep artery

12 Cavities (cavernous
   veins) of corpus
   cavernosum

13 Superficial vein

14 Trabeculae

15 Cavernous urethra

16 Corpus spongiosum

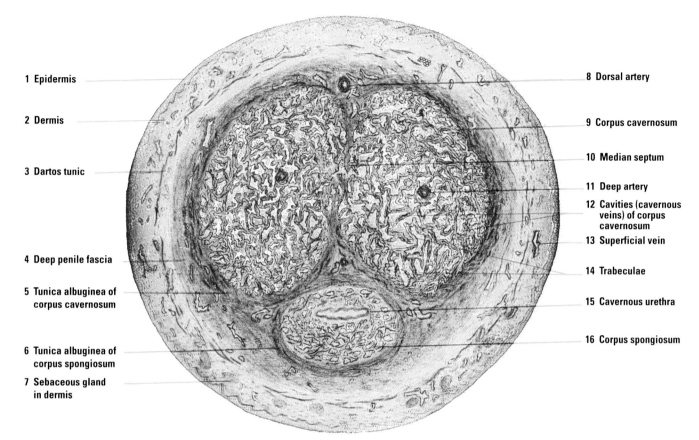

FIG. 1. PENIS (TRANSVERSE SECTION). Stain: hematoxylin-eosin. 12×.

1 Trabecula of the corpus
   spongiosum: smooth
   muscle and connective
   tissue

2 Veins in the corpus
   spongiosum

3 Urethral mucosa:
   lamina propria and
   epithelium

4 Cavernous urethra

5 Stratified columnar
   epithelium

6 Urethral lacuna (of
   Morgagni)

7 Urethral glands (of
   Littré)

8 Cavernous veins
   (venous spaces)

9 Urethral lacunae

10 Cavernous veins
   (venous spaces)

11 Smooth muscle in
   trabeculae

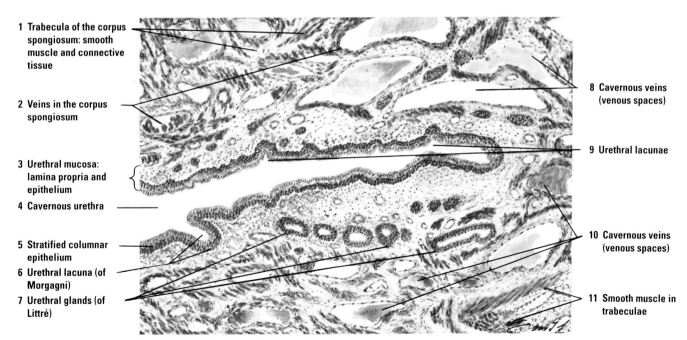

FIG. 2. CAVERNOUS URETHRA (TRANSVERSE SECTION). Stain: hematoxylin-eosin. 80×.

THE FEMALE REPRODUCTIVE SYSTEM

The female reproductive system consists of the ovaries, uterine tubes, uterus, vagina, mammary glands, and external genitalia. The individual organs of this system perform numerous important functions, among which are: secretion of female sex hormones (estrogen and progesterone), production of ova, providing a suitable environment for the developing fetus during pregnancy, and nutrition of the newborn.

During the reproductive life when the female is not pregnant, the reproductive organs exhibit cyclic changes in both structure and function. In humans, these changes are called menstrual cycles and are primarily controlled by the adenohypophyseal (pituitary) hormones, the follicle stimulating hormone (FSH) and the luteinizing hormone (LH), and the ovarian hormones, estrogen and progesterone.

The Ovaries

From the beginning until the end of the reproductive life in humans, the ovaries exhibit different phases of follicular growth, maturation, ovulation, and formation of corpus luteum. The first half of the ovarian cycle is the follicular phase. During this phase, the FSH is the principal circulating gonadotrophic hormone. FSH influences the growth and maturation of different ovarian follicles and stimulates the granulosa and thecal cells of the maturing follicles to produce estrogen. As the levels of circulating estrogens rise during the follicular phase, however, they produce an inhibitory effect on further release of FSH from the pituitary gland. In addition, a hormone called inhibin, produced by the granulosa cells of the follicles, also exerts an inhibitory effect on FSH release.

At midcycle or shortly before ovulation, estrogen secretion reaches a peak. This rise causes a brief surge of LH release and a concomitant smaller release of FSH from the adenohypophysis of the pituitary gland. In conjunction with FSH, the increased levels of LH induce final maturation of the ovarian follicle and its rupture (ovulation), maturation and liberation of the oocyte, and the formation of corpus luteum.

After ovulation of the mature follicle, the ovary enters the luteal phase. During this phase, LH presence induces rapid transformation of the granulosa and theca interna cells of the ruptured ovarian follicle into the granulosa lutein and theca lutein cells of a temporary endocrine gland, the corpus luteum. LH then stimulates the lutein cells to secrete estrogen and large amounts of progesterone.

The development and functional activity of the corpus luteum depends on the presence of LH. The rising level of progesterone produced by the corpus luteum, however, has an inhibitory effect on further release of LH by the adenohypophysis. If fertilization of the oocyte and its implantation in the uterus do not occur, the corpus luteum is not maintained and its function in the woman declines 12 to 14 days after ovulation. The corpus luteum then regresses into a nonfunctional corpus albicans. With the regression of corpus luteum, the inhibitory effects of its hormones on the pituitary gland are removed. This action causes a release of FSH from the adenohypophysis and an initiation of a new ovarian cycle of follicular development.

The Uterine Tubes

The uterine tubes extend from the ovaries to the uterus. One end of the tube opens into the uterine cavity and the other is closely associated with the ovary. The uterine tubes perform several important functions. After ovulation, the uterine tubes capture and conduct the oocyte toward the uterus. This function is accomplished by the gentle peristaltic action of the smooth muscles in the uterine wall and the ciliary action of the ciliated cells in the lining epithelium. The uterine tubes also provide the site of fertilization for the egg, which normally occurs in the ampullary region, and a proper environment for initial development of the embryo.

The epithelium of the uterine wall consists of ciliated and nonciliated (peg) cells. Most cilia beat toward the uterus and play a major role in transporting the ovum through the tube. The nonciliated cells appear to be secretory and contribute nutritive material to the environment of the uterine tubes. The epithelium exhibits cyclic changes that are associated with the ovarian cycle. The height of the epithelium in the uterine tubes is greatest during the follicular phase, at which time the ovarian follicles are maturing and the circulating levels of estrogen are high.

The Uterus

During pregnancy, the uterus provides the site for implantation of the fertilized egg and formation of the placenta, and a suitable environment for the development of a new individual. The wall of the uterus is composed of three layers: an outer perimetrium (serosa or adventitia), a thick middle myometrium (smooth muscle), and an inner endometrium (epithelium and lamina propria). During the reproductive life, the endometrium exhibits cyclic changes in structure and function in response to the ovarian hormones, estrogen and progesterone. These changes prepare the uterus for implantation and nourishment of the embryo and fetus. If implantation of the fertilized egg does not occur, however, the blood vessels in the endometrium deteriorate, rupture, and a portion of the endometrium is shed during menstruation.

The endometrium of the uterus is normally subdivided into two layers, the luminal stratum functionalis and the basal stratum basalis. These layers exhibit different changes during the menstrual cycles. The upper functionalis layer is shed or sloughed off during menstruation, leaving the basalis layer intact and the source of cells for the regeneration of a new functionalis layer.

The arterial supply to the endometrium is important to the menstrual cycle. Branches of uterine arteries divide into straight and spiral arteries in the myometrium. The straight arteries are short and supply the basalis layer of the endometrium, whereas the spiral arteries are long and coiled, and pass to the surface or the functionalis layer of the endometrium. In contrast to the straight arteries, the spiral arteries are highly sensitive to hormonal changes during the menstrual cycle.

During each menstrual cycle, the changes in the endometrium are identified as three continuous phases, each phase gradually passing into the next. The proliferative (follicular) phase starts at the end of menstruation or the menstrual phase. The proliferative phase is characterized by rapid growth and development of the endometrium. Increased mitotic activity of cells in the lamina propria and the remnants of uterine glands in the basalis layer start to cover the raw surface of the mucosa, which was denuded during menstruation. As the endometrium thickens, the uterine glands proliferate, lengthen, and become closely packed. The growth of the endometrium during the proliferative phase closely coincides with the growth of the ovarian follicles and their increased secretion of estrogen.

The secretory (luteal) phase begins shortly after ovulation, corpus luteum formation, and the secretion of progesterone (and estrogen) by the lutein cells of the corpus luteum. During this phase, the endometrium continues to thicken and to accumulate fluid, becoming edematous. In addition, the uterine glands hypertrophy and become tortuous, and their lumina become filled with secretions that are rich in nutrients, especially glycogen. The spiral arteries in the endometrium lengthen, become more coiled, and extend almost to the surface of the endometrium.

The menstrual phase starts when fertilization and implantation of the egg fail to occur. There is a reduction of circulating progesterone (and estrogen) levels as the functional corpus luteum begins to regress. Decreased levels of hormones estrogen and progesterone cause the spiral arteries in the functionalis layer of the endometrium to exhibit intermittent constrictions. This action produces transitory ischemia in and the shrinkage of functionalis layer. After extended periods of vascular constriction, the spiral arteries dilate and their walls rupture, causing the necrotic functionalis layer of the endometrium to be shed in the menstrual flow. Blood, uterine fluid, and stromal and epithelial cells from the functionalis layer mix to form the vaginal discharge. The shedding of the endometrium continues until only the raw surface of the basalis layer is left. The proliferation of cells from the basalis layer, under the influence of estrogen, restores the lost endometrial surface as the next phase of the menstrual cycle begins.

The Placenta

During pregnancy, the fertilized ovum is implanted in the endometrium and forms a placenta. The placenta consists of a fetal portion, formed by the chorionic plate and its branching villi, and a maternal portion, formed by the decidua basalis of the endometrium. Fetal and maternal blood come into close proximity in the placenta, where exchange of nutrients, electrolytes, hormones, gaseous products, and waste metabolites takes place.

The placenta also serves as a temporary endocrine organ, producing essential hormones for the maintenance of pregnancy. The placental cells (syncytial trophoblasts) secrete the hormone chorionic gonadotropin shortly after implantation. The chorionic gonadotropin is similar to LH in function and maintains the corpus luteum during the early stages of pregnancy. In addition, chorionic gonadotropin stimulates the corpus luteum to produce estrogen and progesterone, the two hormones that are essential for the maintenance of pregnancy.

As the pregnancy proceeds, the placenta takes over the production of estrogen and progesterone from the corpus luteum and produces sufficient amounts of progesterone to maintain pregnancy until birth of the individual. The placenta also produces placental lactogen, a hormone that promotes growth and development of the maternal mammary glands.

Cervix and Vagina

The cervical mucosa is not shed during the menstruation as is the functionalis layer in the uterine endometrium. The cervical glands, however, exhibit altered secretory activities during the menstrual cycle. The secretion of the cervical glands is thin and watery during the proliferative phase of the menstrual cycle. This type of secretion allows easier passage of sperm into the uterus. During the luteal phase, however, the cervical secretion becomes highly viscous and hinders the passage of sperm or microorganisms into the uterus.

Like the cervix, the vaginal mucosa is not shed during menstruation. On the other hand, the vaginal epithelium exhibits cyclic changes during the menstrual cycle. During the follicular phase and estrogenic stimulation, the vaginal epithelium becomes thicker. The vaginal cells synthesize and accumulate increased amounts of glycogen as they migrate toward and are desquamated into the lumen. Bacteria in the vagina metabolize the glycogen and increase the acidity of the vaginal canal.

The Mammary Glands

The adult mammary gland consists of individual branched tubuloalveolar glands. The inactive mammary gland consists primarily of duct elements. During different phases of the menstrual cycle, the inactive mammary glands exhibit slight cyclic alterations. Under estrogenic stimulation, the secretory cells increase in height and lumina appear in the ducts as a small amount of secretory material is accumulated.

During pregnancy, extensive growth of mammary glands is promoted by the continuous and prolonged production of estrogen and progesterone initially by the corpus luteum of the ovary, and later by the placenta. In addition, further growth of the mammary glands depends on the hormone prolactin, lactogenic hormone, and adrenal corticoids. Under the hormonal stimulation, the intralobular ducts of the mammary glands undergo rapid proliferation, branch, and form numerous alveoli. The alveoli then hypertrophy and become the active sites of milk secretion during the period of lactation. At the end of pregnancy, the alveoli produce a fluid called colostrum; it is rich in proteins and antibodies. Unlike milk, however, colostrum contains little lipid.

After parturition, the levels of estrogen and progesterone drop and the mammary glands begin active secretion of milk, which is now promoted by the pituitary gland hormone prolactin. Suckling of the mammary glands by the infant promotes further release of prolactin and milk production proceeds as long as suckling continues. In addition, suckling of the mammary gland initiates milk ejection reflex. This reflex causes the release of the hormone oxytocin from the neurohypophysis. Oxytocin induces the contraction of myoepithelial cells around the secretory alveoli and excretory ducts in the mammary glands, causing the ejection or expulsion of milk from the mammary glands toward the nipple.

Decreased nursing and suckling on the mammary glands causes the cessation of milk secretion and regression of the mammary glands to the inactive condition.

PLATE 104

OVARY (PANORAMIC VIEW)

The ovarian surface is covered by a single layer of low cuboidal or squamous cells called the **germinal epithelium (1, 12).** This layer is continuous with the **mesothelium (14)** of the visceral peritoneum. Beneath the germinal epithelium is a dense, connective tissue layer, the **tunica albuginea (2).**

The ovary has a peripheral **cortex (8)** and a central **medulla (24).** The cortex (8) occupies the greater part of the ovary; its connective tissue **stroma (8)** contains large, spindle-shaped fibroblasts. Coursing in all directions in the cortex (8) are compact collagenous and reticular fibers.

The medullary stroma (24) is a typical dense irregular connective tissue, which is continuous with that of the **mesovarium (13).** Numerous **blood vessels (10)** in the medulla distribute smaller vessels to all parts of the cortex. The mesovarium (13) is covered by ovarian germinal epithelium (12) and by peritoneal mesothelium (14).

Numerous **ovarian follicles (3, 4, 7, 9, 16–20, 22, 28, 29)** in various stages of development are located in the stroma of the cortex (8). The detailed structure of some of these follicles is illustrated on Plate 105. The most numerous follicles are the **primordial (3; 29, lower leader),** located in the periphery of the cortex (8) and under the tunica albuginea (2); these follicles are the smallest and simplest in structure. The largest of the ovarian follicles is the **mature follicle (16–20).** Its vari-ous parts are the **theca interna** and **theca externa (16),** the **granulosa cells (17),** a large **antrum (18)** filled with liquor folliculi (follicular fluid), and the **cumulus oophorus (19),** which contains the **primary oocyte (20).** The smaller follicles with stratified granulosa cells around the oocyte are the **growing follicles (4, lower leader).** Larger follicles with antral cavities of various sizes are called **secondary** or **vesicular follicles (7, 9, 28).** These larger follicles are situated deeper in the cortex and are surrounded by modified stromal cells, the **theca folliculi (6).** These cells differentiate into an inner secretory **theca interna (16, upper leader)** and an outer connective tissue **theca externa (16, lower leader).** Most of the illustrated large follicles contain a **primary oocyte (6, 20, 28)** and its nucleus. In the primordial follicles, the oocyte is small but gradually increases in size in the primary, growing, and vesicular follicles.

Most follicles never attain maturity and undergo degeneration (atresia) during various stages of growth, thus becoming **atretic follicles (11, 21, 26, 30;** see also Plate 106); these follicles are gradually replaced by the stroma.

After ovulation, the follicle collapses, its wall exhibits numerous folds, and the corpus luteum is formed (See Plate 106). Successive stages in corpus luteum **regression** are indicated **(5, 15, 23, 27).** Plates 106 and 107 illustrate these changes at a higher magnification.

OVARY (PANORAMIC VIEW)

1 Germinal epithelium

2 Tunica albuginea

3 Primordial follicles

4 Follicular cells of a
  primary and a small
  growing follicle

5 Corpus albicans
  (residue of a corpus
  luteum)

6 Vesicular (secondary)
  follicle: theca folliculi

7 Antrum
  (follicular cavity)
  with fluid

8 Ovarian stroma (cortex)

9 Vesicular (secondary)
  follicle: granulosa cells

10 Blood vessels in the
   medulla

11 Atretic follicles

12 Ovarian germinal
   epithelium

13 Mesovarium

14 Peritoneal
   mesothelium

15 Regressing corpus
   luteum

16 Thecae: interna
   and extrema

17 Granulosa cells

18 Antrum

19 Cumulus
   oophorus

20 Oocyte

21 Atretic follicle

Large vesicular follicle

22 Growing follicle

23 Regressing corpus
   luteum

24 Medulla

25 Follicle sectioned
   near its surface (tg.s.)

26 Atretic follicle

27 Regressing corpus
   luteum

28 Oocyte in a small
   vesicular follicle

29 Primary and primordial
   follicles

30 Atretic follicle

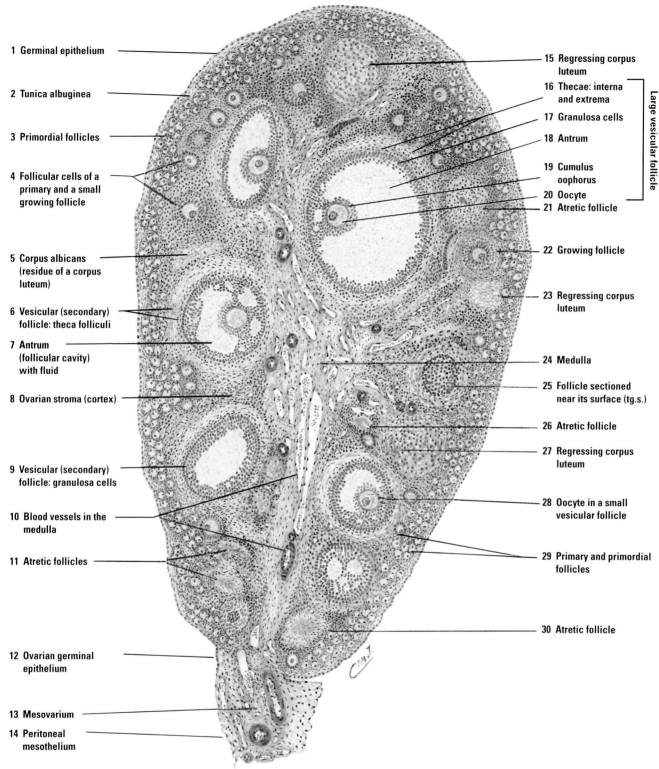

OVARY (DOG). Stain: hematoxylin-eosin. 60×.

275

PLATE 105

■ **FIG. 1**
OVARY: OVARIAN CORTEX, PRIMARY AND GROWING FOLLICLES

The cuboidal **germinal epithelium (1)** lines the ovarian surface. Beneath the surface epithelium is a layer of dense connective tissue, the **tunica albuginea (2)**. Numerous **primordial follicles (5, 6)** are located immediately below the tunica albuginea (2). Each primordial follicle (5, 6) consists of a **primary oocyte (5)** surrounded by a single layer of squamous **follicular cells (6)**. In larger follicles, the **follicular cells (7)** change to cuboidal or low columnar.

In **growing follicles (4)**, the follicular cells proliferate by **mitotis (3)**, form layers of cuboidal cells called the **granulosa cells (10)**, and surround the **primary oocyte (4, 11)**. The innermost layer of the granulosa cells surrounding the oocyte form the **corona radiata (13)**; these cells are more columnar than the other granulosa cells. Between the corona radiata and surrounding oocyte is the noncellular glycoprotein layer, the **zona pellucida (12)**. Stromal cells surrounding the follicular cells differentiate into the **theca interna (9)**; at this stage of follicular development, the cell layer outside of theca interna (9), the theca externa, has not differentiated. The developing oocyte (4) has a large eccentric **nucleus (11)** with a conspicuous nucleolus.

A degenerating, **atretic follicle (15)** is illustrated in the lower right corner of the illustration.

■ **FIG. 2**
OVARY: WALL OF A MATURE FOLLICLE

Figure 2 illustrates a portion of the mature follicle with an **oocyte (11)**. The area represented in this figure is comparable to the area in Plate 104 that illustrates the mature follicle, **cumulus oophorus** with its **oocyte** and the different **thecae layers (Plate 104, 16, 19, 20)**.

The **granulosa cells (6)** enclose the central cavity or **antrum (8)** of the follicle. The antrum (8) is filled with follicular fluid that has been secreted by the surrounding granulosa cells (6). Smaller isolated accumulations of the **follicular fluid (14)** may also occur among the **granulosa cells (6)**. Some of these fluid accumulations appear as clear or faintly acidophilic **vacuoles (3, 7)**; their origin and function are not known.

A local thickening of the granulosa cells on one side of the mature follicle encloses the mature **oocyte (11)** and projects into the antrum (8), forming a hillock called the **cumulus oophorus (12)**. The oocyte is surrounded by a prominent, acidophilic-staining **zona pellucida (10)** and a single layer of radially arranged **corona radiata (9)** cells that are attached to the zona pellucida (10).

The basal row of granulosa cells rests on a thin **basement membrane (5)**. Adjacent to the basement membrane (5) is the **theca interna (4)**, an inner layer of vascularized, secretory cells. Surrounding the theca interna cells (4) is the **theca externa (2)**, a layer of connective tissue cells.

OVARY

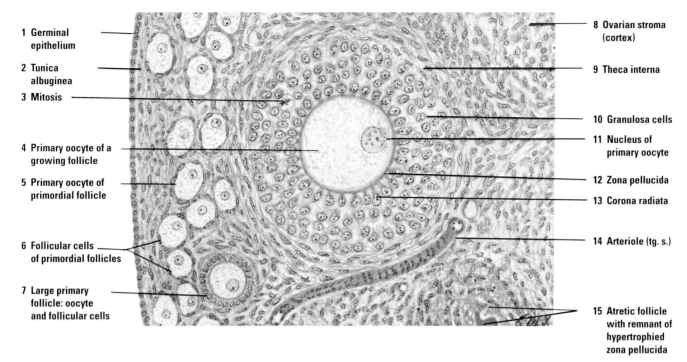

1 Germinal epithelium

2 Tunica albuginea

3 Mitosis

4 Primary oocyte of a growing follicle

5 Primary oocyte of primordial follicle

6 Follicular cells of primordial follicles

7 Large primary follicle: oocyte and follicular cells

8 Ovarian stroma (cortex)

9 Theca interna

10 Granulosa cells

11 Nucleus of primary oocyte

12 Zona pellucida

13 Corona radiata

14 Arteriole (tg. s.)

15 Atretic follicle with remnant of hypertrophied zona pellucida

FIG. 1. CORTEX, PRIMARY AND GROWING FOLLICLES. Stain: hematoxylin-eosin. 320×.

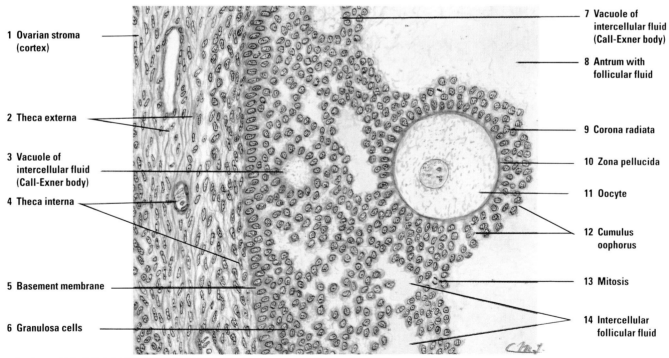

1 Ovarian stroma (cortex)

2 Theca externa

3 Vacuole of intercellular fluid (Call-Exner body)

4 Theca interna

5 Basement membrane

6 Granulosa cells

7 Vacuole of intercellular fluid (Call-Exner body)

8 Antrum with follicular fluid

9 Corona radiata

10 Zona pellucida

11 Oocyte

12 Cumulus oophorus

13 Mitosis

14 Intercellular follicular fluid

FIG. 2. WALL OF A MATURE FOLLICLE. Stain: hematoxylin-eosin. 320×.

277

PLATE 106

HUMAN OVARY: CORPORA LUTEA AND ATRETIC FOLLICLES

This figure illustrates a newly formed corpus luteum, corpora lutea in various stages of regression, and several stages of follicular atresia.

The ovarian surface is covered by a single layer of **germinal epithelium (1)**. Lying directly underneath this layer is a connective tissue layer, the tunica albuginia. The **cortex (2, 18)** constitutes the greater portion of the ovary and contains the follicles and corpora lutea. The **medulla (7)** occupies the central region of the ovary. In the medulla (7) are found larger blood vessels that branch and supply the cortical region (2, 18) of the ovary.

The newly formed **corpus luteum (3)** is a large structure. It is formed after the rupture of the mature follicle and the collapse of its walls. The thin zone of **theca lutein cells (4)**, formed from the theca interna cells of the follicle, is located on the periphery of the corpus luteum (3) and in the contours of its folds. (See Plate 107 for higher magnification and more details.) The mass of the corpus luteum wall (3) is formed from the **granulosa lutein cells (5)**, which are the hypertrophied granulosa cells of the follicle. The **connective tissue (6)** from the theca externa proliferates, forms the stroma for the blood vessels and capillaries in the wall of corpus luteum, and fills the former follicular cavity (6).

Also illustrated in the ovary is a portion of **corpus luteum in moderate regression (10)** with the plane of section passing through its outer wall. The granulosa lutein cells are smaller, the **nuclei pyknotic (10a)**, and larger **blood vessels (10b)** are growing in from the stroma. The theca lutein cells are not visible.

A later stage of **corpus luteum regression (16)** indicates further shrinkage of lutein cells, pyknosis of their **nuclei (16b)**, and a **fibrous central core (16a)**. Connective tissue invades the regressing luteal cells and replaces them as they degenerate. The stroma forms a **capsule (16c)** around the regressing corpus luteum; however, this is not a constant feature. Replacement by the connective tissue of all lutein cells leaves a fibrous, hyalinized scar, the **corpus albicans (15)**.

A large, normal **follicle (17)** exhibits the **theca interna (17a)** and the thick **granulosa cell layer (17b)**; a thin basement membrane separates the **theca interna (17a)** from the granulosa cells (17b). The **cumulus oophorus (17d)** contains a normal **oocyte (17e)**; the **antrum (17c)** is filled with follicular fluid.

Numerous follicles undergo degenerative changes called atresia at any time before reaching maturity. Atresia in large follicles is gradual; however, serial changes of degeneration can be recognized by noting follicles in different stages of atresia. A follicle in an early stage of **atresia (14)** is illustrated. The **theca interna (14a)** and the **granulosa cells (14b)** are intact; however, some of the cells are beginning to slough off into the **antrum (14e)**, which still contains **follicular fluid (14d)**. Also, cumulus oophorus has been disrupted and degeneration of the oocyte is advanced. A remnant of the oocyte, surrounded by thickened **zona pellucida (14c)**, is seen in the antrum.

A follicle in **later atresia (13)** is also illustrated. The **theca interna (13a)** is still visible; however, the cells appear somewhat hypertrophied. The granulosa cells are no longer present; all of the cells have sloughed off and been resorbed. The basement membrane between these two layers has thickened and folded and is now called the **hypertrophied glassy membrane (13b)**. Loose connective tissue is growing in from the **stroma (13e)** and has partially filled the reduced **follicular cavity (13d)**, in which **follicular fluid (13c)** is still present.

With **further atresia (9)**, connective tissue **stroma replaces the theca interna cells (9a)**. The **hypertrophied glassy membrane (9b)** becomes thicker and more folded and the loose connective tissue with small blood vessels **fills the former antrum (9c)**. In the **last stages of atresia (11)**, the entire follicle is replaced by connective tissue; the hypertrophied and folded glassy membrane (11) remains for some time as the only indication of a follicle.

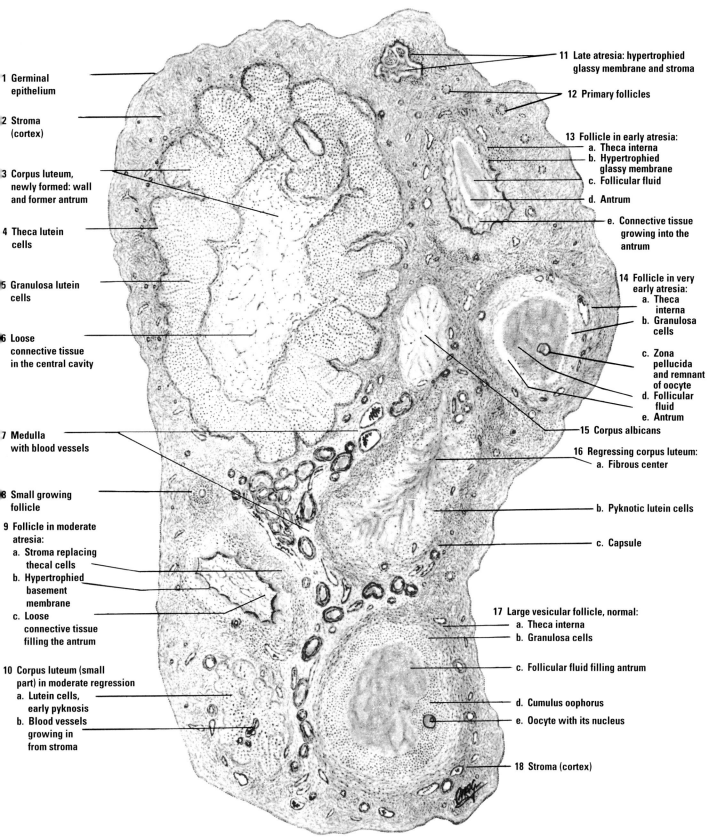

1 Germinal
   epithelium

2 Stroma
   (cortex)

3 Corpus luteum,
   newly formed: wall
   and former antrum

4 Theca lutein
   cells

5 Granulosa lutein
   cells

6 Loose
   connective tissue
   in the central cavity

7 Medulla
   with blood vessels

8 Small growing
   follicle

9 Follicle in moderate
   atresia:
   a. Stroma replacing
      thecal cells
   b. Hypertrophied
      basement
      membrane
   c. Loose
      connective tissue
      filling the antrum

10 Corpus luteum (small
    part) in moderate regression
    a. Lutein cells,
       early pyknosis
    b. Blood vessels
       growing in
       from stroma

11 Late atresia: hypertrophied
    glassy membrane and stroma

12 Primary follicles

13 Follicle in early atresia:
    a. Theca interna
    b. Hypertrophied
       glassy membrane
    c. Follicular fluid
    d. Antrum
    e. Connective tissue
       growing into the
       antrum

14 Follicle in very
    early atresia:
    a. Theca
       interna
    b. Granulosa
       cells
    c. Zona
       pellucida
       and remnant
       of oocyte
    d. Follicular
       fluid
    e. Antrum

15 Corpus albicans

16 Regressing corpus luteum:
    a. Fibrous center
    b. Pyknotic lutein cells
    c. Capsule

17 Large vesicular follicle, normal:
    a. Theca interna
    b. Granulosa cells
    c. Follicular fluid filling antrum
    d. Cumulus oophorus
    e. Oocyte with its nucleus

18 Stroma (cortex)

HUMAN OVARY. Stain: hematoxylin-eosin. 80×.

PLATE 107

■ **FIG. 1**
CORPUS LUTEUM (PANORAMIC VIEW)

At higher magnification, the corpus luteum appears as a highly folded, thick mass of **glandular epithelium (3)**, consisting primarily of **granulosa lutein cells (3, upper leader)** and peripheral **theca lutein cells (3, lower leader)**, which extend along the connective tissue **septa (2, 7)**. The theca externa cells form a poorly defined **capsule (1)** around the developing corpus luteum that also extends inward between the folds (2, 7). The central core of the corpus luteum (the former follicular cavity) contains remnants of follicular fluid, serum, occasional blood cells, and loose **connective tissue (8, 9)** from the theca externa, which has proliferated and penetrated the layers of the glandular tissue. The connective tissue also covers the inner surface of the luteal cells (8) and then spreads throughout the core of the corpus luteum (9).

The **ovarian stroma (4)** around the corpus luteum is highly vascular **(5).**

■ **FIG. 2**
CORPUS LUTEUM (PERIPHERAL WALL)

The **granulosa lutein (7)** cells constitute the mass of the corpus luteum. These cells are the hypertrophied former granulosa cells of the mature follicle. The granulosa cells are large, lightly stained because of lipid inclusions, and have large vesicular nuclei. The **theca lutein cells (2)**, the former theca interna cells, remain external to the granulosa lutein cells on the periphery of the corpus luteum and in the depressions between the folds. Theca lutein cells (2) are smaller than the granulosa lutein cells (7); their cytoplasm stains deeper and the nuclei are smaller and darker.

Numerous **capillaries (4, 8)** and fine connective tissue **septa (6)** from the theca externa are observed between the anatomosing columns of lutein cells.

The connective tissue **capsule (5)** around the corpus luteum is poorly defined and the surrounding **stroma (1, 3, 4)** remains highly vascular.

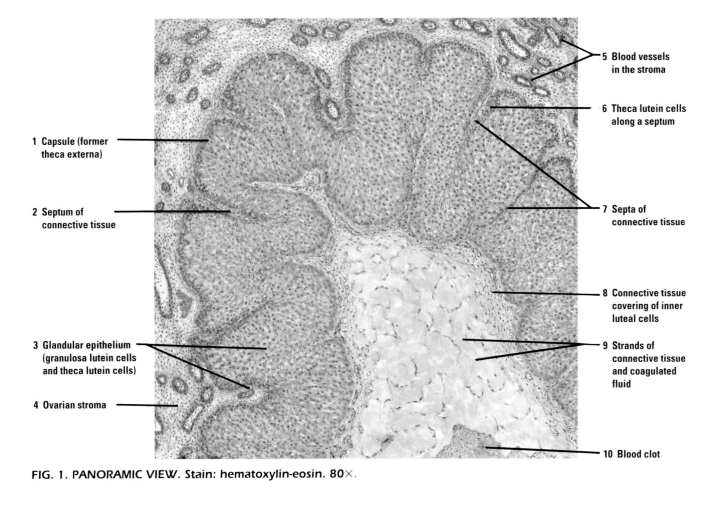

1 Capsule (former theca externa)

2 Septum of connective tissue

3 Glandular epithelium (granulosa lutein cells and theca lutein cells)

4 Ovarian stroma

5 Blood vessels in the stroma

6 Theca lutein cells along a septum

7 Septa of connective tissue

8 Connective tissue covering of inner luteal cells

9 Strands of connective tissue and coagulated fluid

10 Blood clot

FIG. 1. PANORAMIC VIEW. Stain: hematoxylin-eosin. 80×.

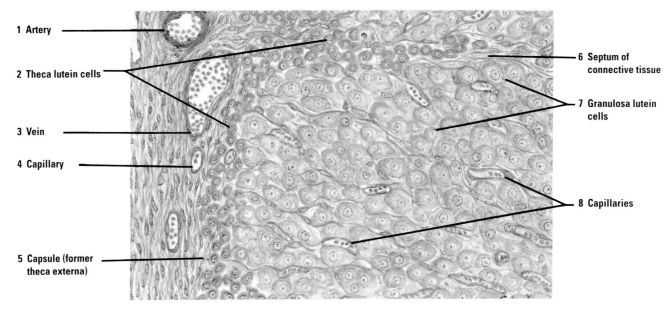

1 Artery

2 Theca lutein cells

3 Vein

4 Capillary

5 Capsule (former theca externa)

6 Septum of connective tissue

7 Granulosa lutein cells

8 Capillaries

FIG. 2. PERIPHERAL WALL. Stain: hematoxylin-eosin. 250×.

PLATE 108

■ FIG. 1
UTERINE TUBE: AMPULLA (PANORAMIC VIEW, TRANSVERSE SECTION)

Extensive ramification of tall, **mucosal folds (9)** forms an irregular lumen in the uterine (Fallopian) tube. The lumen extends between the mucosal folds (9) and forms deep grooves in the tube. The lining **epithelium (10)** is simple columnar and the **lamina propria (8)** is a well vascularized, loose connective tissue. The muscularis consists of two smooth muscle layers, an inner **circular (1)** and an outer **longitudinal layer (6).** The interstitial **connective tissue (2)** is abundant and, as a result, the smooth muscle layers are not distinct, especially the outer layer. The **serosa (7)** forms the outermost layer on the uterine tube.

■ FIG. 2
UTERINE TUBE: MUCOSAL FOLDS, EARLY PROLIFERATIVE PHASE

The lining epithelium is simple but may appear pseudostratified. It consists of **ciliated (1)** and nonciliated, peg or secretory cells. During the early proliferative phase of the menstrual cycle, the ciliated cells hypertrophy, exhibit cilia growth, and become predominant. In addition, there is increased secretory activity in the nonciliated cells. The epithelium of the uterine tube shows cyclic changes and the proportion of ciliated and nonciliated cells vary with different stages of the menstrual cycle.

The **lamina propria (2)** is a highly cellular, loose connective tissue with fine collagenous and reticular fibers.

■ FIG. 3
UTERINE TUBE: MUCOSAL FOLDS, EARLY PREGNANCY

During the luteal phase of the menstrual cycle and early pregnancy, the **peg** or **secretory cells (2)** predominate. These cells appear slender, with elongated nuclei and apices that protrude into tubular lumina. The secretory cells (2) intermix with **ciliated cells (3)** in the uterine tube.

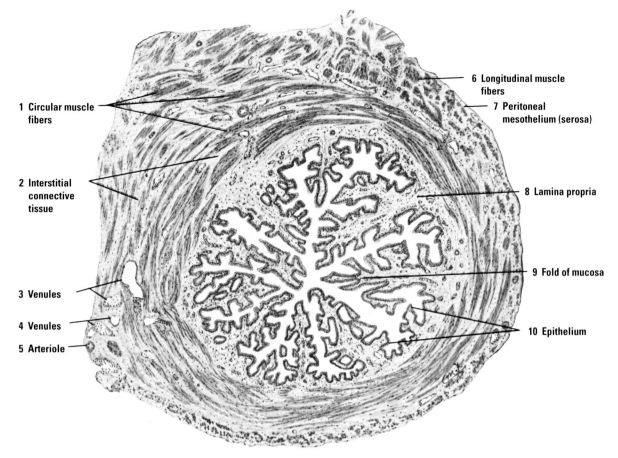

1 Circular muscle
  fibers

2 Interstitial
  connective
  tissue

3 Venules

4 Venules

5 Arteriole

6 Longitudinal muscle
  fibers

7 Peritoneal
  mesothelium (serosa)

8 Lamina propria

9 Fold of mucosa

10 Epithelium

FIG. 1. PANORAMIC VIEW, TRANSVERSE SECTION. Stain: hematoxylin-eosin. 40×.

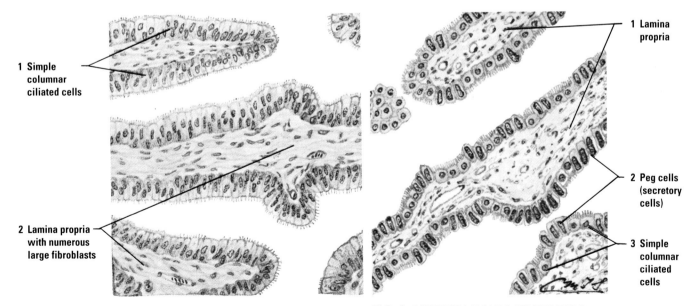

1 Simple
  columnar
  ciliated cells

2 Lamina propria
  with numerous
  large fibroblasts

1 Lamina
  propria

2 Peg cells
  (secretory
  cells)

3 Simple
  columnar
  ciliated
  cells

FIG. 2. MUCOSAL FOLDS (EARLY PROLIFERATIVE PHASE).
Stain: hematoxylin-eosin. 320×.

FIG. 3. MUCOSAL FOLDS (EARLY PREG-
NANCY). Stain: hematoxylin-eosin. 320×.

PLATE 109

UTERUS: PROLIFERATIVE (FOLLICULAR) PHASE

During a normal menstrual cycle, the endometrium exhibits a sequence of changes that are closely correlated with the ovarian function. Cyclic activities in a nonpregnant uterus are divided into three distinct phases: a proliferative or follicular phase, a secretory or luteal phase, and a menstrual phase. The characteristic features of the endometrium during each of these phases are illustrated in detail in Plates 109, 110, and 111, respectively.

The uterine wall consists of three layers: the inner **endometrium (1, 2, 3, 4),** a middle muscular or **myometrium (5, 6),** and the outer serous membrane or the perimetrium (not illustrated). The endometrium is further subdivided into two zones or layers: a narrow, deeper **basalis layer (8)** adjacent to the myometrium (5) and a wider, superficial layer above the basalis layer (8) that extends to the lumen of the uterus, the **functionalis layer (7).**

The surface of the endometrium is lined with a simple columnar **epithelium (1)** overlying the thick **lamina propria (2).** The surface epithelium (1) extends down into the connective tissue of the lamina propria (2) to form numerous long, tubular **uterine glands (4).** The uterine glands (4) are usually straight in the superficial portion of the endometrium, but may exhibit branching in the deeper regions near the myometrium. As a result, numerous uterine glands (4) are seen in cross sections.

During the proliferative phase of the cycle, **coiled (spiral) arteries (3)** in cross section are seen primarily in the deeper regions of the endometrium. At this stage (proliferative phase), the coiled arteries (3) do not normally extend into the superficial third portion of the endometrium, which at this time contains veins and capillaries. The lamina propria (2) of the endometrium is cellular and resembles mesenchymal tissue. The branching fibroblasts are found in the network of reticular and fine collagenous fibers of the ground substance. The connective tissue is more compact in the **basalis layer (8)** and appears somewhat darker in this illustration.

The endometrium is firmly attached to the underlying, highly vascular **(10)** myometrium (5, 6). This layer consists of compact bundles of **smooth muscles (5, 6)** separated by thin strands of **interstitial connective tissue (9).** The bundles of muscles are seen in cross, oblique, and longitudinal sections.

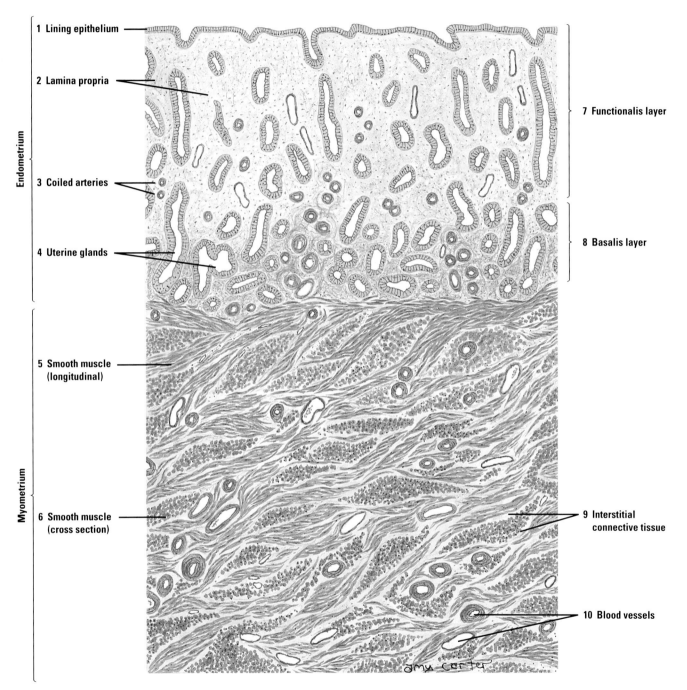

Endometrium

1 Lining epithelium

2 Lamina propria

3 Coiled arteries

4 Uterine glands

Myometrium

5 Smooth muscle (longitudinal)

6 Smooth muscle (cross section)

7 Functionalis layer

8 Basalis layer

9 Interstitial connective tissue

10 Blood vessels

STAIN: hematoxylin and eosin.

285

PLATE 110

UTERUS: SECRETORY (LUTEAL) PHASE

During the secretory phase of the menstrual cycle, the endometrium becomes thicker because of increased glandular secretion and stromal edema. The epithelium of the **uterine glands (4)** hypertrophies because of accumulation of large quantities of secretory product. The **uterine glands** become **tortuous (3, 4, 9)** and their lumina exhibit dilation and **secretory material (5, 10).** In the endometrial **lamina propria (8),** increased accumulation of fluid produces edema. The **coiled arteries (7)** now extend into the superficial portion of the endometrium.

The observed alterations in the uterine glands (4) and lamina propria (8) are characteristic features of the functionalis layer of the endometrium during the secretory or luteal phase of the menstrual cycle. In the **basalis layer (11),** only minimal change is noted.

1 Columnar epithelium

2 Uterine gland: straight portion

3 Uterine glands: tortuous portions

4 Hypertrophied glandular epithelium

5 Bases of uterine glands filled with secretion

6 Myometrium

7 Coiled arteries

8 Interglandular lamina propria (stroma)

9 Tortuous uterine glands

10 Dilated uterine glands with secretion

11 Basal lamina propria (stroma)

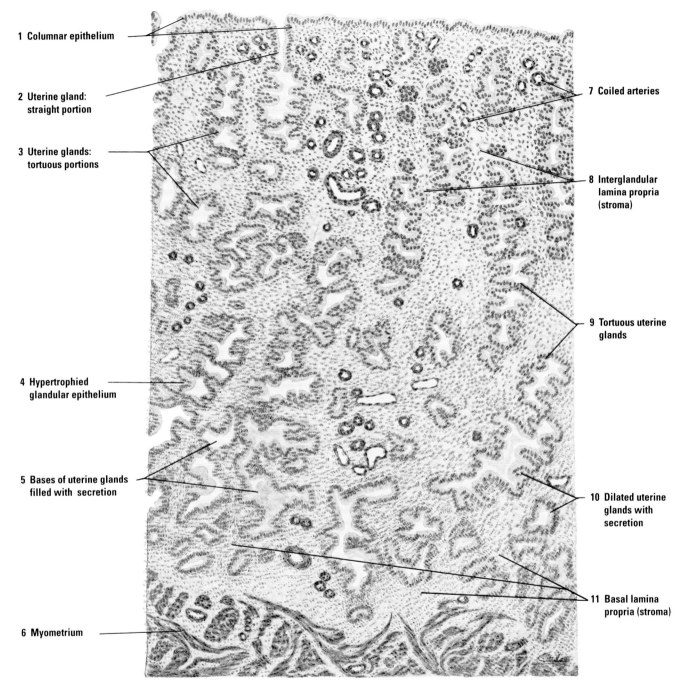

Stain: hematoxylin-eosin. 45×.

PLATE 111

UTERUS: MENSTRUAL PHASE

During every menstrual cycle, the **endometrium (1)** in the functionalis layer is shed or sloughed off during the menstrual phase. The endometrium that is shed contains **fragments of disintegrated stroma (6), blood clots (7),** and uterine glands. Some of the intact **uterine glands (2)** are filled with blood. In the deeper layers of the endometrium or the **basalis layer (4),** the **fundi or the bases of the uterine glands (9)** remain intact during the menstrual flow.

The endometrial stroma of most of the functionalis layer contains aggregations of **erythrocytes (8);** these have been extruded from the torn and disintegrating blood vessels. In addition, endometrial stroma (6) exhibits moderate infiltration of lymphocytes and neutrophils.

The basalis layer (4) of the endometrium remains generally unaffected during this phase because the distal or superficial portions of the **coiled arteries (3)** become necrotic and the deeper parts of these vessels remain intact.

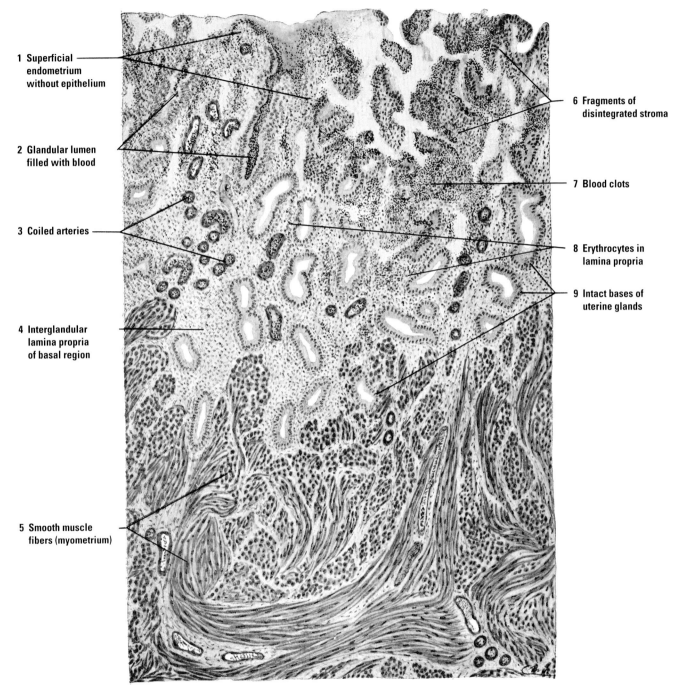

1 Superficial endometrium without epithelium

2 Glandular lumen filled with blood

3 Coiled arteries

4 Interglandular lamina propria of basal region

5 Smooth muscle fibers (myometrium)

6 Fragments of disintegrated stroma

7 Blood clots

8 Erythrocytes in lamina propria

9 Intact bases of uterine glands

Stain: hematoxylin-eosin. 45×.

PLATE 112

■ **FIG. 1**
PLACENTA: FIVE MONTHS' PREGNANCY (PANORAMIC VIEW)

The upper region in the figure illustrates the fetal portion of the **placenta (10, 11).** This includes the **chorionic plate (10)** and the **villi (4, 5, 7)** arising from it. The maternal placenta is the **decidua basalis (8)** and includes the functionalis layer of the **endometrium (12-14),** which lies directly beneath the fetal placenta (10, 11). Below this region is the basalis layer of the endometrium, containing the basal parts of the **uterine glands (15);** this region is not shed during parturition. A portion of the **myometrium (17)** is seen in the lower right field of the figure.

The surface of the **amnion (1)** is lined by the squamous epithelium. The underlying layer represents the merged **connective tissue (2)** of the amnion and chorion. Below the connective tissue layer (2) is the **trophoblast of the chorion (3, 10),** details of which are not distinguishable at this magnification. The trophoblast (3, 10) and the underlying connective tissue (2) form the chorionic plate (10).

The **anchoring villi (4, 7)** arise from the chorionic plate (10), extend to the uterine wall, and embed in the decidua basalis (8). This continuity is not seen in this illustration; however, larger units in the fetal placenta

probably represent sections of the anchoring villi (4, lower leader). These increase in size and complexity during the pregnancy.

Numerous **floating villi (chorion frondosum) (5, 11)** are seen, sectioned in various planes because of their outgrowth in all directions from the anchoring villi (7). These villi "float" in the **intervillous spaces (6),** which are bathed in maternal blood. The detailed structures of these villi are illustrated in Figure 2.

The maternal portion of the placenta or the decidua basalis (8) exhibits embedded anchoring villi (7), groups of large **decidual cells (8),** and typical stroma. Also seen in the decidual basalis (8) are the distal portions of the uterine glands (14) in various stages of regression and **maternal blood vessels (9),** recognized by their size or by red blood cells in their lumina. A maternal blood vessel is seen opening into an **intervillous space (13).**

Coiled arteries (16) and basal portions of the **uterine glands (15)** are present deep in the endometrium. **Fibrin deposits (12)** appear on the surface of the decidua basalis (8) and which increase in volume and extent as the pregnancy continues.

■ **FIG. 2**
CHORIONIC VILLI: PLACENTA AT FIVE MONTHS

Several chorionic villi are illustrated at a higher magnification from a placenta at 5 months of pregnancy. The trophoblast epithelium consists of an outer layer of syncytial cells, the **syncytiotrophoblast (1),** and an inner layer of cells, the **cytotrophoblast (2).** The core of the villus contains **embryonic connective tissue (3)** and **fetal blood vessels (5),** which are branches of umbilical

arteries and veins; both nucleated and non-nucleated erythrocytes may be present. The **intervillous spaces (4)** are bathed by maternal blood and the erythrocytes are non-nucleated. One of the illustrated villi is **attached to the endometrium (6)** and several **decidual cells (7)** are seen in the stroma.

■ **FIG. 3**
CHORIONIC VILLI: PLACENTA AT TERM

Several chorionic villi are illustrated from a placenta at term. In contrast to the villi in Figure 2, the chorionic epithelium in these villi is observed only as **syncytiotrophoblast (1);** its syncytial character is more pronounced than in Figure 2. The **connective tissue (2)** is

more differentiated, illustrating more fibers, fewer typical fibroblasts, and numerous, large, round **macrophages (Hofbauer) cells (4). Fetal blood vessels (3)** are numerous, having increased in complexity during pregnancy.

PLACENTA

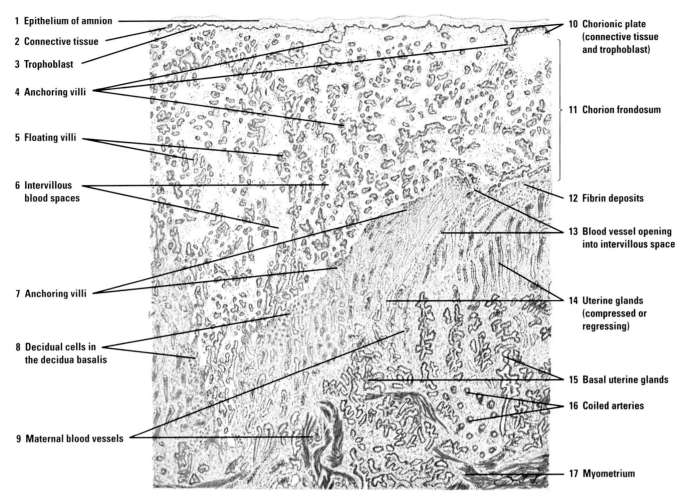

1 Epithelium of amnion

2 Connective tissue

3 Trophoblast

4 Anchoring villi

5 Floating villi

6 Intervillous blood spaces

7 Anchoring villi

8 Decidual cells in the decidua basalis

9 Maternal blood vessels

10 Chorionic plate (connective tissue and trophoblast)

11 Chorion frondosum

12 Fibrin deposits

13 Blood vessel opening into intervillous space

14 Uterine glands (compressed or regressing)

15 Basal uterine glands

16 Coiled arteries

17 Myometrium

FIG. 1. PLACENTA: FIVE MONTHS' PREGNANCY (PANORAMIC VIEW). Stain: hematoxylin-eosin. 10×.

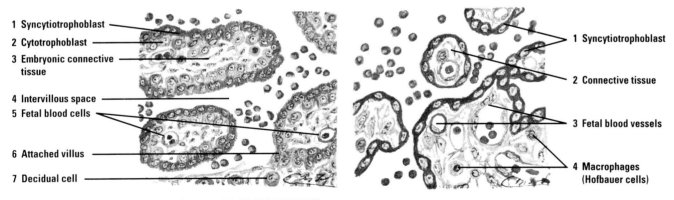

1 Syncytiotrophoblast

2 Cytotrophoblast

3 Embryonic connective tissue

4 Intervillous space

5 Fetal blood cells

6 Attached villus

7 Decidual cell

1 Syncytiotrophoblast

2 Connective tissue

3 Fetal blood vessels

4 Macrophages (Hofbauer cells)

FIG. 2. CHORIONIC VILLI (PLACENTA AT FIVE MONTHS). Stain: hematoxylin-eosin. 350×.

FIG. 3. CHORIONIC VILLI (PLACENTA AT TERM). Stain: hematoxylin-eosin. 350×.

PLATE 113

CERVIX (LONGITUDINAL SECTION)

The cervix is the lower part of the uterus. The endo-cervix (cervical canal) is lined with tall, mucus-secreting **columnar epithelium (1).** This epithelium differs from the uterine epithelium, with which it is continuous. Similar epithelium also lines the numerous, highly branched tubular **cervical glands (2)** which extend deep into the wide **lamina propria (4).** The lamina propria (4) in the cervix is more fibrous than in the uterus.

The lower end of the cervix or the **os cervix (5)** bulges into the lumen of the vaginal canal. The columnar epithelium of the cervical canal abruptly changes to **stratified squamous (6).** This epithelium then lines the vaginal portion of the cervix, the **portio vaginalis (6)** and the **external surface (8)** in the **vaginal fornix (7).** At the base of the fornix (7), the epithelium reflects back to line the vaginal canal.

The **muscularis (3, 10)** is not as compact as in the body of the uterus; however, both the muscularis (3, 10) and the lamina propria (4) are well vascularized **(11).**

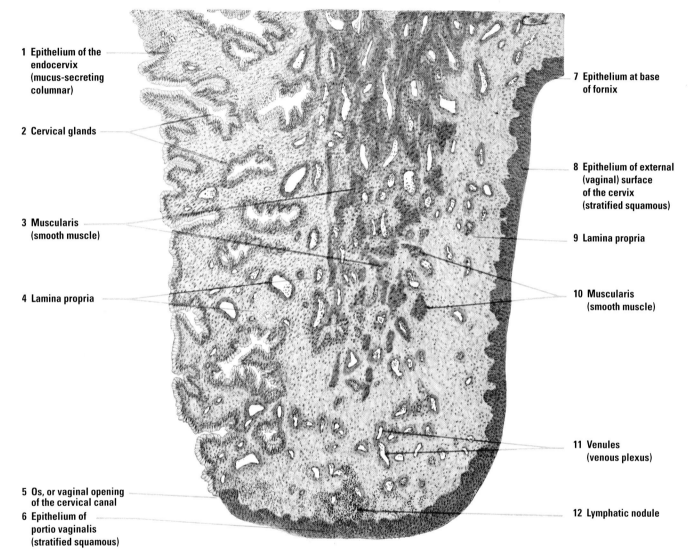

1 Epithelium of the
  endocervix
  (mucus-secreting
  columnar)

2 Cervical glands

3 Muscularis
  (smooth muscle)

4 Lamina propria

5 Os, or vaginal opening
  of the cervical canal

6 Epithelium of
  portio vaginalis
  (stratified squamous)

7 Epithelium at base
  of fornix

8 Epithelium of external
  (vaginal) surface
  of the cervix
  (stratified squamous)

9 Lamina propria

10 Muscularis
   (smooth muscle)

11 Venules
   (venous plexus)

12 Lymphatic nodule

Stain: hematoxylin-eosin. 20×.

PLATE 114

■ FIG. 1
VAGINA (LONGITUDINAL SECTION)

The vaginal mucosa is highly irregular and exhibits numerous **folds (1).** The epithelium lining the surface of the vaginal canal is noncornified **stratified squamous (2).** Connective tissue **papillae (3)** below the epithelium are prominent and vary in height.

The wide **lamina propria (7)** contains moderately dense, irregular connective tissue that is rich in elastic fibers. Fibers from lamina propria extend down and pass into the muscularis layer as **interstitial fibers (10).** Diffuse **lymphatic tissue (8),** a **lymphatic nodule (4),** and numerous small **blood vessels** (arterioles and venules) **(9)** are usually observed in the lamina propria (7).

The muscularis consists predominantly of **longitudinal (5a)** and oblique bundles of smooth muscle fibers. The **transverse muscle fibers (5b)** are less numerous but more frequently found in the inner layers. The interstitial connective tissue (10) is rich in elastic fibers and the **adventitia (6, 12)** contains **blood vessels (11)** and nerve bundles.

■ FIG. 2
GLYCOGEN IN HUMAN VAGINAL EPITHELIUM

Glycogen is a prominent component of the vaginal epithelium except in the deepest layers, where its content is minimal or lacking. During the follicular phase of the menstrual cycle, glycogen accumulates in the vaginal epithelium, reaching its maximum level before ovulation. Glycogen can be demonstrated by iodine vapor or iodine solution in mineral oil (Mancini's method); glycogen stains a reddish purple.

The vaginal specimens in illustrations a and b were fixed in absolute alcohol and formaldehyde. The amount of glycogen in the vaginal epithelium during the interfollicular phase of the cycle is illustrated in a. During the follicular phase, glycogen content increases in the cells of the intermediate and the more superficial layers (b).

The tissue sample illustrated in c is from the same specimen as in b, but was fixed by the Altmann-Gersch method (freezing and drying in a vacuum). This method produces less tissue shrinkage and illustrates abundant glycogen during the follicular phase and its diffuse distribution throughout the vaginal epithelium.

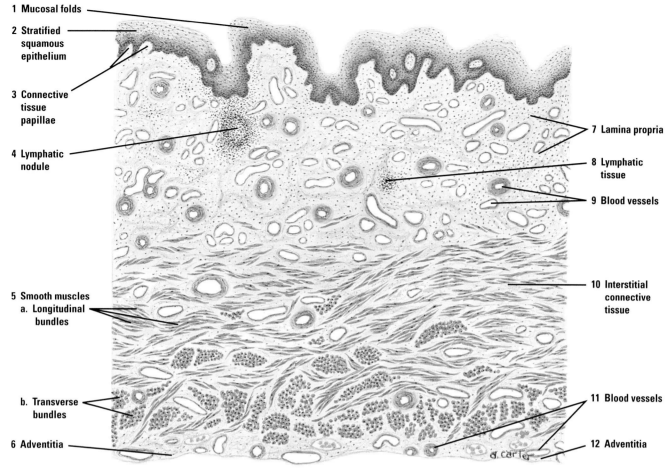

1 Mucosal folds

2 Stratified squamous epithelium

3 Connective tissue papillae

4 Lymphatic nodule

5 Smooth muscles
   a. Longitudinal bundles

   b. Transverse bundles

6 Adventitia

7 Lamina propria

8 Lymphatic tissue

9 Blood vessels

10 Interstitial connective tissue

11 Blood vessels

12 Adventitia

FIG. 1. VAGINA: LOGITUDINAL SECTION. PLASTIC SECTION AND HEMATOXYLIN AND EOSIN STAIN.

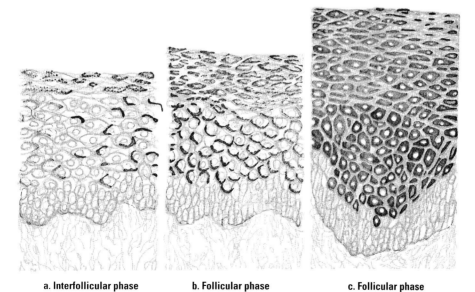

a. Interfollicular phase   b. Follicular phase   c. Follicular phase

FIG. 2. GLYCOGEN IN HUMAN VAGINAL EPITHELIUM. Stain: Mancini's iodine technique.

PLATE 115

VAGINA: EXFOLIATE CYTOLOGY, VAGINAL SMEARS

This plate illustrates different cells in vaginal smears obtained from normal woman during the menstrual cycle, early pregnancy, and menopause. The Shorr trichrome stain (Bierbrich Scarlet, Orange G, and Fast Green) plus Harris hematoxylin facilitates recognition of different cell types.

Figure 7 illustrates individual cell types observed in a normal vaginal smear. The superficial **acidophilic cell (a)** of the vaginal mucosa appears flat and somewhat irregular in outline, measures from 35 to 65 μm in diameter, exhibits a small nucleus, and contains ample cytoplasm stained light orange. Adjacent to the acidophilic cell (a) is a similar superficial **basophilic cell (b)** with blue-green cytoplasm. Illustrated at **c** is a cell from the **intermediate stratum** of the vaginal epithelium. It is flattened like the superficial cells but is smaller, measuring 20 to 40 μm, and has a basophilic blue-green cytoplasm. The nucleus is somewhat larger and often vesicular. The cells illustrated at **d** are **intermediate cells** in profile, characterized by their elongated form with folded borders and elongated, eccentric nucleus. At **e** are illustrated cells of the internal basal layers of the vaginal epithelium, the **basal cells.** The larger cells are from the external portion of the basal layers and the more superficial are the parabasal cells. All cells are oval, measure from 12 to 15 μm in diameter, and exhibit a large nucleus with a more prominent chromatin. Most of these cells exhibit basophilic staining.

In Figure 1 is illustrated a vaginal smear taken during the fifth day of the menstrual cycle (postmenstrual phase). Predominant are the **intermediate cells (1)** from the outer layers of the intermediate layer (transitions to the deeper superficial cells). A few **superficial acidophilic and basophilic (2)** cells and leukocytes are present.

Figure 2 represents a vaginal smear collected during the ovulatory phase (14th day) of the menstrual cycle. This phase is characterized by predominance of large superficial **acidophilic cells (8)**, the scarcity of superficial **basophilic cells (10)**, and **intermediate cells (9)**, and the absence of leukocytes. This smear is characteristic of the high estrogenic stimulation normally observed before ovulation and is called the "follicular smear." The superficial cells (8) "mature" with increased estrogen levels and become acidophilic. A similar type of smear can be obtained from a menopausal woman treated with high doses of estrogen.

In Figure 3 is a representative vaginal smear observed during the luteal (progestational) phase (21st day of the menstrual cycle). This phase is indicative of increased levels of progesterone. Predominant are large cells from the **intermediate layers (3)** (precornified superficial cells) with folded borders that aggregate into clumps. Superficial **acidophilic cells (4),** superficial **basophilic cells (5),** and leukocytes are scarce.

The cells in Figure 4 represent the vaginal smear during the premenstrual phase (28th day of the menstrual cycle). This stage is characterized by a great predominance of grouped **intermediate cells (13, 14)** with folded borders, an increase of **neutrophilic cells (12),** a scarcity of **superficial cells (11),** and an abundance of mucus, which blurs the preparations.

Figure 5 illustrates a vaginal smear taken from a 3-month pregnancy, illustrating predominantly cells from the intermediate layers, many with **folded borders (6).** These cells typically form dense groups or **conglomerations (7).** Cells from superficial layers and neutrophilic cells are scarce.

The vaginal smear during menopause (Fig. 6) is different from all other phases. In a typical "atrophic" smear, the predominant cells are the oval **basal cells (17)** of various sizes. Cells from the **intermediate layers (15)** are scarce, whereas the **neutrophilic cells (16)** are abundant. The menopausal smears, however, vary according to the stage of menopause and the estrogen levels.

The vaginal exfoliate cytology is closely correlated with the ovarian cycle. Understanding its characteristic features permits recognition of follicular activity during normal menstrual phases or after estrogenic and other therapy. Also, exfoliate cytology provides important information (together with cells from the endocervix) for detecting regional pathologic or malignant conditions.

VAGINA: EXFOLIATE CYTOLOGY (VAGINAL SMEARS)

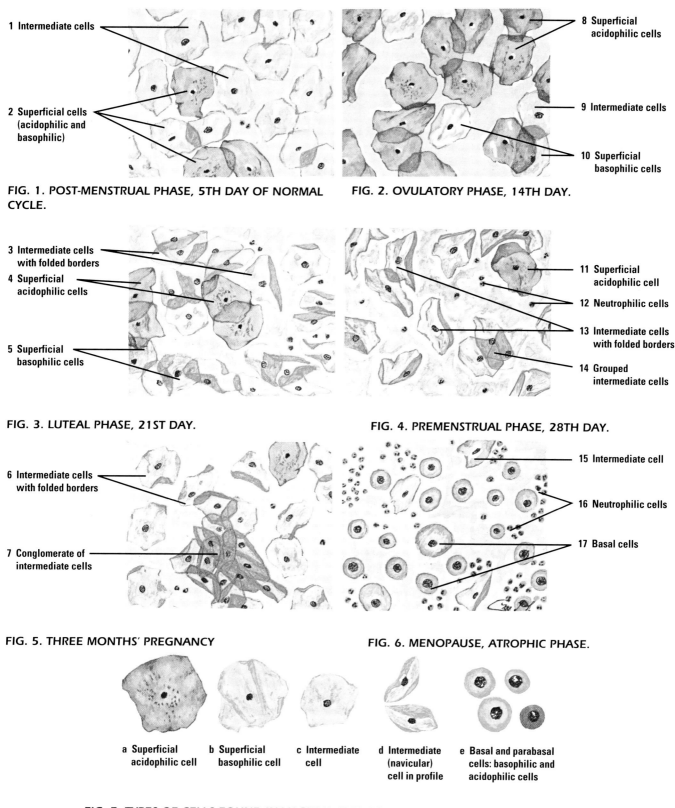

1 Intermediate cells

2 Superficial cells
(acidophilic and
basophilic)

8 Superficial
acidophilic cells

9 Intermediate cells

10 Superficial
basophilic cells

FIG. 1. POST-MENSTRUAL PHASE, 5TH DAY OF NORMAL CYCLE.

FIG. 2. OVULATORY PHASE, 14TH DAY.

3 Intermediate cells
with folded borders
4 Superficial
acidophilic cells

5 Superficial
basophilic cells

11 Superficial
acidophilic cell

12 Neutrophilic cells

13 Intermediate cells
with folded borders

14 Grouped
intermediate cells

FIG. 3. LUTEAL PHASE, 21ST DAY.

FIG. 4. PREMENSTRUAL PHASE, 28TH DAY.

6 Intermediate cells
with folded borders

7 Conglomerate of
intermediate cells

15 Intermediate cell

16 Neutrophilic cells

17 Basal cells

FIG. 5. THREE MONTHS' PREGNANCY

FIG. 6. MENOPAUSE, ATROPHIC PHASE.

a Superficial
acidophilic cell

b Superficial
basophilic cell

c Intermediate
cell

d Intermediate
(navicular)
cell in profile

e Basal and parabasal
cells: basophilic and
acidophilic cells

FIG. 7. TYPES OF CELLS FOUND IN VAGINAL SMEARS DURING DIFFERENT AND NORMAL REPRODUCTIVE PHASES. Stain: Shorr's trichrome. 250× and 450×.

PLATE 116

PLATE 116

■ **FIG. 1**
MAMMARY GLAND, INACTIVE

The mammary gland (breast) consists of 15 to 25 lobes, each of which is an individual compound tubulo-alveolar type of gland (see Plate 7 and accompanying text). Each glandular lobe is separated by interlobar stroma and has its own lactiferous duct, which emerges independently onto the surface of the nipple. The interlobar stroma consists of dense connective tissue and varying amounts of fat. (11) Each lobe contains **interlobular connective tissue (2, 4)** between individual lobules. Figure 1 illustrates one complete mammary gland lobule and a **portion of another lobule (1).**

The inactive mammary gland is characterized by an abundance of connective tissue and a minimum of glandular elements. The lobule contains groups of small **tubules (3, 10)** that are lined with cuboidal or low columnar epithelium. These tubules resemble ducts and remain in this state as long as the mammary gland remains inactive. Some cyclic changes may be seen in the mammary gland; however, these regress at the end of the menstrual cycle. Occasionally a better defined tubule is seen; this is a small **intralobular duct (6)** or a large **intralobular excretory (8)** duct that emerges from the lobule to join the interlobular duct. Potential tubules may be present as undifferentiated solid **cords of cells (5).**

The excretory tubules are surrounded by a loose, fine connective tissue, the intralobular connective tissue (4), which contains fibroblasts, lymphocytes, plasma cells, and eosinophils. Surrounding this region is the dense interlobular connective (2) and **adipose tissue (11).**

■ **FIG. 2**
MAMMARY GLAND DURING FIRST HALF OF PREGNANCY

The mammary gland exhibits extensive structural changes in preparation for lactation. During the first half of the pregnancy, the intralobular ducts undergo rapid proliferation and form terminal buds, which differentiate into **alveoli (2, 6).** Most of the alveoli are empty; however, some may contain a **secretory product (5).** At this stage of mammary gland development, it is difficult to distinguish between small **intralobular ducts (9)** and alveoli (2, 6). The ducts appear more regular in outline and have a more distinct epithelial lining **(9).**

The glandular lobules contain numerous alveoli (2, 6) and the **loose intralobular connective tissue (7)** appears reduced. On the other hand, there is an increased infiltration of lymphocytes and other cells. The **interlobular dense connective tissue (3)** appears as septa between the developing lobules. The **interlobular ducts (4)** that are lined with taller columnar cells course in the interlobular septa (3) and empty into the large **lactiferous ducts (8),** which are usually lined with low pseudostratified columnar epithelium. Each lactiferous duct (8) collects the secretory product of a lobe and transports it to the nipple.

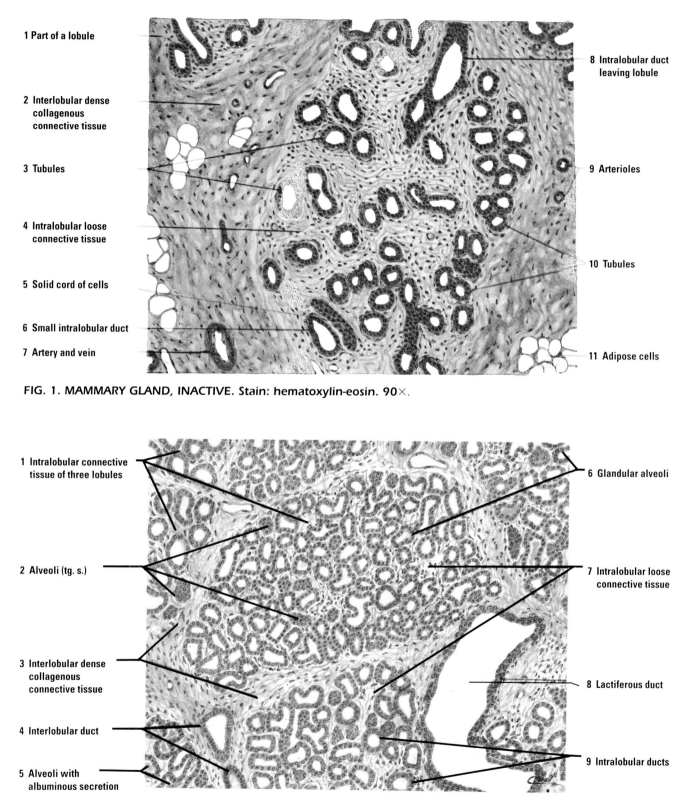

1 Part of a lobule

2 Interlobular dense collagenous connective tissue

3 Tubules

4 Intralobular loose connective tissue

5 Solid cord of cells

6 Small intralobular duct

7 Artery and vein

8 Intralobular duct leaving lobule

9 Arterioles

10 Tubules

11 Adipose cells

FIG. 1. MAMMARY GLAND, INACTIVE. *Stain: hematoxylin-eosin. 90×.*

1 Intralobular connective tissue of three lobules

2 Alveoli (tg. s.)

3 Interlobular dense collagenous connective tissue

4 Interlobular duct

5 Alveoli with albuminous secretion

6 Glandular alveoli

7 Intralobular loose connective tissue

8 Lactiferous duct

9 Intralobular ducts

FIG. 2. MAMMARY GLAND DURING THE FIRST HALF OF PREGNANCY. *Stain: hematoxylin-eosin. 90×.*

PLATE 117

■ **FIG. 1**
MAMMARY GLAND DURING SEVENTH MONTH OF PREGNANCY

At 7 months of pregnancy, the glandular alveoli enlarge, the alveolar cells become secretory, and the secretory product is observed in some **alveolar lumina (1)**. Because the intralobular ducts also contain secretory material, the distinction between the alveoli and ducts remains difficult. In some sections, the round **alveoli (7)** can be seen opening directly into an elongated **intralobular excretory duct (6)**.

In later stages of pregnancy, there is a further relative reduction in the amount of **intralobular (3)** and **interlobular connective tissue (5)**. The interlobular connective tissue (5) contains the **interlobular ducts (2)** and a **lactiferous duct (4)** with secretory product in its lumen.

■ **FIG. 2**
MAMMARY GLAND DURING LACTATION

This figure depicts a lactating mammary gland at lower (left) and higher (right) magnification. The depicted structures are generally similar to those in Figure 1.

The major difference in the lactating mammary gland is the presence of a large number of distended alveoli filled with **milk secretion (2)** and showing irregular **branching patterns (3)**. Also, there is a reduction of **interlobular connective tissue septa (4)**.

During lactation, the histology of individual alveoli varies; all of the alveoli do not exhibit the same state of secretory activity. The active alveoli are lined by low epithelium and their lumina are filled with milk; milk appears as eosinophilic material with large vacuoles of dissolved **fat droplets (2, 9)**. Some alveoli accumulate secretory product in their **cytoplasm (8)**, and their apices appear vacuolated because of the removal of fat during the routine tissue preparation. Other alveoli appear **inactive (6, 11)** with empty lumina and taller epithelium.

In the mammary gland, the myoepithelial cells (not illustrated) are present between the alveolar cells and the basal lamina (see Plates 56, 57, and 58). The contraction of the myoepithelial cells assists in expelling the milk from the alveoli into the excretory ducts. The **interlobular ducts (5, 7)** are embedded in the connective tissue septa, which contain numerous **adipose cells (1, 12)**.

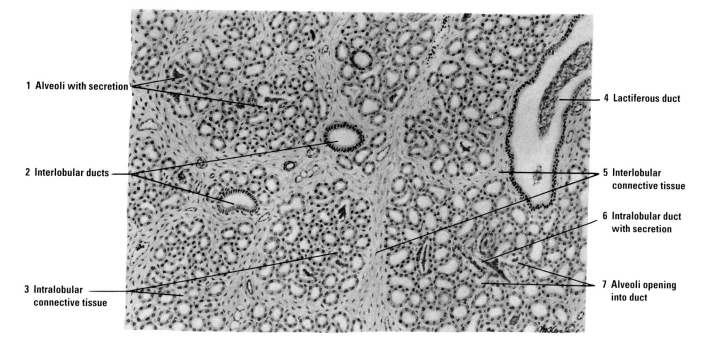

1 Alveoli with secretion

2 Interlobular ducts

3 Intralobular connective tissue

4 Lactiferous duct

5 Interlobular connective tissue

6 Intralobular duct with secretion

7 Alveoli opening into duct

FIG. 1. MAMMARY GLAND, SEVENTH MONTH OF PREGNANCY. Stain: hematoxylin-eosin. 90×.

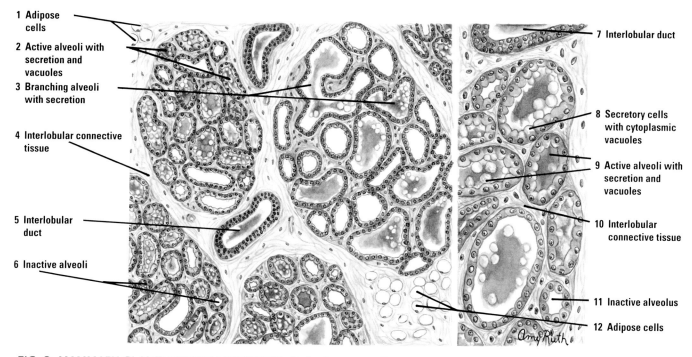

1 Adipose cells

2 Active alveoli with secretion and vacuoles

3 Branching alveoli with secretion

4 Interlobular connective tissue

5 Interlobular duct

6 Inactive alveoli

7 Interlobular duct

8 Secretory cells with cytoplasmic vacuoles

9 Active alveoli with secretion and vacuoles

10 Interlobular connective tissue

11 Inactive alveolus

12 Adipose cells

FIG. 2. MAMMARY GLAND DURING LACTATION. Stain: hematoxylin-eosin. 90× and 200×.

ORGANS OF SPECIAL SENSES

The Eye

The eye is a highly specialized sense organ for vision and photoreception. Each eye contains a layer of cells that are sensitive to light, the photoreceptors, a lens for focusing the incoming light, and nerves that conduct the impulses from the photoreceptors in the eye to the brain.

The eyeball is surrounded by three layers. The outer layer is the sclera; it is modified anteriorly into the transparent cornea, through which light enters the eye. Inside the sclera is the pigmented layer called the choroid; this layer contains numerous blood vessels that nourish the photoreceptor cells and the structures of the eyeball. Lining most of the posterior compartment of the eye and terminating at the ora serrata is the layer with the photosensitive cells, the retina. Anterior to the ora serrata, the retina is not photosensitive.

The photosensitive retina is composed of three main types of neurons: the photoreceptive rods and cones, the bipolar cells, and the ganglion cells. The rods and cones synapse with the bipolar cells, which then connect the receptor cells with the ganglion cells. The axons that leave the ganglion cells converge posteriorly at the optic papilla (disk) and leave the eye as the optic nerve. The optic papilla is also called the blind spot because this area lacks photoreceptor cells. Because the rods and cones are situated next to the choroid layer, the light rays must first pass through the ganglion and bipolar cell layers to reach the photosensitive cells. The pigmented layer of choroid next to the retina absorbs the light rays and prevents them from reflecting back through the retina.

The rods are sensitive to light and function best during low light, such as at dusk or during the night. The cones are less sensitive to low light and respond to high light intensity; they function as sensors for high visual acuity and color vision (red, green, or blue).

The posterior region of the eye contains a yellowish pigmented spot called macula lutea. In its center is a depression called the fovea centralis. The center of the fovea centralis is devoid of rods and blood vessels, but contains densely packed cones. In this region, the light rays fall directly on the cones. As a result, this region of the eye produces the greatest visual acuity and sharpest color discrimination.

The Ear

The ear serves two important purposes: it is an organ for hearing and an organ for balance and equilibrium. The external ear, the middle ear, and the inner ear form the integral components of the auditory system.

The external ear collects the sound waves and directs them through the external auditory canal to the tympanic membrane or ear drum. The middle ear or the tympanic cavity is located in the temporal bone of the skull and is spanned by three very small bones, the ossicles. The middle ear is separated from the external auditory canal by the tympanic membrane. The sound waves that enter through the external auditory canal vibrate the tympanic membrane. These vibrations activate the three ossicles in the middle ear. The ossicles then transmit the vibrations across the air-filled middle ear to the fluid-filled inner ear.

The inner ear, lying deep in the temporal bone, contains the sensory components in the semicircular canals and cochlea. The semicircular canals contain receptor cells that are responsible for maintaining the balance and equilibrium; however, their function is independent of the external ear and middle ear.

The cochlea houses the organ of Corti, in which are located the auditory receptors or hair cells responsible for hearing. The hair cells in the organ of Corti convert the vibrations into nerve impulses. The sound impulses then pass along the nerve processes of the ganglion cells that are located in the spiral ganglia of the inner ear. The axons from the spiral ganglia form the auditory nerve, which carries the impulses from the inner ear to the brain for sound interpretation.

PLATE 118

EYELID (SAGITTAL SECTION)

The exterior layer of the eyelid (illustrated on the left) is the thin skin. The **epidermis (4)** consists of a stratified squamous epithelium with papillae. In the underlying **dermis (6)** are found **hair follicles (1, 3)** with their associated **sebaceous glands (3).** Also seen in the dermis are the **sweat glands (5).**

The interior layer of the eyelid (illustrated on the right) is a mucous membrane, the **palpebral conjunctiva (15);** it lies adjacent to the eyeball. The lining epithelium of the palpebral conjunctiva (15) is a low stratified columnar type with a few goblet cells. The stratified squamous epithelium (4) of the skin continues over the margin of the eyelid and then transforms into the stratified columnar type of the palpebral conjunctiva (15). The thin lamina propria of the palpebral conjunctiva (15) contains elastic and collagenous fibers. Beneath the lamina propria is a plate of dense, collagenous connective tissue, the **tarsus (16).** This region contains large, specialized sebaceous glands, the **tarsal (Meibomian)** glands **(17).** The secretory acini of these glands open into a long **central duct (19),** which runs parallel to the palpebral conjunctiva (15) and opens at the eyelid margin.

The free end of the eyelid contains **eyelashes (10),** which arise from large, long **hair follicles (9).** Associated with the eyelashes (10) are small **sebaceous glands (11).** Between the hair follicles of the eyelashes are large **sweat glands** (of Moll) **(18).**

The eyelid contains three sets of muscles: the extensive palpebral portion of the skeletal muscle, the **orbicularis oculi (8),** the skeletal **ciliary muscle (of Roilan) (20)** in the region of the hair follicles of the eyelashes (10) and tarsal glands (17), and in the upper region of the eyelid, the strands of the smooth muscle, the **superior tarsal muscle (of Müller) (12).**

The **connective tissue (7)** of the eye lid also contains **adipose tissue (2), blood vessels (14),** and **lymphatic tissue (13).**

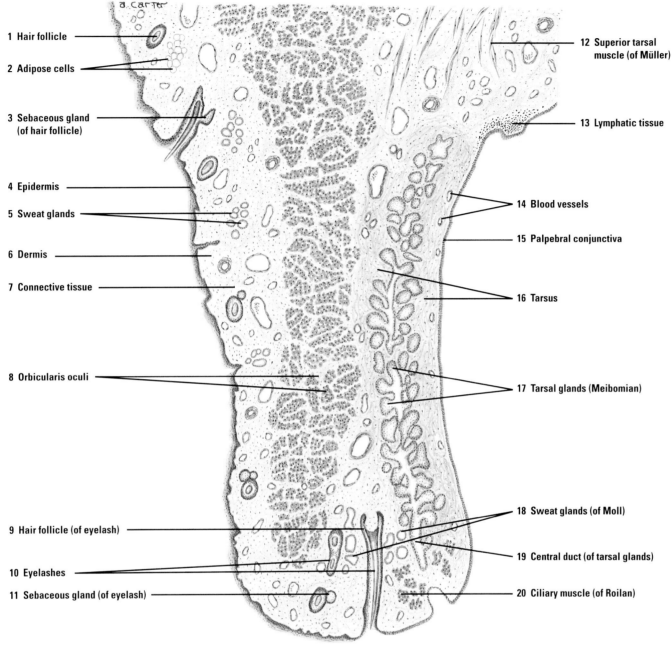

1 Hair follicle

2 Adipose cells

3 Sebaceous gland (of hair follicle)

4 Epidermis

5 Sweat glands

6 Dermis

7 Connective tissue

8 Orbicularis oculi

9 Hair follicle (of eyelash)

10 Eyelashes

11 Sebaceous gland (of eyelash)

12 Superior tarsal muscle (of Müller)

13 Lymphatic tissue

14 Blood vessels

15 Palpebral conjunctiva

16 Tarsus

17 Tarsal glands (Meibomian)

18 Sweat glands (of Moll)

19 Central duct (of tarsal glands)

20 Ciliary muscle (of Roilan)

Stain: Hematoxylin and eosin

PLATE 119

■ FIG. 1
LACRIMAL GLAND

The lacrimal gland secretes tears and is composed of several tubuloacinar glands. The secretory **acini (1, 8)** vary in size and shape and resemble the serous type; however, their lumina are larger. Some acini may exhibit irregular **outpocketings of cells (5)** in the lumina. The **acinar cells (1, 8)** are more columnar than pyramidal, contain large secretory granules and lipid droplets, and stain light. **Myoepithelial cells (basket cells) (3)** surround individual acini.

■ FIG. 2
CORNEA (TRANSVERSE SECTION)

The anterior surface of the cornea is covered with nonpapillated, stratified squamous nonkeratinized **epithelium (1, 6, 7).** The lowest or basal cell layer is columnar and rests on thin basement membrane (not illustrated). Beneath the corneal epithelium is a thick, homogeneous **anterior limiting membrane (Bowman's) (2),** which is derived from the underlying **corneal stroma** or **substantia propria (3).** The corneal stroma (3) forms the body of the cornea. It consists of parallel bundles of collagenous fibers which form thin **lamellae**

The smaller intralobular **excretory ducts (2, lower leader)** are lined with simple cuboidal or columnar epithelium. The larger intralobular ducts **(2, upper leader)** and the **interlobular ducts (7, 11)** are lined with two layers of low columnar cells or pseudostratified epithelium.

The interalveolar (intralobular) **connective tissue (9)** is sparse; however, **interlobular connective tissue (4)** is abundant and may contain adipose cells.

(9) and layers of flat, branching fibroblasts, the **keratocytes (8),** between the collagenous fibers. The corneal keratocytes (8) are modified fibroblasts.

The posterior surface of the cornea is covered with a low cuboidal epithelium, the **posterior epithelium (5, 10),** which is also the corneal endothelium. The **posterior limiting membrane (Descemet's membrane) (4)** is wide and constitutes the basement membrane of the posterior corneal epithelium (5, 10). It rests on the posterior portion of the corneal stroma (3).

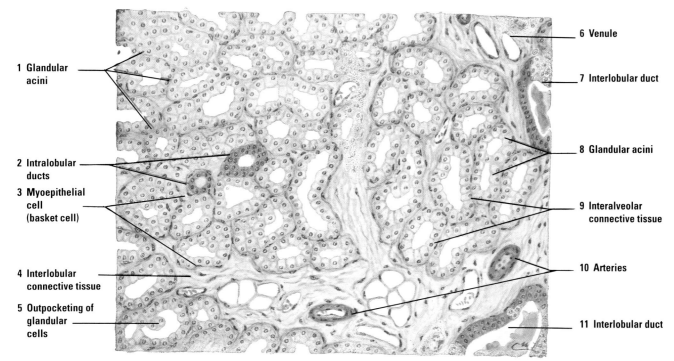

1 Glandular acini

2 Intralobular ducts

3 Myoepithelial cell (basket cell)

4 Interlobular connective tissue

5 Outpocketing of glandular cells

6 Venule

7 Interlobular duct

8 Glandular acini

9 Interalveolar connective tissue

10 Arteries

11 Interlobular duct

FIG. 1. LACRIMAL GLAND. Stain: hematoxylin-eosin. 180×.

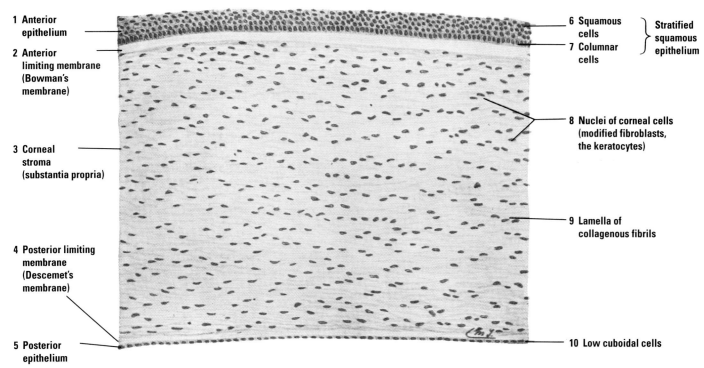

1 Anterior epithelium

2 Anterior limiting membrane (Bowman's membrane)

3 Corneal stroma (substantia propria)

4 Posterior limiting membrane (Descemet's membrane)

5 Posterior epithelium

6 Squamous cells

7 Columnar cells

} Stratified squamous epithelium

8 Nuclei of corneal cells (modified fibroblasts, the keratocytes)

9 Lamella of collagenous fibrils

10 Low cuboidal cells

FIG. 2. CORNEA (TRANSVERSE SECTION). Stain: hematoxylin-eosin. 180×.

PLATE 120

WHOLE EYE (SAGITTAL SECTION)

The eyeball is surrounded by three major concentric layers: an outer, tough, fibrous tissue layer composed of **sclera (18)** and **cornea (1)**; a middle layer or uvea composed of the highly vascular, pigmented **choroid (7)**, the **ciliary body (consisting of ciliary processes and ciliary muscle) (4, 14, 15)**, and the **iris (13)**; and the innermost layer composed of the photosensitive nerve tissue, the **retina (8).** The histology of the cornea (1) is illustrated in greater detail on Plate 119, Figure 2.

The sclera (18) is the white, opaque, and tough connective tissue layer composed of densely woven collagenous fibers. It aids in maintaining the rigidity of the eyeball and appears as the "white" of the eye. The junction between the cornea and sclera occurs at the transition area called the **limbus (12),** located in the anterior region of the eye. In the posterior region of the eye, where the **optic nerve (10)** emerges from the ocular capsule, is the transition site between the sclera (18) of the eyeball and the connective tissue **dura mater (23)** of the central nervous system.

The choroid (7) and the ciliary body (4, 14, 15) are situated adjacent to the sclera (18). In a sagittal section of the eyeball, the ciliary body (4, 14, 15) appears triangular in shape and is composed of the **ciliary muscle (14)** and the **ciliary processes (4, 15).** The ciliary muscle (14) is a smooth muscle; its fibers exhibit longitudinal, circular, and radial directions. The folded and highly vascular extensions of the ciliary body constitute the ciliary processes (4, 15). These processes attach to the equator of the **lens (16)** by the suspensory ligament or **zonular fibers (5)** of the lens. Contraction of the ciliary muscle reduces the tension on the suspensory ligament and allows the lens (16) to assume a more convex shape.

The **iris (13)** partially covers the lens and is the colored portion of the eye. The circular and radial distribution of the smooth muscle fibers forms a round opening in the iris called the **pupil (11).** The interior portion of the eye located in front of the lens is subdivided into two compartments. The **anterior chamber (2)** is situated between the iris (13) and the cornea (1), and **the posterior chamber (3)** lies between the iris (13) and lens (16). Both the anterior (2) and posterior (3) chambers are filled with a watery fluid, the aqueous humor. The large posterior compartment in the eyeball located behind the lens is the **vitreous body (19).** It is filled with a gelatinous material, the transparent vitreous humor.

The inner layer or retina (8) of the eyeball is the photosensitive region of the eye; however, not all retina is photosensitive. Behind the ciliary body (4, 14, 15) is the **ora serrata (6, 17),** the sharp, anteriormost boundary of the photosensitive portion of the retina. Anterior to the ora serrata (6, 17) lies the nonphotosensitive region of the retina, which continues forward in the eyeball to form the inner lining of the ciliary body (4, 14, 15) and posterior part of the iris (13). Posterior to the ora serrata (6, 17) is the photosensitive optic retina (8). It consists of numerous cell layers, one of which contains the light-sensitive cells, the rods and cones. The histology of the retina is presented in greater detail on Plate 121, Figures 1 and 2.

The posterior wall of the eye contains the **macula lutea (20)** and the **optic papilla (9)** or optic disk. The macula lutea (20) is a small yellow-pigmented spot in whose center is a shallow depression called the **fovea (20).** This region represents the area of greatest visual acuity in the eye. The center of the fovea (20) is devoid of the rod cells and blood vessels. Instead, this region contains only cone cells.

The optic papilla (9) is the area where the **optic nerve (10)** leaves the eyeball. The optic papilla lacks both light-sensitive cells, the rods and cones, and thus constitutes the "blind spot" of the eye.

The outer sclera is adjacent to the orbital tissue, which contains loose connective tissue, **adipose cells (21)** of the orbital fatty tissue, nerve fibers, **blood vessels (22),** lymphatics, and glands.

EYE (SAGITTAL SECTION)

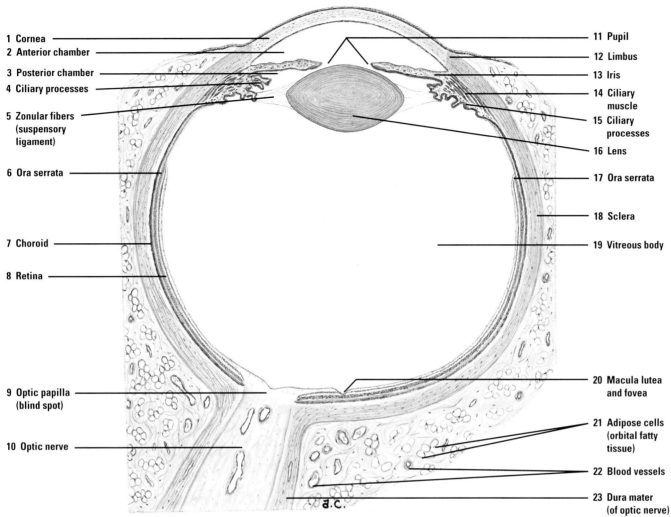

1 Cornea
2 Anterior chamber
3 Posterior chamber
4 Ciliary processes
5 Zonular fibers (suspensory ligament)
6 Ora serrata
7 Choroid
8 Retina
9 Optic papilla (blind spot)
10 Optic nerve

11 Pupil
12 Limbus
13 Iris
14 Ciliary muscle
15 Ciliary processes
16 Lens
17 Ora serrata
18 Sclera
19 Vitreous body
20 Macula lutea and fovea
21 Adipose cells (orbital fatty tissue)
22 Blood vessels
23 Dura mater (of optic nerve)

EYE (SAGITTAL SECTION). Stain: hematoxylin-eosin.

PLATE 121

■ FIG. 1
RETINA, CHOROID, AND SCLERA

The wall of the eyeball is composed of the **sclera (1)**, **choroid (2)**, and **retina (3)**, which contain the photosensitive receptor cells. In this illustration, only the deeper portion of the sclera (1) is illustrated. The stroma of the sclera (1) contains dense **collagenous fibers (4)**, which course parallel to the surface of the eyeball. Between the collagen bundles is a delicate network of elastic fibers. Flattened or elongated fibroblasts are present throughout the sclera (1), and the **melanocytes (5)** are found in the deepest layer.

The layers of the choroid and retina are described in greater detail in Figure 2.

■ FIG. 2
LAYERS OF THE CHOROID AND RETINA IN DETAIL

The choroid is subdivided into numerous layers. These are the: **suprachoroid lamina (17)**, **vascular layer (18)**, **choriocapillary layer (19)**, and the transparent limiting membrane, the glassy membrane (Bruch's membrane).

The suprachoroid lamina (17) consists of lamellae of fine collagenous fibers, a rich network of elastic fibers, fibroblasts, and numerous large melanocytes. The vascular layer (18) contains numerous medium-sized and large **blood vessels (1)**. In the loose connective tissue layer between the blood vessels (1) are numerous, large flat **melanocytes (2)**, which give this layer its characteristic dark color. The choriocapillary layer (19) contains a network of capillaries with large lumina in a stroma of fine collagenous and elastic fibers. The innermost layer of the choroid, the glassy membrane, lies adjacent to the **pigmented cells (3)** of the retina.

The outermost layer of the retina is the pigment epithelium (3); its basement membrane forms the innermost layer of the glassy membrane of the choroid. The cuboidal pigment cells (3) contain melanin granules in apical regions of the cytoplasm while their processes with pigment granules extend between the rods and cones **(20)** of the retina.

Adjacent to the pigment cells (3) is a layer of slender **rods (4, 22)** and thicker **cones (5, 21)** situated next to the **outer limiting membrane (6, 23)**, which is formed by the processes of the neuroglial cells, the **Müller's cells (30)**.

The outermost nuclear layer contains **nuclei of the rods (8, 25)** and **cones (7, 24)** and the **outermost processes of Müller's cells (26)**. In the **outer plexiform layer (9)**, the axons of rods and cones synapse with the **bipolar (28)** and **horizontal cells (27)**. The inner **nuclear layer (10)** contains the nuclei of **bipolar (29)**, horizontal, **amacrine (31)**, and neuroglial Müller's cells (30). The horizontal and amacrine cells are association cells. In the **inner plexiform layer (11)**, the axons of bipolar cells (29) synapse with the dendrites of the ganglion and amacrine cells **(32)**.

The **ganglion cell layer (12)** contains the cell bodies of **ganglion cells (33)** and neuroglial cells. Dendrites from the ganglion cells synapse in the inner plexiform layer (32).

The **nerve fiber layer (13, 14)** contains the axons of the ganglion cells (14) and the inner **fiber network of Müller's cells (13, 37)**. **Axons of the ganglion cells (14, 33)** converge toward the optic disk and form the optic nerve. The terminations of the inner fibers of Muller's cells expand to form the **inner limiting membrane (15, 36)** of the retina.

Blood vessels of the retina course in the nerve fiber layer and penetrate as far as the **inner nuclear layer (10)**. Sections of the vessels in various planes can be seen (unlabeled) in this layer.

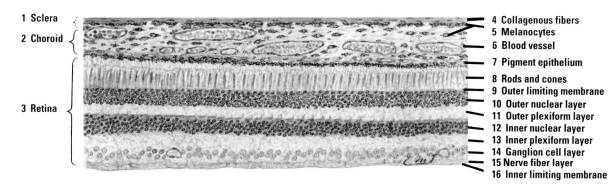

1 Sclera
2 Choroid
3 Retina

4 Collagenous fibers
5 Melanocytes
6 Blood vessel
7 Pigment epithelium
8 Rods and cones
9 Outer limiting membrane
10 Outer nuclear layer
11 Outer plexiform layer
12 Inner nuclear layer
13 Inner plexiform layer
14 Ganglion cell layer
15 Nerve fiber layer
16 Inner limiting membrane

FIG. 1. PANORAMIC VIEW. Stain: hematoxylin-eosin. 130×.

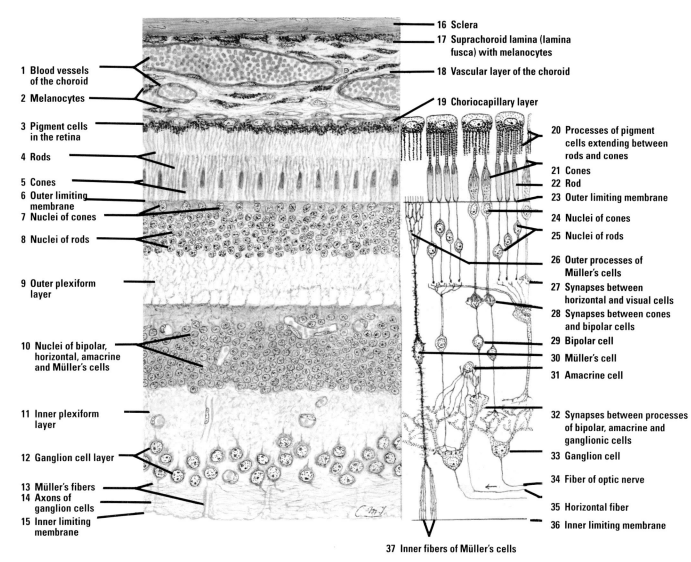

1 Blood vessels of the choroid
2 Melanocytes
3 Pigment cells in the retina
4 Rods
5 Cones
6 Outer limiting membrane
7 Nuclei of cones
8 Nuclei of rods
9 Outer plexiform layer
10 Nuclei of bipolar, horizontal, amacrine and Müller's cells
11 Inner plexiform layer
12 Ganglion cell layer
13 Müller's fibers
14 Axons of ganglion cells
15 Inner limiting membrane

16 Sclera
17 Suprachoroid lamina (lamina fusca) with melanocytes
18 Vascular layer of the choroid
19 Choriocapillary layer
20 Processes of pigment cells extending between rods and cones
21 Cones
22 Rod
23 Outer limiting membrane
24 Nuclei of cones
25 Nuclei of rods
26 Outer processes of Müller's cells
27 Synapses between horizontal and visual cells
28 Synapses between cones and bipolar cells
29 Bipolar cell
30 Müller's cell
31 Amacrine cell
32 Synapses between processes of bipolar, amacrine and ganglionic cells
33 Ganglion cell
34 Fiber of optic nerve
35 Horizontal fiber
36 Inner limiting membrane

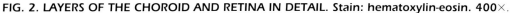

37 Inner fibers of Müller's cells

FIG. 2. LAYERS OF THE CHOROID AND RETINA IN DETAIL. Stain: hematoxylin-eosin. 400×.

311

PLATE 122

■ FIG. 1
INNER EAR: COCHLEA (VERTICAL SECTION)

The bony or osseous labyrinth of the **cochlea (16, 18)** spirals around a central axis of a spongy bone, the **modiolus (17)**. Embedded within the modiolus (17) is the **spiral ganglion (14)**, which is composed of bipolar afferent neurons. Long axons from these bipolar cells join to form the **cochlear nerve (9)**; the shorter dendrites innervate the hair cells in the hearing apparatus, the **organ of Corti (13)**.

The bony labyrinth is divided into two major cavities by the **osseous spiral lamina (8)** and the **basilar membrane (7)**. The osseous spiral lamina (8) projects from the modiolus about halfway into the lumen of the cochlear canal. The basilar membrane (7) continues from the osseous spiral lamina (8) to the **spiral ligament (6)**, which is a thickening of the periosteum on the outer **bony wall (5)** of the cochlear canal. The cochlear canal is subdivided into two large compartments, the lower **scala tympani (4)** and the upper **scala vestibuli (2)**. Both compartments pursue a spiral course to the apex of the cochlea, where they communicate through a small opening called the **helicotrema (1)**.

The **vestibular (Reissner's) membrane** (10) separates the scala vestibuli (2) from the **cochlear duct (scala media) (3)** and forms the roof of the cochlear duct (3). The sensory cells specialized for receiving sound vibrations and transmitting them as nerve impulses to the brain are located in the organ of Corti (13); this organ rests on the basilar membrane (7) on the floor of the cochlear duct (3). A **tectorial membrane (12)** overlies the cells in the **organ of Corti (13)**.

■ FIG. 2
INNER EAR: COCHLEAR DUCT (SCALA MEDIA)

The **cochlear duct (9)**, the **organ of Corti (12)**, and the associated cells are illustrated at higher magnification and in greater detail.

The outer wall of the cochlear duct (9) is formed by the vascular area called the **stria vascularis (16)**. The stratified epithelium covering the stria vascularis (16) is unique in that it contains intraepithelial capillary network formed from the vessels that supply the connective tissue of the **spiral ligament (17)**. The lamina propria in this region is the **spiral ligament (17, 19)**; it consists of collagenous fibers, pigmented fibroblasts, and numerous blood vessels.

The roof of the cochlear duct (9) is formed by the **vestibular membrane (6)**, which separates it from the **scala vestibuli (7)**. The vestibular membrane (6) extends from the spiral ligament (17) of the outer wall of the cochlea, located at the upper extent of the stria vascularis **(15, 16)**, to the thickened **periosteum of the osseous spiral lamina (4)** near the **spiral limbus (5)**.

The spiral limbus (5) forms part of the floor of the **cochlear duct (9)**. The limbus (5) is a thickened mass of periosteal connective tissue (4) of the **osseous spiral lamina (1)** that extends into the cochlear duct (9). It is supported by a lateral extension of the osseous spiral lamina (1). The limbus (5) is covered by an epithelium that appears columnar. The lateral extracellular extension of this epithelium beyond the limbus is the **tectorial membrane (10)**. The tectorial membrane (10) overlies the **inner spiral sulcus (8)** and a portion of the **organ of Corti (12)**, including its **hair cells (11)**.

The **basilar membrane (13)** consists of vascularized connective tissue underlying a thinner plate of basilar fibers. The organ of Corti (12), resting on these basilar fibers, extends from the spiral limbus (5) to the spiral ligament (17, 19). The highly specialized sensory or hair cells (11), several types of supporting cells, and spaces and tunnels constitute the organ of Corti (12).

Peripheral (afferent) processes (2) from the bipolar cells of the **spiral ganglion (3)** course through the channels in the osseous spiral lamina (1) and synapse with the hair cells (11) in the organ of Corti (12).

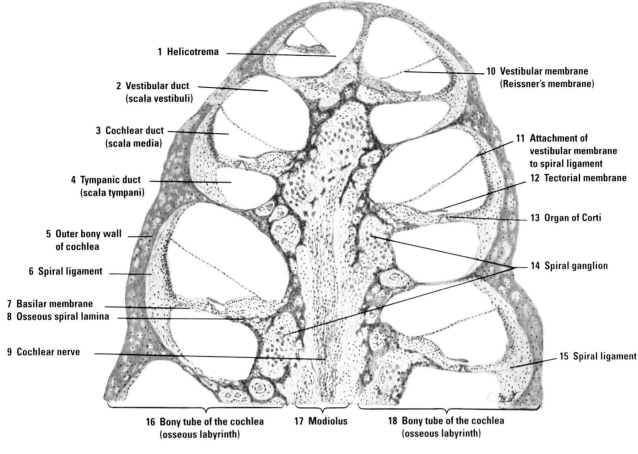

1 Helicotrema

2 Vestibular duct
(scala vestibuli)

3 Cochlear duct
(scala media)

4 Tympanic duct
(scala tympani)

5 Outer bony wall
of cochlea

6 Spiral ligament

7 Basilar membrane
8 Osseous spiral lamina

9 Cochlear nerve

10 Vestibular membrane
(Reissner's membrane)

11 Attachment of
vestibular membrane
to spiral ligament

12 Tectorial membrane

13 Organ of Corti

14 Spiral ganglion

15 Spiral ligament

16 Bony tube of the cochlea
(osseous labyrinth)

17 Modiolus

18 Bony tube of the cochlea
(osseous labyrinth)

FIG. 1. COCHLEA (VERTICAL SECTION). Stain: hematoxylin-eosin. 55×.

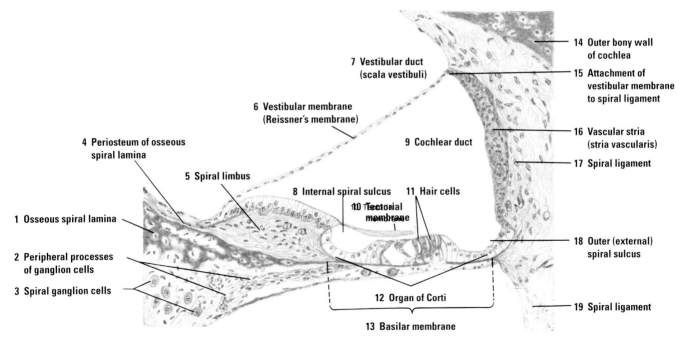

14 Outer bony wall
of cochlea

7 Vestibular duct
(scala vestibuli)

15 Attachment of
vestibular membrane
to spiral ligament

6 Vestibular membrane
(Reissner's membrane)

9 Cochlear duct

16 Vascular stria
(stria vascularis)

17 Spiral ligament

4 Periosteum of osseous
spiral lamina

5 Spiral limbus

8 Internal spiral sulcus

11 Hair cells

10 Tectorial
membrane

1 Osseous spiral lamina

2 Peripheral processes
of ganglion cells

3 Spiral ganglion cells

18 Outer (external)
spiral sulcus

12 Organ of Corti

19 Spiral ligament

13 Basilar membrane

FIG. 2. COCHLEAR DUCT (SCALA MEDIA). Stain: hematoxylin-eosin. 200×.

Oocytes, 274–279
Optic nerve, 308, 309
Optic papilla, 308, 309
Ora serrata, 308, 309
Orbicularis oculi muscle, 304, 305
Orbicularis oris muscle, 136, 137
Orbital conjunctiva, 304, 305
Orcein stain
    for elastic fibers, aorta, 102, 103
Organ of Corti, 312, 313
Os cervix, 292, 293
Osmic acid stain
    for bile canaliculi, 200, 201
    for myelin sheath, 80, 81
Ossification
    bone collar, 42, 43
    endochondral, 42-45
    epiphyseal, 48, 49
    fetal, 40–50
    intramembranous, 40, 41
    osteon development, 46, 47
    secondary centers of, 48, 49
    zone of, 42, 43
Osteoblasts, 37, 40–47
Osteoclasts, 37, 44–47
Osteocytes, 37, 40, 41, 44–47
Osteogenic (osteoprogenitor) cells, 37, 42, 43
Osteoid, 40, 41
Osteons, 38–41
    formation of, 46, 47
Ovary(ies), 271, 274–281
    cortex of, 276, 277
    follicles of, 274–279
    medulla of, 278, 279
Oxyphil cells, parathyroid, 248, 249

P
Pacinian corpuscles
    connective tissue, 26–27
    in pancreas, 206, 207
    subcutaneous tissue, 130–133, 206, 207
Palpebral conjunctiva, 304, 305
Pancreas, 196, 206, 207
    function of, 196
Paneth cells, 175, 180, 181
Papillae, of tongue, 138–143
Pappenheim's stain
    for blood smears, 54, 55
Parafollicular cells, thyroid, 246, 247
Parasympathetic ganglia, of appendix, 188, 189
Parathyroid glands, 240, 248, 249
Parietal cells, 155, 162, 163, 164, 165, 166–169
Parotid glands, 148, 149
Pars distalis, adenohypophysis, 242–245
Pars intermedia, adenohypophysis, 242, 243
Pars nervosa, neurohypophysis, 242, 243
Pars tuberalis, adenohypophysis, 242, 243
PAS hematoxylin (PASH) stain
    for dermal glomus, 132, 133
Peg cells, 282, 283
Penis, 268, 269
Perichondrium
    in endochondral ossification, 44, 45
    in epiglottis, 214, 215
    in thyroid cartilage, 216
    in trachea, 32, 33, 218, 219
Perimysium, 68, 69
Perineurium, 80–83
Perinuclear sarcoplasm, myocardium, 62
Periosteum, 42–45, 48, 49
Peripheral nerve(s), 80, 81
Peripheral nervous system, 71
Peritoneum, visceral, 164, 165, 178, 179

Peyer's patches, 182, 183
Phagocytes, in hepatic sinusoids, 200, 201
Pia mater, 86–89, 92, 93
Pigment cells, 22, 23
Pituicytes, 242–245
Pituitary gland, 239–240, 242–245
    adenohypophysis
        pars distalis, 242–245
        pars intermedia, 242, 243
        pars tuberalis, 242, 243
    neurohypophysis, 242, 243
        infundibular stalk, 242, 243
        pars nervosa, 242, 243
Placenta, 272, 290, 291
Plasma cells, in connective tissue, 19, 22, 23
Plasmablasts, 120, 121
Platelets, 51–53, 58, 59
Pleura, visceral, 220, 221
Plica circulares, 180, 181
Polymorphous cells, cerebral cortex, 92, 93
Portal canals, 198, 199
Portal vein, 198–201
Portio vaginalis, 292, 293
Pregnancy, 271–273
    mammary gland and, 273, 298–301
    placenta, 290, 291
    uterine tubes in, 282, 283
    vaginal smears and, 296, 297
Principal cells
    in parathyroid glands, 248, 249
    in stomach, 166–169
Proerythroblasts, 58, 59
Proplasmacytes, 120, 121
Prostate gland, 264, 265
Protargol and aniline blue stain
    for nervous tissue, 82, 83
Pulmonary artery(ies), 106, 107, 220–223
Pulmonary valve, 106, 107
Pulp cavity, tooth, 144, 145
Pupil, eye, 308, 309
Purkinje
    cells, cerebellum, 90, 91
    fibers, 62, 104–107
    layer, of cerebellum, 90, 91
Pyloric-duodenal junction, 172, 173
Pyloric glands, 170–173
Pyloric sphincter, 172, 173
Pylorus, 170–173
Pyramidal cells, 92, 93
Pyramids, of kidney, 228, 229
Pyriform cells, 90, 91

R
Ranvier nodes, 72, 81–83
Rectum, 190, 191
Reissner's membrane, 312, 313
Renal sinus, 228, 229
Reproductive system
    female, 271–301
    male, 253–269
        accessory, 254
Respiratory system, 209–223
    conducting portion, 209, 214–219
    olfactory portion, 209, 212–213
    passage linings, 10, 11
    respiratory portion, 209–210, 220–223
Rete testis, 256, 257
Reticular cells, 56, 57, 116–119
Reticular fibers, in hepatic lobules, 202, 203
Reticulocytes, 58, 59
Retina, 303, 308–311
Retzius growth lines, tooth, 144, 145